Oral Medicine: The Basis of Diagnosis and Treatment

Oral Medicine: The Basis of Diagnosis and Treatment

Editor: Philip Chiders

FOSTER ACADEMICS
www.fosteracademics.com

www.fosteracademics.com

FOSTER
ACADEMICS

Cataloging-in-Publication Data

Oral medicine : the basis of diagnosis and treatment / edited by Philip Chiders.
p. cm.
Includes bibliographical references and index.
ISBN 978-1-63242-516-4
1. Oral medicine. 2. Dentistry. I. Chiders, Philip.
RC815 .O73 2018
617.522--dc23

Foster Academics,
118-35 Queens Blvd., Suite 400,
Forest Hills, NY 11375, USA

ISBN 978-1-63242-516-4 (Hardback)

Printed and bound in China.

Contents

Preface

Oral health refers to the study and treatment, diagnosis, and prevention of diseases and disorders related to teeth, gum, oral cavity and temperomandibular joint. The main diseases that are treated under this subject are tooth decay, gum diseases, or periodontal disease. This book is meant for students who are looking for an elaborate reference text on oral health. It is compiled in such a manner that it will provide in-depth understanding of this field to all. The topics covered in this text offer readers new insights in the field of dentistry. It attempts to assist those with a goal of delving into this field. The text aims to serve as a resource guide for students and experts alike and contribute to the growth of the discipline.

The information shared in this book is based on empirical researches made by veterans in this field of study. The elaborative information provided in this book will help the readers further their scope of knowledge leading to advancements in this field.

Finally, I would like to thank my fellow researchers who gave constructive feedback and my family members who supported me at every step of my research.

Editor

1

Oral health-related quality of life and early childhood caries among preschool children in Trinidad

Rahul Naidu[1*], June Nunn[2] and Erica Donnelly-Swift[2]

Abstract

Background: Early childhood caries (ECC) is a public health problem in developed and developing countries. The purpose of this study was to describe the relationship between oral health-related quality of life (OHRQoL) and ECC among preschool children in a Caribbean population.

Method: Parents/primary caregivers of children attending nine, randomly selected preschools in central Trinidad were invited to complete an oral health questionnaire and have their child undertake an oral examination. The questionnaire included the Early Childhood Oral Health Impact Scale (ECOHIS). Visible caries experience was assessed using WHO criteria. Logistic regression models were used to determine the factors associated with OHRQoL and ECC.

Results: Three hundred nine parents/caregivers participated in the study (age-range 25–44 years) and 251 children (mean age 3.7 years) completed oral examinations. Adjusting for other factors, the odds for a child aged 4 years of having dental caries were greater than the odds for a child aged 3 years (OR 3.61; 95% CI (1.76, 6.83). The odds for children having difficulty drinking hot or cold drinks were greater for those with dental caries than the odds for children who have no such difficulty. Similarly, the odds for children who had difficulty eating were greater for those with dental caries than the odds ratios for children who had no difficulty eating (OR 8.29; 95% CI (2.00, 43.49). Adjusting for the effects of other factors, the odds of parents/caregivers feeling guilty were greater if their child had experienced dental caries in comparison to parents/caregivers whose child did not have dental caries (OR 3.50; 95% CI (1.32, 9.60). Adjusting for other factors, the odds of parents/primary caregivers having poor quality of life was increased when they had a child with a dmft in the range 1–3 (OR 2.68; 95% CI (1.30, 5.64) dmft > 4 (OR 8.58; 95%CI (3.71, 22.45), in comparison to those whose child had a dmft = 0.

Conclusion: In this sample of preschool children OHRQoL was associated with ECC. More negative impacts were found in children with a greater severity of visible caries experience. This suggests the need for strategies to prevent and manage ECC in this Caribbean population.

Keywords: Early childhood caries, Quality of life, Preschool children, Caribbean

Background

Early Childhood Caries (ECC) has been defined by the American Academy of Pediatric Dentistry as 'the presence of one or more decayed, missing due to caries, or filled tooth surfaces in any primary teeth in children under 6 years of age [1]. In children younger than 3 years of age, any sign of smooth-surface caries is indicative of severe early childhood caries (S-ECC) [1].

Beyond the immediate distress caused by toothache, early childhood caries (ECC) can also have longer term negative, health outcomes [2, 3]. Untreated decay in infancy and early childhood is believed to affect weight gain and overall growth and development [4]. Along with these patho-physiological effects, ECC can impact on oral health related quality of life (OHRQoL) [2, 3]. As parents and caregivers have the main responsibility for

* Correspondence: rsnaidu937@gmail.com
[1]School of Dentistry, The University of the West Indies, Saint Augustine, Trinidad and Tobago
Full list of author information is available at the end of the article

their preschool-aged children, ECC can also affect them indirectly, for example, work-loss and financial impact due to having to stay at home to take care of the child [5]. ECC is therefore recognized as a public health problem due to its high prevalence in some populations and the potential for negative health impacts if left untreated [6, 7].

The few studies that have been undertaken in the English-speaking Caribbean suggest that caries prevalence among infants and preschool children in the region is high [8, 9]. In central Trinidad, the prevalence of ECC among 251 preschool children was reported as 29.1% with the majority of this being untreated, decayed teeth and 12% of children were in need of urgent care or referral [10]. Affordability and access to dental care for people from lower socioeconomic groups and those living in rural locations is a challenge in Trinidad and Tobago as most of the county's registered dentists work in private practices, generally clustered in urban centers.

Although there are international reports on OHRQoL of preschool children [11–16], nothing is known about the effect of ECC on OHRQoL among preschool children in the Caribbean.

Understanding the impact of dental caries in young children and their families can guide the development of treatment and preventive protocols as part of dental service planning.

The aim of this study was to describe the relationship between OHRQoL and ECC among preschool children in Trinidad.

Method

A cross-sectional oral health survey of preschool children was undertaken in the Caroni region of central Trinidad. The accessible population were children aged 3 to 5 years of age, attending preschools in the Caroni Education District. Based on the list of registered preschools, there were 27 government/government-assisted and 57 non-government preschools in the district at the time of the survey, with an enrolled population of approximately 2000 children. Previous data from Anguilla [9] (which estimated prevalence at 30%) was used to determine that 340 children were required to assess caries prevalence within the preschool population in the district. This figure accounted for 6% precision and 20% non-response rate.

Sampling consisted of cluster sampling within the Caroni Education District. A total of ten schools were selected by systematic random sampling from the school lists (three government/assisted schools and seven non-government preschools). Each cluster consisted of all registered children within the preschool. Each preschool was assumed to have an average of 30 registered children. Very small schools (<15) and very large schools (>60) were excluded, in order to enable inclusion of preschools of similar sizes and enable data collection by a single examiner. Stratification was not employed.

Ethical approval for the study was obtained from The University of the West Indies, Faculty of Medical Sciences Research Ethics Committee. Permission for the selected preschool's inclusion in the study was obtained from individual head teachers and written positive consent was requested from parents and caregivers for the oral examinations. Self-administered oral health questionnaires were provided to participating preschools. These questionnaires were then given to all parents and caregivers by the school administration, along with a consent form.

OHRQoL was measured using the Early Childhood Oral Health Impact Scale (ECOHIS) [3], included as part of the oral health questionnaire. The ECOHIS is a short, condition-specific tool, to be completed by the child's parent or primary caregiver. It has been validated in the English language and translated versions are reported to have good psychometric properties [3]. The ECOHIS consists of questions relating to quality of life domains for both the child and the family. These domains include: symptoms, function, psychological effects, self-image, parent distress and family function [3]. Responses are based on the scale: *Never, Hardly ever, Occasionally, Often, Very often, Don't know*. Scores for the instrument are calculated from the sum of responses for the child (0–36) and family sections (0–16) and reported as mean impacts per item/section (maximum overall score of 52). Higher mean ECOHIS score represents worse OHRQoL.

The ECOHIS instrument was piloted among 30 parents and caregivers of young children attending a dental hospital clinic in Trinidad. The instrument was found to have acceptable face and content validity and thus did not require any modification. The 'don't know' response were treated as 'missing' for the analyses.

Dental examinations were undertaken by a single, trained and calibrated dentist (RN) using WHO criteria [17]. Training and calibration was achieved by use of clinical slides on CD ROM, representing all categories of caries to be assessed and recorded. This was done under the supervision of a dental epidemiologist (JN). Examinations took place in classrooms using natural light, with the child in a seated position on a small chair/bench with the examiner positioned behind. Teeth were assessed visually with the use of a disposable mouth mirror, with the examiner wearing disposable gloves and facemask. New gloves and a mouth mirror were used for each child. Teeth were not air dried but soft debris on tooth surfaces was removed with a cotton roll or gauze square.

Examiner reliability was assessed by re-examination of children at one preschool (25 children). These re-examinations took place on the same day as data collection. The Kappa statistic for intra-examiner reliability was 0.9. Data collection was undertaken over a three-month period.

In the field, oral examination data were entered onto a record sheet by a research assistant. This information was subsequently transferred to a computer database (SPSS v 16) for storage and processing. Data were cleaned and checked for transcription errors before processing using SPSS version 16 for Windows and STATA version 10.

Statistical analysis

Logistic regression models were adopted to determine the family and child related factors associated with dmft and ECOHIS. Specifically, models examining factors relating to dmft were used to examine the odds of children having a dmft > 0 compared to the odds of children with a dmft = 0. Similarly, the odds of a parent/primary caregiver having an ECOHIS score >0 was compared to the odds of parents/primary caregivers with an ECOHIS score = 0, taking sociodemographic factors into account. Child and/or parent-primary caregiver characteristics were included as fixed effects in the models and a random intercept was included to account for cluster variation (i.e. variation within preschools). Akaike's information criteria and likelihood ratio tests were used to evaluate goodness of fit. In addition to variables retained in the final model, all models were adjusted for age and sex. Model sensitivity and specificity were examined using receiver operating characteristic curves and area under the curve (AUC). If a model achieves perfect sensitivity and specificity, then the AUC would have a value of 1. If the AUC has a value of 0.5 then the model achieves poor sensitivity and specificity. Despite estimation of AUC, the models developed for this research are for descriptive purposes, they are not intended for prediction. Generalised variance inflation factors (GVIF) and adjusted GVIF were used to determine the presence of multicollinearity. Model results are displayed in terms of odds ratios (ORs) and corresponding 95% confidence interval (CI). ORs have a range from 0 to infinity. An OR equal to one, denotes that there is no difference in odds whereas an OR greater than 1 indicates, for instance, that the ratio of those with a dmft > 0 versus a dmft = 0 in the selected group is greater than the baseline group. If there is no evidence to suggest that the ratio of those with dmft > 0 (versus dmft = 0) for the selected group are different from the baseline group, then the 95% CI for the OR will contain 1 in the interval.

Statistical analysis was performed using statistical software R (version 3.2.3) [18].

Results

From an enrolment of 340 children, 314 parents gave consent for the oral examination (91% response rate). Of these children, 36 (11.5%) were absent on the day and 27 (8.6%) refused examination. Three hundred and nine parents completed the questionnaire (Table 1). The mean age of the parents and primary caregivers was not determined as the questionnaire only recorded respondent age-range. Among these 309 respondents, 90% of parents/primary caregivers were in the age range 25–44 years. Parent/primary caregiver ethnicity was 74.4% Indian,

Table 1 Socio-demographic information for all parents and caregivers (*N* = 309)

	n	Percent
Age group		
18–24	17	5.5
25–34	183	59.2
35–44	95	30.7
45–54	8	2.6
55–64	2	0.7
65+	1	0.3
Missing	3	1.0
Ethnic group		
African	35	11.3
Indian	230	74.4
Mixed	41	13.3
White	1	0.3
Other	2	0.7
Occupation		
Professional	11	3.6
Managerial/lower professional	48	15.5
Non-manual	44	14.2
Manual -skilled	107	34.6
Manual- semi-skilled	6	1.9
Manual –unskilled	43	13.9
Housewife/unemployed	15	4.9
Retired/old-age pensioner	7	2.3
Missing	28	9.1
Education		
None	1	0.3
Primary	29	9.4
Secondary	255	50.2
Technical college	54	17.5
University	49	15.9
Other	15	4.9
Missing	6	1.9

Table 2 Socio-demographic information for parents/caregivers whose child completed the oral health assessment ($N = 251$)

	ECOHIS = 0		ECOHIS > 0		dmft = 0		dmft > 0	
	Count	%	Count	%	Count	%	Count	%
Parent/primary caregiver characteristics								
Age								
< 25 years	8	3.19	7	2.79	12	4.78	3	1.20
25–34	83	33.07	64	25.50	102	40.64	45	17.93
35–44	46	18.33	32	12.75	54	21.51	24	9.56
45+	7	2.79	2	0.80	8	3.19	1	0.40
Unknown	2	0.80	0	0.00	2	0.80	0	0.00
Sex								
Male	16	6.37	14	5.58	24	9.56	6	2.39
Female	130	51.79	91	36.25	154	61.35	67	26.69
Education								
Primary or lower	13	5.18	11	4.38	15	5.98	9	3.59
Secondary	47	18.73	38	15.14	85	33.86	40	15.94
Third level	74	29.48	51	20.32	64	25.50	21	8.37
Other	9	3.59	4	1.59	11	4.38	2	0.80
Unknown	3	1.20	1	0.40	3	1.20	1	0.40
Visits to the dentist								
Never	27	10.76	19	7.57	30	11.95	16	6.37
1–2 per year	82	32.67	55	21.91	101	40.24	36	14.34
Only when in pain	23	9.16	14	5.58	25	9.96	12	4.78
Other	14	5.58	16	6.37	22	8.76	8	3.19
Unknown	0	0.00	1	0.40	0	0.00	1	0.40
Child characteristics								
Age (years)								
3	56	22.31	29	11.55	71	28.29	14	5.58
4	74	29.48	64	25.50	87	34.66	51	20.32
5	16	6.37	12	4.78	20	7.97	8	3.19
Sex								
Male	70	27.89	56	22.31	89	35.46	37	14.74
Female	76	30.28	49	19.52	89	35.46	36	14.34
DMFT								
0	122	48.61	56	22.31				
1–3	16	6.37	20	7.97				
> 4	8	3.19	29	11.55				

11.3% African, 13.3% mixed and 1% white or other (Table 1).

The ECOHIS showed good internal consistency with a Cronbach alpha reliability coefficient of 0.94. For the child and family sections Cronbach alpha was 0.92 and 0.85, respectively.

Overall, quality of life impacts were low, with median score being 0. Mean impacts scores for the whole instrument were 2.29 (sd 5.52) and for the child and family sections 1.09 (sd 3.62) and 0.80 (sd 2.16), respectively. Examination of responses relating to the child's quality of life indicated that approximately 10.4% (32/309) reported that their child experienced pain in the teeth, mouth or jaw.

Approximately 5.2% (16/309) and 4.2% (13/309) reported that their child experienced difficulty eating some foods or difficulty drinking hot or cold drinks.

Examination of responses relating to family function indicated that approximately 10% (31/309) of parents/primary caregivers reported that they felt guilty, 5.2%

(16/309) had been upset and 4.9% (15/309) reported that they had taken time off work due to their child's oral health problems.

Despite 309 parent/primary caregivers completing the questionnaire, approximately 18% (58/309) of children did not complete the oral examination, thus a total of 251 children completed the oral examination. Of these children, 50.2% were male, with an age range of 3 to 5 years-old and mean age of 3.7 years (sd 0.67). Full results for visible caries experience have been reported previously [10]. Socio-demographic characteristic for parents/primary caregivers, together with information on ECOHIS and dmft for those children who completed the oral health assessment, are shown in Table 2.

Table 3 shows the frequency of oral health impacts for children with some caries experience (dmft > 0) and for those with no caries experience (dmft = 0) for the child and family levels, respectively.

Regression analysis was performed on the complete dataset excluding all missing and unknown observations. As previously stated, initially, there were 340 children to be involved in the study. The final sample was reduced to 245 (after excluding 7.6% (26/340) of those who did not give consent and missing observations (69/340). This accounted for approximately 28% (95/340) not being available for statistical analysis. Thus as a result of this reduced data set, a number of categories had low numbers. Logistic models without a random effect were adequate in all three models as the estimated standard deviation for unexplained variation within each cluster had a value <0.0001. In the principle of parsimony, models with lowest AIC were utilised. With reference to the model examining family perspectives associated with dmft > 0, the AIC for the model, including random effects, was 284.14 and was 283.69 for the simplified model. Similarly, the model examining child related factors associated with dmft > 0, the AIC for the model including random effects was 274.87 and was 273.09 for the less complex model. Examining factors associated with ECOHIS > 0 resulted in the model including random effect having an AIC of 318.19 and the simplified model having an AIC of 316.19. The factors included in all models were free from multicollinearity as all adjusted GVIF values had values less than 2. Factors that could not be included for statistical analysis were 'child avoided talking' and 'child being irritable or frustrated', as these factors had excessively high adjusted GVIF values. The factor 'child smiling' was also omitted from the analysis due to zero observations for this factor with dmft = 0. Crude and adjusted ORs for children with dmft > 0 compared to those with dmft = 0 can be seen in Tables 4 and 5.

Table 6 shows the crude and adjusted ORs for parents/primary caregivers with ECOHIS > 0 compared to those with ECOHIS = 0. Model evaluations indicate that the three models are adequate in terms of sensitivity, with AUC being estimated as 0.68, 0.64 and 0.74, respectively. However, as previously stated, these models were not developed for predictive purposes and caution must be exercised in model interpretation due to wide confidence intervals.

Table 3 Oral health impacts for children with no visible caries dmft = 0 and some visible caries dmft > 0

	Never/hardly ever				Occasionally/often/very often				Don't know/NA			
	dmft = 0		dmft > 0		dmft = 0		dmft > 0		dmft = 0		dmft > 0	
	n	%	n	%	n	%	n	%	n	%	n	%
Child impacts												
Pain in the teeth, mouth or jaw	170	76.9	51	23.1	6	22.2	21	77.8	2	66.6	1	33.3
Difficulty drink hot or cold drinks	174	73.7	62	26.3	2	18.2	9	81.8	2	50.0	2	50.0
Difficulty eating some foods	175	74.5	60	25.5	3	20.0	12	80.0	0	0	1	100
Difficulty pronouncing some words	175	72.6	66	27.4	3	42.9	4	57.1	0	0	3	100
Missed preschool	176	72.1	68	27.9	1	20.0	4	80.0	1	50.0	1	50.0
Trouble sleeping	175	72.9	65	26.4	2	22.2	7	77.8	1	50.0	1	50.0
Been irritable or frustrated	177	74.7	60	25.3	1	8.3	11	91.7	0	0	2	100
Avoided smiling or laughing	176	73.3	64	26.7	1	14.3	6	85.7	1	25.0	3	75.0
Avoided talking	176	72.1	68	27.9	1	20.0	4	80.0	1	50.0	1	50.0
Family impacts												
Felt upset	173	73.3	63	26.7	4	30.8	9	69.2	1	50.0	1	50.0
Felt guilty	169	75.1	56	24.9	8	33.3	16	66.7	1	50.0	1	50.0
Taken time off work	175	74.5	60	25.5	3	21.4	11	78.6	0	0	1	100
Had a financial impact on your family	177	72.8	66	27.8	1	14.3	6	85.7	0	0	1	100

309 parents/caregiver observations were recorded, of whom 187 had children with dmft = 0, 73 dmft > 0 and 58 unknown dmft

Table 4 Child factors associated with DMFT >0

	Crude OR	95% CI	Adjusted OR	95% CI
Child's age				
3	1.0		1.0	
4	3.08	(1.59, 6.34)	3.61	(1.76, 7.95)
5	2.12	(0.74, 5.79)	2.26	(0.71, 6.83)
Child's sex				
Male	1.0		1.0	
Female	0.89	(0.51, 1.54)	1.04	(0.57, 1.91)
Pain in the teeth, mouth or jaw				
No	1.0		——	
Yes	0.76	(0.31, 1.71)		
Difficulty drinking hot or cold drinks				
No	1.0		1.0	
Yes	12.55	(3.13, 83.85)	7.14	(1.36, 55.13)
Difficulty eating some foods				
No	1.0		1.0	
Yes	10.51	(3.16, 47.63)	8.29	(2.00, 43.49)
Difficulty pronouncing some words				
No	1.0		——	
Yes	3.42	(0.74, 17.76)		
Missed preschool				
No	1.0		——	
Yes	10.38	(1.5, 205.20)		
Trouble sleeping				
No	1.0		——	
Yes	9.76	(2.21, 64.62)		

Note: 'Yes' denotes occasionally/often/very often; 'No' denotes never/hardly ever
Model adjusted for other factors in the model
As confidence intervals are large, caution must be exercised when interpreting results

In Model 1: child related factors associated with dmft > 0, statistically significant factors include child's age, difficulty drinking hot or cold drinks, difficulty eating some foods, missing preschool and trouble sleeping (Table 4). Adjusting for the effects of other factors the odds for a child aged 4 years were greater for having dmft > 0 (in comparison to dmft = 0) than the odds for a child aged 3 years (OR 3.61; 95% CI (1.76, 6.83)). The odds for children who had difficulty drinking hot or cold drinks were greater for those with dmft > 0 than the odds for children who had no such difficulty (OR 7.14; 95% CI (1.36, 55.13)). Similarly, the odds of a dmft >0 were increased for children who have difficulty eating than the odds for children who have no difficulty eating (OR 8.29; 95% CI (2.00, 43.49)).

In Model 2: family perspectives associated with child's dmft > 0, statistically significant factors include parent/primary caregiver feeling upset, guilty and having to take time off work (Table 5). Adjusting for the effects of other factors, the odds of parents/primary caregivers who felt guilty were greater for those with a child with a dmft > 0 in comparison to parents/primary caregivers who did not feel guilty (OR 3.50; 95% CI (1.32, 9.60)). Similarly, the odds of parents/primary caregivers who had to take time off work were greater with a child with dmft > 0, in comparison to parents/primary caregivers who did not

Table 5 Family factors associated with child's DMFT > 0

	Crude OR	95% CI	Adjusted OR	95% CI
Parent/primary caregiver age				
< 25 years	0.61	(0.13, 2.16)	0.35	(0.05, 1.53)
25–34	1.12	(0.61, 2.07)	1.06	(0.56, 2.04)
35–44	1.0		1.0	
45+	0.31	(0.02, 1.81)	0.40	(0.02, 2.40)
Parent/guardian sex				
Male	1.0			
Female	1.66	(0.68, 4.67)	1.34	(0.53, 3.85)
Parent/primary caregiver highest level of education				
Primary or below	1.92	(0.71, 5.07)		
Secondary	1.38	(0.74, 2.60)		
Third level	1.0		——	
Other/unknown	0.54	(0.08, 2.25)		
Parent/guardian visits to dentist				
Never	1.49	(0.70, 3.07)		
1–2 per year	1.0		——	
Only when in pain	1.33	(0.59, 2.89)		
Other	1.11	(0.43, 2.67)		
Felt upset				
No	1.0		——	
Yes	6.13	(1.92, 23.30)		
Felt guilty				
No	1.0		1.0	
Yes	5.52	(2.28, 14.38)	3.50	(1.32, 9.60)
Taken time off work				
No	1.0		1.0	
Yes	9.29	(2.74, 42.45)	7.27	(1.76, 41.11)
Had a financial impact on your family				
No	1.0		——	
Yes	13.03	(2.05, 252.15)		
Type of pre-school				
Private school	1.0		——	
Government school	0.98	(0.54, 1.78)		

Note: 'Yes' denotes occasionally/often/very often; 'No' denotes never/hardly ever
Model adjusted for other factors in the model
As confidence intervals are large, caution must be exercised when interpreting results

Table 6 Factors associated with ECOHIS > 0

	Crude OR	95% CI	Adjusted OR	95% CI
Parent/guardian age				
< 25 years	1.27	(0.43, 1.08)	1.59	(0.46, 5.44)
25–44	1.12	(0.41, 3.90)	1.11	(0.60, 2.07)
45–64	1.0		1.0	
65+	0.41	(0.05, 1.85)	0.55	(0.23, 1.28)
Parent/guardian sex				
Male	1.0		1.0	
Female	0.75	(0.35, 1.66)	0.55	(0.23, 1.28)
Parent/guardian highest level of education				
Primary or below	1.11	(0.44, 2.81)		
Secondary	0.82	(0.47, 1.43)		
Third level	1.0		——	
Other/unknown	0.54	(0.14, 1.79)		
Parent/guardian visits to dentist				
Never	0.68	(0.48, 0.95)		
1–2 per year	1.0		——	
Only when in pain	0.90	(0.42, 1.88)		
Other	1.70	(0.75, 3.89)		
Child's age				
3	1.0		1.0	
4	1.63	(0.93, 2.88)	1.30	(0.70, 2.43)
5	1.37	(0.55, 3.35)	1.04	(0.38, 2.76)
Child's sex				
Male	1.0		1.0	
Female	0.79	(0.47, 1.31)	0.83	(0.48, 1.47)
Child's DMFT				
0	1.0		1.0	
1–3	2.68	(1.30, 5.64)	2.55	(1.19, 5.50)
> 4	8.58	(3.71, 22.45)	8.70	(3.54, 23.13)

Model adjusted for other factors in the model

have to take time off work (OR 7.27; 95% CI (1.76, 41.11)).

In Model 3: factors associated with ECOHIS > 0, a child's dmft value were found to be statistically significantly related (Table 6). Adjusting for parental age/sex and child's age and sex, model results indicate that the odds of parents/primary caregivers having ECOHIS >0 (in comparison to ECOHIS = 0), was increased when a child's dmft was in the range 1–3 (OR 2.68; 95% CI (1.30, 5.64) or dmft > 4 (OR 8.58; 95% CI (3.71, 22.45)) compared with those whose child had a dmft = 0.

Discussion

Overall, the frequency of oral health impacts for this Trinidadian sample was low for both Child and Family sections of the instrument, which is similar to data reported from the US [3]. As the majority of respondents had no impacts this may have resulted in a high 'floor effect'. This can reduce the ability of the instrument to measure the interaction between the items in the child and family domains and OHRQoL. Unlike several other instruments, for the ECHOHIS the parent is asked to consider lifetime experience rather than the previous three months, to take account of lower disease levels in some populations.

The most frequent child impacts in this sample were similar to ECOHIS data from Australia, Canada, Iran, Hong Kong, Brazil and Turkey, which included English and non-English-speaking populations in developed and developing countries [11–16]. These main impacts were: *pain in the mouth, teeth or jaw, difficulty with eating some foods, drinking hot or cold beverages and being irritable or frustrated.* This suggests that OHRQoL impacts due to ECC are consistent across developed and developing countries. In a multiethnic population in a developing country, Malaysia, the main impacts were again similar, however, the prevalence of these impacts was much higher than in the present study [19]. This may have been due to the slightly older age groups (4–6 years) and differences in social/cultural backgrounds. These main impacts are consistent with symptoms from untreated dental caries in children and confirms the negative effect on quality of life that ECC can have in preschool children. Findings in the family section were also consistent with several other countries, where ECOHIS has been used, with *feeling guilty or upset* being the most common impacts (4,11,12,14,15,16). Interestingly, data from a Turkish study [16] differed from the present study findings, with most frequent family impacts being *financial* and *having to take time off work*, although this study was among a sample of older children with a higher severity of caries experience.

The issue of feelings of guilt about the oral health of their preschool aged child was explored by Carvalho et al. who defined guilt as *"a feeling that occurs when one assesses one's specific action as a failure or when the particular action has led to failure"* [20]. The authors suggest that these feelings may be due to some parents having knowledge about prevention and dental care but are unable to act on it, effectively, with respect to their child.

In the present study the odds of having negative OHRQoL impacts for both the child and family were significantly associated with having visible caries experience. These odds increased with greater caries severity, indicating that families of children with untreated dental caries suffer the majority of the disease burden and should be prioritized for treatment and preventive care.

These findings highlight the need to develop oral health promotion strategies that support parents and caregivers and that go beyond merely increasing oral health knowledge. Changing behavior requires approaches that impart practical advice and enhance motivation, as well as developing coping skills, enabling families to overcome barriers to preventive dental care. In this regard, patient-centered counselling approaches and brief counselling techniques such as motivational interviewing (MI) have shown promise in relation to improving preschool children's oral health [21, 22] and found to be an acceptable as part of health promotion for families of preschool children in Trinidad [23].

Limitations of the study

1. This was a cross-sectional study from one education district and therefore limits the generalizability of the findings to the rest of Trinidad. However, the Caroni district does have a mixed of urban and rural population and a varied SES profile, similar to the national demographic profile.
2. Sampling was not stratified, which may have influenced the findings and masked differences by SES. Also, not all children under 5-years of age attend preschool and some of those children are likely to have had worse oral health than those in the sampling frame.
3. The findings for OHRQoL of preschool children are limited due to the use of proxy reports. Proxy reports on children's oral health may underestimate the severity of oral health impacts.
4. Re-examination of children for intra examiner reliability took place on the same day, however, to avoid the bias due to memory of the initial examination, ideally, these should have been done on a return visit to the preschools.
5. Exclusion of very large preschools may have limited the representativeness of the sample.

Conclusion

Although overall oral health impacts were low in this sample of preschool children, OHRQoL was found to be related to ECC. More impacts were found in children with greater severity of visible caries experience. The burden of dental disease and its impacts appears concentrated in a minority of young children, suggesting the need for strategies to address oral health in early childhood in Trinidad. Measuring the effect on OHRQoL in families with young children may enable prioritization and evaluation of interventions. Such interventions should support families in implementing positive dental care practices for their young children and include caries risk assessment, early establishment of the dental home and access to regular fluoride therapy for children at high risk for ECC, along with consistent information from dental health professionals, family physicians, pediatricians, community nurses, and preschool staff.

Abbreviations

AAPD: American Academy of Paediatric Dentistry; ECC: Early childhood caries; ECOHIS: Early Childhood Oral Health Impact Scale; OHRQoL: Oral health related quality of life

Acknowledgements

The authors would like to acknowledge the late Dr. Alan Kelly (Trinity College Dublin), Dr. Donald Simeon and Miss Shelly Hunte for statistical advice.

Funding

This research was supported by a grant from the University of the West Indies Campus Research and Publication Fund.

Authors' contributions

RN and JN contributed to the design and conduct of this research. EDS contributed to the data analyses. All authors contributed to the writing of the manuscript. All authors read and approved the final manuscript.

Competing interests

The authors declare that they have no competing interests.

Consent for publication

Not applicable.

Ethics approval and consent to participate

Ethical approval for this research was obtained from the University of the West Indies Campus Research Ethics Committee. Written positive consent was requested from parents and caregivers for the oral examinations.

Author details

[1]School of Dentistry, The University of the West Indies, Saint Augustine, Trinidad and Tobago. [2]School of Dental Sciences, Trinity College Dublin, Dublin 2, Ireland.

References

1. American Academy of Pediatric Dentistry and American Academy of Pediatrics. Policy on early childhood caries (ECC): classifications, consequences and preventive strategies. Reference Manual. (Revised 2014): http://www.aapd.org/media/policies_guidelines/p_eccclassifications.pdf. Accessed Sept 2016.
2. Abanto J, Carvalho TS, Mendes FM, Wanderley MT, Bonecker M, Raggio DP. Impact of oral disease and disorders on oral health-related quality of life of preschool children. Community Dent Oral Epidemiol. 2011;139:105–14.
3. Pahel BT, Rozier RG, Slade GD. Parental perceptions of children's oral health: The Early Childhood Oral Health Impact Scale (ECOHIS). Health Qual Life Outcomes. 2007;5:6. http://www.hqlo.com/content/pdf/1477-7525-5-6.pdf.
4. Sheiham A. Dental caries affects body weight, growth and quality of life in preschool children. Br Dent J. 2006;20:625–6.
5. Gift H, Reisine S, Larch D. The social impact of dental problems and visits. Am J Public Health. 1992;82:1163–8.
6. O' Mullane D, Parnell C. Early childhood caries: a complex problem requiring a complex solution. Community Dent Health. 2011;28:254.
7. Seow W. Environmental, maternal and child factors which contribute to early childhood caries: a unifying conceptual model. Int J Paediatr Dent. 2012;2:157–68.
8. Vignarajah S, Williams GA. Prevalence of dental caries and enamel defects in the primary dentition of Antiguan preschool children aged 3–4 years including an assessment of their habits. Community Dent Health. 1992;9:349–60.
9. Adewakun A, Beltran-Aguilar ED. Early childhood caries in Anguilla, British West Indies. Am J Gen Dent. 2003;5:42–7.

10. Naidu R, Nunn J, Kelly A. Socio-behavioral factors and early childhood caries: a cross-sectional study of preschool children in central Trinidad. BMC Oral Health. 2013;13:30. http://www.biomedcentral.com/1472-6831/13/30.
11. Arrow P, Klobas E. Evaluation of the Early Childhood Oral Health Impact Scale in an Australian preschool population. Aust Dent J. 2015;60:375–81.
12. Li S, Veronneau J, Allison PJ. Validation of a French language version of the early childhood oral health impact scale (ECOHIS). Health Qual Life Outcomes. 2014;6:9. http://www.hqlo.com/content/pdf/1477-7525-6-9.pdf.
13. Jabbarifar S, Ahmady N, Sahafian SA, Samei F, Soheillipour S. Association of parental stress and early childhood caries. Dent Res J. 2009;6:65–70.
14. Wong H, McGrath CPJ, King NM, Lo ECM. Oral health-related quality of life in Hong Kong preschool children. Caries Res. 2011;45:370–6.
15. Scarpelli A, Oliveira BH, Tesch FC, Leao AT, Pordeus Paiva SM. Psychometric properties of the Brazilian version of the Early Childhood Oral Health Impact Scale (B-ECOHIS). BMC Oral Health. 2011;11:19. http://www.biomedcentral.com/content/pdf/1472-6831-11-19.pdf.
16. Peker K, Uysal O, Bermek G. Cross-cultural adaptation and preliminary validation of the Turkish version of the Early Childhood Oral Health Impact Scale among 5–6 year-old children. Health Qual Life Outcomes. 2011;9:118. http://www.ncbi.nlm.nih.gov/pmc/articles/PMC3310831/pdf/1477-7525-9-118.pdf.
17. World Health Organisation. Oral health surveys. Basic methods. Geneva: WHO; 1997.
18. R software. https://cran.r-project.org/. Accessed Sept 2016.
19. Hashim AN, Tuysof ZY, Esa R. The Malay version of the Oral Health Impact Scale (Malay-ECOHIS) assessing validity and reliability. Health Qual Life Outcomes. 2015;13:190. http://www.ncbi.nlm.nih.gov/pmc/articles/PMC4660630/pdf/12955_2015_Article_386.pdf.
20. Carvalho TS, Abanto J, Mendes FM, Raggio DP, Bonecker M. Association between parental guilt and oral health problems in preschool children. Braz Oral Res. 2012;26:557–63.
21. Yevlahova D, Satur J. Models for individual oral health promotion and their effectiveness: a systematic review. Aust Dent J. 2009;54:190–7.
22. Borreli B, Tooley EM, Lori AJ, Scott-Sheldon LAJ. Motivational interviewing for parent–child health interventions: a systematic review and meta-analysis. Pediatr Dent. 2015;37:254–65.
23. Naidu RS, Nunn JH, Irwin JD. The effect of motivational interviewing on oral health knowledge, attitudes and behaviors of parents of preschool children. An exploratory cluster randomised controlled study. BMC Oral Health. 2015; 15:101. http://www.biomedcentral.com/content/pdf/s12903-015-0068-9.pdf.

2

Effectiveness of bovine-derived xenograft versus bioactive glass with periodontally accelerated osteogenic orthodontics in adults: a randomized, controlled clinical trial

Maha A. Bahammam

Abstract

Background: Periodontally accelerated osteogenic orthodontics (PAOO) combines periodontal therapy with orthodontic therapy, which minimises treatment time. This study compared the effectiveness of a bovine-derived xenograft with that of bioactive glass when combined with PAOO for the treatment of adult patients with moderate crowding of the teeth.

Methods: In this prospective, single-masked clinical trial, 33 orthodontic patients (20 women, 13 men; mean age 21.2 ± 1.43 [18 – 27] years), were randomly allocated to one of three groups. Group 1 underwent a modified corticotomy technique on the labial side only, whereas group 2 was treated with the same technique combined with PAOO using a bovine-derived xenograft and group 3 was treated in the same way but combining PAOO with bioactive glass. The total treatment duration was recorded from the start of active orthodontic treatment, immediately after corticotomy, and at the time of debonding. Probing depth was evaluated clinically and bone density and root length were evaluated radiographically on the day of surgery (baseline, T1), post-treatment at debonding (T2), and 9 months post-treatment (T3).

Results: The duration of orthodontic treatment was markedly reduced to an average of 11.4 ± 0.14 weeks in all groups. All probing depths were < 3 mm, the interdental papillae were well preserved, there was no loss of tooth vitality, and there was no evidence of significant apical root resorption at any time interval. All groups showed a decrease in mean bone density at T2 followed by an increase at T3. The net percentage change that occurred between baseline and 9 months post-treatment was significantly different between the three groups. Groups 2 and 3, where grafts were incorporated, demonstrated a statistically significant greater increase in bone density than group 1 at T3.

Conclusion: Combination of orthodontic treatment and periodontal surgery is an effective treatment for adult patients that decreases the duration of active treatment and reduces the risk of root resorption. Use of a bovine-derived xenograft with modified corticotomy provided superior benefits in terms of increased bone density than did the use of bioactive glass.

Trial registration: The study was retrospectively registered at ClinicalTrials.gov under Clinical Trial Registration Number: NCT02796911.

Keywords: Alveolar bone density, Bone grafts, Corticotomy-assisted orthodontic treatment, Root resorption

Correspondence: mbahammam@kau.edu.sa
Department of Periodontology, Faculty of Dentistry, King Abdulaziz University, P. O. Box 80209, Jeddah 21589, Kingdom of Saudi Arabia

Background

There has been a significant increase in the number of adult patients seeking orthodontic treatment [1]. The average duration of routine orthodontic treatment for adults is considerably longer than for adolescent patients, ranging from 18.7 to 31 months, and even more time is required for extraction cases [2, 3]. Adult patients are also more vulnerable to root resorption and periodontal pathologies during or after active orthodontic treatment, given their narrow, aplastic, poorly vascularised periodontal membrane, and alveolar bone morphology [1, 4]. Hence, it is imperative to modify treatment modalities to reduce the treatment time and achieve optimal clinical results in adults.

Corticotomy and osteotomy have been used in orthodontics primarily to resolve crowding of teeth as rapidly as possible. In published case reports, moderate or severe crowding has been treated without extraction by corticotomy/osteotomy-assisted orthodontics, and in shorter time periods [5, 6]. It has been reported that this approach was efficient for reducing the treatment time to as little as a quarter of that usually required for conventional orthodontics [5, 7–9]. Additional applications for this technique have reportedly facilitated several orthodontic modalities in a short period of time, with greater post-orthodontic stability [7, 10].

A temporary stage of remodelling of localised soft and hard tissue, termed the "regional acceleratory phenomenon" (RAP), results in rebuilding of the sites injured in corticotomy/osteotomy to a normal state by recruitment of osteoclasts and osteoblasts via local intercellular mediator mechanisms that involve precursors, supporting cells, blood capillaries, and lymph. RAP begins within a few days of the insult, typically peaks at 1 – 2 months, and may take as long as 2 years to subside completely [11, 12].

Periodontally accelerated osteogenic orthodontics (PAOO) is a technique involving combination of a selective decortication-facilitated orthodontic technique and alveolar augmentation. Thus, teeth can be moved 2 – 3 times further in one third to one quarter of the time required by traditional orthodontic therapy. Moreover, PAOO provides an increased net alveolar volume after orthodontic treatment and is associated with low morbidity [9, 13]. The greater alveolar volume eliminates bony dehiscence and fenestrations under most circumstances [5]. Likewise, the additional alveolar bone width may be the cause of the enhanced long-term orthodontic stability noted with this technique [13, 14].

Hong et al. conducted a study in 2011 using a Beagle animal model for histologic assessment of the biological effects of PAOO. In the group that underwent corticotomy, no osteoclasts were found on the cementum or dentin, although numerous osteoclasts were detected around the alveolar bone facing the palatal side of the retracted incisor. In addition, a more intact periodontal ligament space of consistent thickness was noted between the surrounding alveolar bone and the root surface. The compression side of the retracted incisor showed no evidence of root resorption [7, 15].

Interestingly, current therapies in both traumatology and tissue regeneration dentistry are based on the use of artificial or natural materials, which produce stimulating signals that trigger physiological regeneration, a process that depends on three mechanisms: osteogenesis, osteoinduction, and osteoconduction [16]. Xenografts and bioactive glass offer such alternatives. A number of previous studies have demonstrated the effectiveness of xenografts as osteoconductive matrices [17–21]. On the other hand, bioactive glass is an alloplastic bone graft and a possible choice for alveolar augmentation in corticotomy-assisted orthodontic treatment (CAOT) [16–25]. Results from clinical studies have indicated that treatment of intrabony defects with bone grafts alone may result in improved clinical outcomes, as evidenced by improvements in probing depth (PD) and clinical attachment [23].

In spite of the advantages of PAOO, assessment of this technique remains challenging in clinical trials, and evidence of the success of these grafts has been evaluated only in a few case reports [5, 8, 26, 27]. Accordingly, the purpose of this study was to evaluate the effectiveness of a bovine-derived xenograft versus that of bioactive glass, using a modified corticotomy procedure, in the orthodontic treatment of adult patients with moderate crowding.

Methods

Sample

The study protocol was approved by the ethics committee of King Abdulaziz University in accordance with the guidelines published by the CONSORT group and the World Medical Association's Declaration of Helsinki, (proposal number 029-16). All research procedures were explained to the patients, who provided signed consent to participate in the study. The study was retrospectively registered at ClinicslTrials.gov under Clinical Trial Registration No. (NCT02796911).

Thirty-three adult orthodontic patients (23 female, 10 male) of mean age 21.2 ± 1.43 (range 18 – 27) years were included in this randomised, prospective, single-masked trial that was conducted between February 2015 and March 2016. The study participants were selected from patients seeking orthodontic treatment at the outpatient clinic in the Orthodontic Department, Faculty of Dentistry, King Abdulaziz University. The criteria for inclusion in the study were as follows: good oral hygiene and systemic health; PD values (measured as the distance from the bottom of the sulcus to the most apical portion of the gingival margin) not exceeding 3 mm; no radiographic evidence of bone loss; no regular administration of any medication that affects bone metabolism, such as prolonged use of corticosteroids, bisphosphonates, or non-steroidal anti-inflammatory drugs; moderate crowding of the lower anterior teeth only, ranging from 4 – 5 mm; and no previous orthodontic treatment.

Cephalometric analyses were performed to limit patient selection to those with a Class I skeletal pattern and a favourable mandibular incisor plane angle. Orthodontic study cast analyses were used to limit the selection to cases of moderate crowding. Standardised digital periapical radiographs from the left mandibular canine to the right mandibular canine were used and the exposure parameters were fixed for all patients, both initially and during the follow-up period.

Each patient was randomly assigned to one of three groups, masked with respect to assignment and each containing 11 patients. Group 1 (seven women, four men) was treated with a modified technique of CAOT alone, group 2 (six women, five men) was treated with CAOT combined with a bovine-derived xenograft (Bio-Oss, Geistlich, Princeton, NJ, USA), and group 3 (seven women, four men) was treated with CAOT combined with bioactive glass (GlassBone, NORAKER, Villeurbanne, France). Randomisation was performed using a commercially available computer software package (NCSS-PASS, Number Cruncher Statistical Systems, Kaysville, UT, USA).

The proposed treatment procedures along with their advantages and disadvantages were explained in detail to all patients and informed consent was obtained. Initial prophylaxis and periodontal therapy, consisting of full mouth scaling utilising both hand and ultrasonic instruments, were performed under local anaesthesia.

Each participant received orthodontic treatment with a mandibular fixed appliance inserted during the week preceding surgery. In accordance with the treatment plan, the standardised treatment protocol used a pre-adjusted appliance that included direct bond brackets (Roth Prescription) 0.022" × 0.028" in size (Integra Brackets, Rocky Mountain Orthodontics Inc, Denver, CO, USA) from the right mandibular second premolar to the left mandibular second premolar, using a chemical cure orthodontic adhesive (Transbond XT; 3 M Unitek, Monrovia, CA, USA) and banding of the mandibular first molars (Rocky Mountain Orthodontics Inc). The appliance was not activated presurgically. Orthodontic tooth movement was started 2 weeks after the corticotomy procedure; the interval allowed between routine orthodontic adjustments was 2 weeks, which is in line with previous recommendations [5, 9, 27].

During orthodontic treatment, the mandibular arch was initially levelled and aligned using nickel titanium arch wires of increasing size (0.012", 0.014", 0.016", and 0.018"). Thereafter, rectangular stainless steel wires (0.016" × 0.022") were placed. Stainless steel arch wires up to size 0.019" × 0.025" were used for finishing. During the active tooth movement phase, patients were assessed by the periodontist at monthly intervals.

Periodontal surgical procedure

The PAOO technique used for the three groups in the current study was performed under local anaesthesia and is a modification of the basic corticotomy technique described by Wilcko et al. [8, 9, 27]. Intra-crevicular full-thickness flaps were reflected labially only from the distal surface of the lower right canine to the distal surface of the lower left canine while preserving the interdental papilla. The labial flap was reflected beyond the apices of the lower anterior teeth. Selective alveolar decortication was then performed in the form of vertical grooves through the labial cortical plate of bone, using a small round stainless steel surgical bur (number 2) in a low-speed hand piece, under copious irrigation, and extended through the entire thickness of the cortical plate, barely reaching the medullary bone. The vertical grooves started 1 – 2 mm below the alveolar crest and extended 1 – 2 mm below the apices of the teeth (Fig. 1). The lingual flap was not elevated and no horizontal subapical cuts were performed [28].

In groups 2 and 3, after completion of the corticotomy procedure, a bovine xenograft and/or bioactive glass were mixed with blood from the surgical site in a sterile Dappen dish until a sandy consistency was obtained. The resulting coagulum was transferred in increments and applied directly over the decorticated areas (Fig. 1). Next, the flap was carefully repositioned at the original

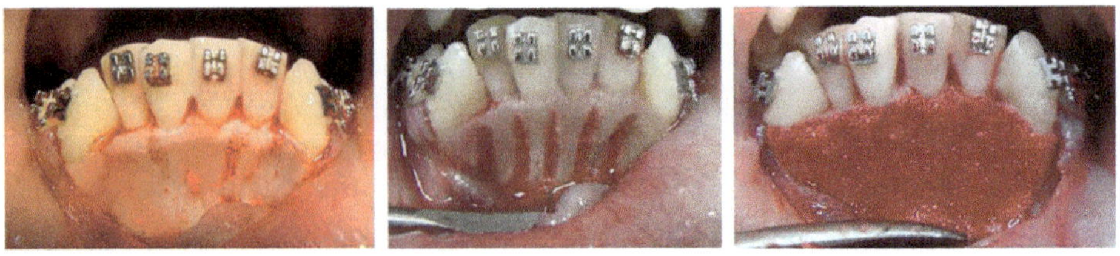

Fig. 1 Surgical procedures

pre-surgical site and sutured with nonresorbable 4-0 silk using the interrupted technique [23, 29].

All patients were provided with oral hygiene instructions and closely monitored to prevent inflammation of the gingival tissues. Antibiotic, diuretic, and analgesic agents were prescribed for 7 days. The efforts to control plaque formation were augmented by antiseptic mouthwash (0.12% chlorhexidine gluconate, for 1 min twice daily for 2 weeks), and the sutures were removed after 10 days. Figure 2 shows representative intraoral images taken before and after treatment.

Data analysis

The total duration of active orthodontic treatment was estimated in weeks for the three study groups from the time of starting active orthodontic treatment, immediately following the corticotomy procedure, to the time of debonding.

Clinical and radiographic parameters were recorded on the day of surgery (T1), post-treatment (at time of debonding) (T2), and 9 months post-treatment (T3) for all three groups. PD measurements were taken using a William's probe 26 from the gingival margin to the base of the sulcus and recorded to the nearest millimetre. Six readings for each tooth were recorded (mesial, distal, and midpoint for both the labial and lingual surfaces).

Radiographic measurements were obtained from standardised digital periapical radiographs from the left mandibular canine to the right mandibular canine using Digora system software (Orion Corp, Sordex Medical System, Helsinki, Finland). The radiographic images for each patient were saved and analysed to record bone density and root length, and the mean of the readings was calculated (Fig. 2).

To measure the bone density, the mean grey value in each region of interest was calculated (256 grey levels of colour resolution) by assigning the grey value of 0 to black, and a grey value of 256 to white. Linear density was measured by drawing a line parallel to the root surface, extended from the apex of the alveolar crest to the level of the apex of the root. A line was drawn midway between every two lower anterior teeth. Five lines were drawn (between the lower right canine and lateral incisor, between the lower right lateral incisor and central incisor, between the two lower central incisors, between the lower left lateral incisor and central incisor, and between the lower left canine and lateral incisor).

The grey level along each line was recorded at the beginning, middle, and end of the line, and the average of the three readings was calculated to obtain the mean average density (grey level) along this line. The mean value of the readings of the five lines was calculated to present the density value.

The root length was assessed by measuring the distance between the cemento-enamel junction (as a reference point) and the apex of the root in millimetres.

One operator (MB) performed all the surgeries and was informed of group assignment after corticotomy just before placing the graft material. Another calibrated operator, who was not involved in the study, performed all the clinical and radiographic measurements without knowledge of group assignment. Intra-examiner calibration was evaluated before starting the study by examination of 30 sites on two separate occasions 48 h apart.

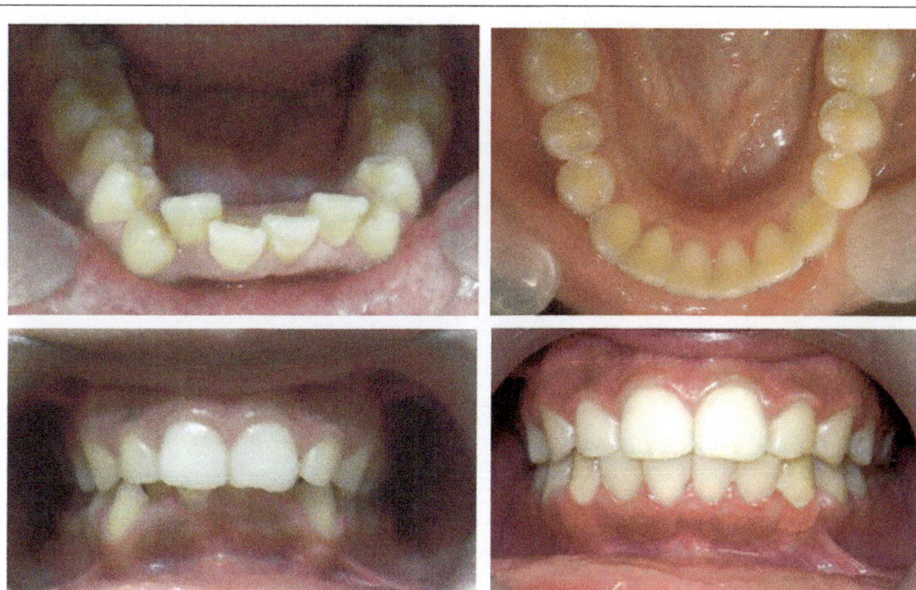

Fig. 2 Occlusal and frontal Pre and post treatment intraoral pictures

Calibration was only accepted if 90% of the readings could be reproduced within a 1 mm difference.

The primary outcome of the study was duration of orthodontic treatment from baseline to the time of debonding. Secondary outcomes included changes in PD, bone density, and root length up to 9 months post-treatment.

Statistical analysis

The collected data were tabulated and statistically analysed using Statistical Package for the Social Sciences version 20 (IBM Corp., Armonk, NY USA). Descriptive statistics (mean, standard deviation, range) are presented. One-way analysis of variance was used to compare data between the three groups, and a post-hoc (Tukey's) test was used for pair-wise comparisons between the groups when analysis of variance test were significant. The Student's *t*-test was used to compare the mean differences within each group for each time interval.

Results

The total treatment time was calculated in weeks from the time of activation of the orthodontic appliance immediately following the corticotomy procedure to the time of debracketing. The treatment duration for patients in all groups ranged from 12 to 20 weeks, with a mean of 15 weeks for group 1, 16.8 weeks for group 2, and 14.4 weeks for group 3. Figure 3 shows representative intraoral images before and after treatment.

Clinical parameters

Probing depth

There was no significant difference in PD at baseline between the three groups ($P > 0.05$; Table 1). Within each group, there was a significant difference between the participants in terms of the net amount of change in PD that occurred between the start of treatment and 9 months post-treatment ($P > 0.05$; Table 2).

There was a statistically significant difference between the three groups regarding the change that occurred in PD during each time interval. Nine months post-treatment (during the retention period), group 1 demonstrated a mean PD of 1.18 ± 0.19 mm, while group 2 demonstrated a mean PD of 1.20 ± 0.20 mm and group 3 demonstrated a mean PD of 1.19 ± 0.18 ($P > 0.05$; Table 1).

Bone density

Within the three groups, there were significant differences in the amount of change that occurred in bone density during the different time intervals. During the period of active tooth movement (from pre-treatment to post-treatment), all groups demonstrated a decrease in bone density; the mean decrease was -29.82% in group 1, -14.43% in group 2, and -24.04% in group 3. The amount of increase in bone density from post-treatment to 9 months post-treatment was also significantly different between the three groups; the mean increase was 0.87% in group 1, 31.99% in group 2, and 13.71% in group 3 (Table 1). The net percentage increase in bone density from the start of treatment to 9 months post-treatment (97.53% ± 6.33%) was greater in group 2 than in groups 1 and 3.

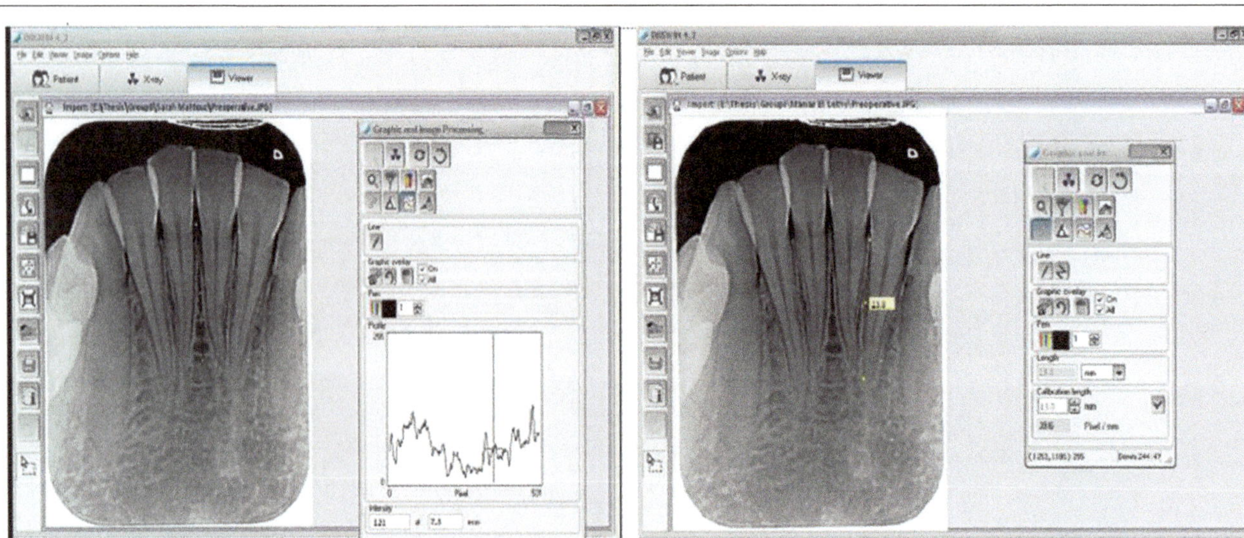

Fig. 3 Radiographic assessment

Table 1 Mean probing depth, bone density, and root length between the groups at each time interval

Parameter	Time	Group 1 (CAOT without graft)		Group 2 (CAOT with xenograft)		Group 3 (CAOT with bioactive glass)		*P*-value
		Mean	SD	Mean	SD	Mean	SD	
Probing depth (mm)	T1	1.54	0.17	1.57	0.13	1.56	0.14	0.054
	T2	1.17[b]	0.16	1.19[a]	0.14	1.19[a]	0.17	0.047*
	T3	1.18[b]	0.19	1.20[a]	0.20	1.19[a,b]	0.18	0.012*
Bone density	T1	63.24[c]	7.21	65.54[b]	6.41	66.41[a]	6.32	<0.000*
	T2	33.42[c]	6.81	51.11[a]	6.21	42.32[b]	6.43	<0.000*
	T3	64.11[c]	6.22	97.53[a]	6.33	80.12[b]	6.31	<0.000*
Root length (mm)	T1	12.81[b]	0.73	12.82[a]	0.54	12.82[a]	0.51	0.037*
	T2	12.79	0.71	12.79	0.64	12.80	0.53	0.968
	T3	12.78	0.64	12.78	0.53	12.79	0.52	0.060

Notes: *P*, probability level; $*P \leq 0.05$; different superscript letters in the same row are significantly different. *n* number; T1, before CAOT (baseline); T2, after debonding (post-treatment); T3, 9 months after debonding. *Abbreviations*: *CAOT* corticotomy-assisted orthodontic treatment, *SD* standard deviation

Root resorption

There was no significant difference between the three groups in terms of the average root length values obtained pre-treatment, post-treatment, and 9 months post-treatment. The difference in the net amount of root resorption between the three groups was also statistically insignificant. The average net decrease in root length was -0.02 ± 0.02 mm in group 1, -0.03 ± 0.11 mm in group 2, and -0.01 ± 0.01 mm in group 3 (Table 1).

Discussion

Most orthodontic patients, and particularly adults, are interested in the possibility of reducing their treatment time. Given this constant demand for shorter treatments, orthodontists have increasingly sought ways and new approaches to shorten the treatment duration without compromising results. CAOT has been suggested for reducing the orthodontic treatment time [5, 6, 8, 9, 28–30]. PAOO can play a major role in the comprehensive treatment of occlusal and esthetic needs in some patients. PAOO is an extension of previously described techniques involving surgical alteration of the alveolar bone to decrease treatment time [5].

In this study there was a significant reduction in the treatment time for adult patients demonstrating moderate crowding to an average of 11.4 (range 10 – 13) weeks. This is in agreement with other reports of CAOT [5–9, 30–32] and agrees with the findings of Wilcko et al., who presented cases treated over short periods with a combination of CAOT and periodontal alveolar augmentation [5, 8, 9, 27].

Table 2 Comparison of mean probing depth (mm) in each group at different time intervals

Group	Time interval	Mean difference	SD difference	*P*-value
Group 1	T1–T2	0.37	0.08	0.002*
	T1–T3	0.36	0.09	0.004*
Group 2	T1–T2	0.38	0.07	0.001*
	T1–T3	0.37	0.08	0.000*
Group 3	T1–T2	0.37	0.08	0.001*
	T1–T3	0.37	0.08	0.002*

Notes: *P*, probability level; $*P \leq 0.05$; T1, before CAOT; T2, after debonding; T3, 9 months after debonding
Abbreviation: *SD* standard deviation

Thirty-three patients were initially enrolled in the present study, but four were excluded because of multiple missed appointments and failure to maintain good oral hygiene, when a considerable amount of patient cooperation was necessary. After 9 months, only 27 patients were available for clinical and radiographic reevaluation; these patients had a good clinical outcome and did not experience any relapse.

Interestingly, the current results also showed that the total orthodontic treatment time was markedly reduced when compared with the average treatment time (31 months) for extraction therapy [2, 33]. In a clinical trial, Hajji [7] investigated the effects of resolving mandibular anterior dental crowding by comparing non-extraction, extraction, and CAOT approaches. The mean active treatment time for the CAOT group was 6.1 months versus 18.7 months in a non-extraction orthodontic group and 26.6 months in an extraction group, which is consistent with the findings of the present study.

Several theories have been proposed in an attempt to explain the rapid tooth movement observed after corticotomy. The initial concept, which prevailed in several subsequent reports, was based on "bony block movement". According to this theory, the tooth embedded within a block of medullary bone serves as the handle by which the bands of less dense medullary bone surrounding the teeth are moved block by block [33]. However, the latest concept concerning the rapid tooth movement after corticotomy is supported by RAP, described as accelerated bone turnover and decreased regional bone density [8, 9, 12, 33, 34]. RAP is a local response to a stimulus, and describes a process by which tissue forms more rapidly than during the normal regional regeneration process. The term "regional" refers to the demineralisation of both the cut site and the adjacent bone and the term "accelerated" refers to an exaggerated or intensified bone response in cuts that extend to the marrow. It is explained as a temporary phase of localised soft and hard tissue remodelling that results in rebuilding of the injured sites to a normal state. By enhancing the various healing stages, this phenomenon causes healing to occur 2–10 times more rapidly than normal physiological healing. The RAP mechanism potentiating tissue healing has been shown to occur in the mandible as well as in the long bones [12, 34, 35].

No hazardous effects on the periodontium were observed after corticotomy in this study. PD in particular was not significantly different between the study groups (Table 1). Not only was there no deterioration in periodontal depth, but patients demonstrated a slight improvement in PD values.

Unlike most of the corticotomy procedures described earlier, the present cortical cuts were made in the labial cortical plate of bone only, without making subapical cuts, and the lingual flap was not reflected. This was performed to support the blood supply of the mandibular dentoalveolar region via the lingual mucosa and to protect the thin roots of the incisors in the region where access is difficult and there is a possibility of damaging the teeth. Labial subapical horizontal cuts were omitted to protect the overlying cortical bone and to maintain the blood supply to the incisors, because the spongiosa bone was not left intact. Furthermore, it was assumed that RAP induced by the buccal corticotomy would readily involve the non-corticotomised lingual side [28, 36]. Moreover, the main purposes of using the present conservative technique were to reduce the duration and extent of surgery and the postoperative discomfort by eliminating exposure of the patient to the risks of additional lingual surgery [28, 36]. In addition, using the current corticotomy technique, the vertical cuts were started 1 - 2 mm below the alveolar crest in an attempt to protect the crestal bone and periodontal membrane, as per previous recommendations [28].

Several reports have speculated that, by avoiding the crest of the marginal bone during vertical corticotomies, there would be less risk of damage to the marginal periodontium [5, 6, 28, 33, 37]. These surgical conservative criteria could explain the absence of detrimental clinical side effects on the periodontium in this study.

The current results are in accordance with other reports of rapid tooth movement and reduced treatment times without clinically noticeable adverse periodontal effects [8, 30, 38]. The fact that the teeth can be moved more rapidly, thus resulting in shortened treatment times, is certainly advantageous for periodontal health, because a reduction of the time that the patient needs a fixed appliance reduces patient "burnout" and substantially reduces the time available for relatively benign commensal bacterial biofilms to undergo qualitative changes and convert to a destructive cytotoxic ("periodontopathic") type, which is often seen when fixed appliances have remained on the teeth for more than a year [9].

The present study revealed a reduction in alveolar bone density at the time of debonding (T2) in all three groups (Table 1). This is in agreement with other reports that have attributed this to the trauma caused to cortical bone, which has been shown to be a potentiating factor in producing localised osteoporosis or reversible osteopenia. For bone, this temporary condition means increased mobilisation of calcium, decreased bone density, and increased bone turnover, all of which would facilitate more rapid tooth movement [28, 39–41]. After an initial reduction, the bone density had increased again at 9 months post-treatment in all three groups (Table 2), which adds further support to the view that the dynamics of tooth movement in these patients might be more appropriately described as a demineralisation/remineralisation process, rather than bony block movement [8, 9, 15, 16, 28, 36, 39–41].

PAOO with bone augmentation was performed in the present study to increase alveolar volume and to avoid the possible risks of the procedure [8, 9]. It was considered that the roots would still have sufficient support if very large expansions were implemented to resolve severe crowding. The reshaped alveolar bone provides additional support for the roots of the teeth after completion of treatment and diminishes potential dehiscence [8, 9, 36]. Two different types of bone grafts, a xenograft (bovine xenograft) and an alloplast (bioactive glass), were utilised in this study. Numerous studies have shown the biocompatibility and effectiveness of a variety of xenografts that incorporate biomaterials derived from bovine bone. Other studies have reached the conclusion that this material has a system of interconnected pores, the structure of which is similar to that of human spongy bone, which may contribute to promoting the close interrelationship between hydroxyapatite and bone during growth [17–25]. Bioactive glass was selected as the second bone graft material because a number of in vivo and in vitro studies have highlighted its potential as a regenerative scaffold [18, 21, 22]. Moreover, highly bioactive glass particles have good clinical manageability and certain haemostatic properties, and showed both osteoproduction and osteoconduction [22].

It is interesting to note that, at the end of the study period, there was a significantly greater increase in bone density in the two groups that had been treated with bone grafting when compared with the group that had been treated with a modified CAOT alone (Table 1). Moreover, patients who were treated with the bovine-derived xenograft showed a greater (albeit not statistically significant) increase in bone density than those who were treated with bioactive glass. This could be attributed to a different ability of the two biomaterials to promote bone formation. In addition, the composition of animal bone is morphologically more similar than any synthetic product to human bone; a previous analysis of the results of clinical testing and the clinical take-up of different products developed by the biomedical industry has shown the overall superiority of bone substitutes of natural origin over derivative substitutes [40, 42].

In terms of root resorption, the current study revealed no significant difference in root length values between the three study groups (Table 1). Root resorption is a complex process, involving the combination of a multitude of biological and mechanical factors. It is generally accepted that some root resorption is expected with any orthodontic tooth movement [43] Thus, it is believed that the absence of any significant root resorption in this study might be, in part, attributed to the short treatment duration, which is in agreement with previous reports of this advantage of CAOT [22, 29, 31, 32, 44]. However, incorporation of bone grafting appears to have little effect on the incidence or amount of root resorption because of the absence of any statistically significant difference between the three groups regarding the amount of root resorption (Table 1).

Conclusions

The results of this study suggest that PAOO is an effective and promising treatment approach that can decrease the active treatment duration, the risk of root resorption, and/or adverse periodontal effects in adult patients. PAOO may improve the state of the periodontium by increasing bone density and decreasing the risk of root resorption. Use of bovine-derived xenografts provided better results than bioactive glass in terms of increasing bone density. However, further randomised testing in humans is required to shed more light on an expanded use of PAOO, as well as to confirm the claimed advantages of this technique and evaluate the long-term effects and stability of such treatment.

Abbreviations

CAOT: Corticotomy-assisted orthodontics; PAOO: Periodontally accelerated osteogenic orthodontics; PD: Probing depth; RAP: Regional acceleratory phenomenon

Acknowledgment

The author would like to thank the Deanship of Scientific Research for technical and financial support.

Funding

This study was funded by the Deanship of Scientific Research (DSR), King Abdulaziz University, Jeddah, Kingdom of Saudi Arabia (Grant No. D-180-165-1437).

Author information

Bahammam MA is an Associate Professor in the Department of Periodontology, Faculty of Dentistry, King Abdulaziz University.

Competing interests

Bahammam MA has no conflict of interests, and the work was not supported or funded by any bone graft/pharmaceutical company.

Consent to publish

Signed consent was obtained from all participants to publish their personal details and images.

Ethics approval and consent to participate

The study protocol was submitted and approved by the ethical committee of King Abdulaziz University (proposal number 029-16). All research procedures were explained to the patients, who provided signed consent to participate in the study. The study was retrospectively registered at ClinicslTrials.gov under Clinical Trial Registration Number NCT02796911.

References

1. Mathews DP, Kokich VG. Managing treatment for the orthodontic patient with periodontal problems. Semin Orthod. 1997;3(1):21–38.
2. Kocadereli I. Changes in soft tissue profile after orthodontic treatment with and without extractions. Am J Orthod Dentofacial Orthop. 2002;122(1):67–72.
3. Vig PS, Weintraub JA, Brown C, Kowalski CJ. The duration of orthodontic treatment with and without extractions: a pilot study of five selected practices. Am J Orthod Dentofacial Orthop. 1990;97(1):45–51.
4. Ong MM, Wang HL. Periodontic and orthodontic treatment in adults. Am J Orthod Dentofacial Orthop. 2002;122(4):420–8.
5. Chung KR, Oh MY, Ko SJ. Corticotomy-assisted orthodontics. J Clin Orthod. 2001;35(5):331–9.
6. Wilcko MT, Wilcko WM, Pulver JJ, Bissada NF, Bouquot JE. Accelerated osteogenic orthodontics technique: a 1-stage surgically facilitated rapid orthodontic technique with alveolar augmentation. J Oral Maxillofac Surg. 2009;67(10):2149–59.
7. Hajji SS. The influence of accelerated osteogenic response on mandibular de- crowding; 2000
8. Wilcko T, Wilcko WM, Bissada NF. An evidence-based analysis of periodontally accelerated orthodontic and osteogenic techniques' A synthesis of Scientific perspectives. Semin Orthod. 2008;14(4):305–16.
9. Wilcko WM, Ferguson DJ, Bouquot JE, Wilcko T. Rapid orthodontic decrowding with alveolar augmentation: case report. J Orthod. 2003;4:197–205.
10. Kole H. Surgical operations on the alveolar ridge to correct occlusal abnormalities. Oral Surg Oral Med Oral Pathol. 1959;12(4):413–20.
11. Frost HM. The regional acceleratory phenomenon: a review. Henry Ford Hosp Med J. 1983;31(1):3–9.
12. Yaffe A, Fine N, Binderman I. Regional accelerated phenomenon in the mandible following mucoperiosteal flap surgery. J Periodontol. 1994;65(1):79–83.
13. Dinesh MR, Gupta S, Yannawar V, Sharma K, Agarwal A, Lagali P, et al. Periodontally accelerated osteogenic tooth movement in orthodontics: A review. Int J Adv Health Sci. 2011;1(11):32–7.
14. Rothe LE, Bollen AM, Little RM, Herring SW, Chaison JB, Chen CS, et al. Trabecular and cortical bone as risk factors for orthodontic relapse. Am J Orthod Dentofacial Orthop. 2006;130(4):476–84.
15. Kim H-S, Lee Y-J, Park Y-G, K-R C, Kang TG, Choo HR, et al. Histologic assessment of the biological effects after speedy surgical orthodontics

in a beagle animal model: a preliminary study. Korean J Orthod. 2011;41(5):361–70.
16. Esposito M, Grusovin MG, Coulthard P, Worthington HV. The efficacy of various bone augmentation procedures for dental implants: a Cochrane systematic review of randomized controlled clinical trials. Int J Oral Maxillofac Implants. 2006;21(5):696–710.
17. Richardson CR, Mellonig JT, Brunsvold MA, McDonnell HT, Cochran DL. Clinical evaluation of Bio-Oss: a bovine-derived xenograft for the treatment of periodontal osseous defects in humans. J Clin Periodontol. 1999;26(7):421–8.
18. Sculean A, Pietruska M, Schwarz F, Willershausen B, Arweiler NB, Auschill TM. Healing of human intrabony defects following regenerative periodontal therapy with an enamel matrix protein derivative alone or combined with a bioactive glass. A controlled clinical study. J Clin Periodontol. 2005;32(1):111–7.
19. Tadic D, Epple M. A thorough physicochemical characterisation of 14 calcium phosphate-based bone substitution materials in comparison to natural bone. Biomaterials. 2004;25(6):987–94.
20. Tamai N, Myoui A, Tomita T, Nakase T, Tanaka J, Ochi T, et al. Novel hydroxyapatite ceramics with an interconnective porous structure exhibit superior osteoconduction in vivo. J Biomed Mater Res. 2002;59(1):110–7.
21. Trombelli L, Heitz-Mayfield LJ, Needleman I, Moles D, Scabbia A. A systematic review of graft materials and biological agents for periodontal intraosseous defects. J Clin Periodontol. 2002;29 Suppl 3:117–35. discussion 60-2.
22. Froum SJ, Weinberg MA, Tarnow D. Comparison of bioactive glass synthetic bone graft particles and open debridement in the treatment of human periodontal defects. A clinical study. J Periodontol. 1998;69(6):698–709.
23. Keles GC, Cetinkaya BO, Albayrak D, Koprulu H, Acikgoz G. Comparison of platelet pellet and bioactive glass in periodontal regenerative therapy. Acta Odontol Scand. 2006;64(6):327–33.
24. Sculean A, Nikolidakis D, Schwarz F. Regeneration of periodontal tissues: combinations of barrier membranes and grafting materials - biological foundation and preclinical evidence: a systematic review. J Clin Periodontol. 2008;35(8 Suppl):106–16.
25. Wenz B, Oesch B, Horst M. Analysis of the risk of transmitting bovine spongiform encephalopathy through bone grafts derived from bovine bone. Biomaterials. 2001;22(12):1599–606.
26. Vercellotti T, Podesta A. Orthodontic microsurgery: a new surgically guided technique for dental movement. Int J Periodontics Restorative Dent. 2007;27(4):325–31.
27. Wilcko WM, Wilcko T, Bouquot JE, Ferguson DJ. Rapid orthodontics with alveolar reshaping: two case reports of decrowding. Int J Periodontics Restorative Dent. 2001;21(1):9–19.
28. Germec D, Giray B, Kocadereli I, Enacar A. Lower incisor retraction with a modified corticotomy. Angle Orthod. 2006;76(5):882–90.
29. De Rouck T, Eghbali R, Collys K, De Bruyn H, Cosyn J. The gingival biotype revisited: transparency of the periodontal probe through the gingival margin as a method to discriminate thin from thick gingiva. J Clin Periodontol. 2009;36(5):428–33.
30. Hasan E. Orthodontic maxillary canine retraction after partial corticotomy of the buccal plate; Clinical and radiographic investigations. Cairo: Faculty of Dental Medicine, Al-Azhar University; 2005.
31. Moon CH, Wee JU, Lee HS. Intrusion of overerupted molars by corticotomy and orthodontic skeletal anchorage. Angle Orthod. 2007;77(6):1119–25.
32. Ren A, Lv T, Kang N, Zhao B, Chen Y, Bai D. Rapid orthodontic tooth movement aided by alveolar surgery in beagles. Am J Orthod Dentofacial Orthop. 2007;131(2):160. e1-10.
33. Suya H. Corticotomy in orthodontics. In: Hosl E, Baldauf A, eds. Mechanical and Biological Basics in Orthodontic Therapy. Heidelberg, Germany: Hutlig Buch; 1991:207-26. Quoted in: Germec D, Giray B; Kocadereli I, Enacart A. Lower incisor retraction with a modified corticotomy. Angle Orthod. 2006;76:882–90.
34. Frost HM. The biology of fracture healing. An overview for clinicians. Part I. Clin Orthop Relat Res. 1989;248:283–93.
35. Frost HM. The biology of fracture healing. An overview for clinicians. Part II. Clin Orthop Relat Res. 1989;248:294–309.
36. Mostafa YA, Mohamed Salah Fayed M, Mehanni S, ElBokle NN, Heider AM. Comparison of corticotomy-facilitated vs standard tooth-movement techniques in dogs with miniscrews as anchor units. Am J Orthod Dentofacial Orthop. 2009;136(4):570–7.
37. Gantes B, Rathbun E, Anholm M. Effects on the periodontium following corticotomy-facilitated orthodontics. Case reports. J Periodontol. 1990;61(4):234–8.
38. Iino S, Sakoda S, Miyawaki S. An adult bimaxillary protrusion treated with corticotomy-facilitated orthodontics and titanium miniplates. Angle Orthod. 2006;76(6):1074–82.
39. Lee W, Karapetyan G, Moats R, Yamashita DD, Moon HB, Ferguson DJ, et al. Corticotomy-/osteotomy-assisted tooth movement microCTs differ. J Dent Res. 2008;87(9):861–7.
40. Sebaoun JD, Kantarci A, Turner JW, Carvalho RS, Van Dyke TE, Ferguson DJ. Modeling of trabecular bone and lamina dura following selective alveolar decortication in rats. J Periodontol. 2008;79(9):1679–88.
41. Wang L, Lee W, Lei DL, Liu YP, Yamashita DD, Yen SL. Tisssue responses in corticotomy- and osteotomy-assisted tooth movements in rats: histology and immunostaining. Am J Orthod Dentofacial Orthop. 2009;136(6):770. e1-11 discussion -1.
42. Santos FA, Pochapski MT, Martins MC, Zenobio EG, Spolidoro LC, Marcantonio Jr E. Comparison of biomaterial implants in the dental socket: histological analysis in dogs. Clin Implant Dent Relat Res. 2010;12(1):18–25.
43. Owman-Moll P, Kurol J, Lundgren D. Continuous versus interrupted continuous orthodontic force related to early tooth movement and root resorption. Angle Orthod. 1995;65(6):395–401. discussion -2.
44. Machado I, Ferguson DJ, Wilcko WM, Wilcko MT, Alkadhara T. Root resorption following orthodontics with and without alveolar corticotomy. J Dent Res. 2002;80(301):301.

3

Prevalence of and factors affecting malocclusion in primary dentition among children in Xi'an, China

Zhifei Zhou[1†], Fen Liu[1,2†], Shuning Shen[1,3], Linjuan Shang[1,4], Lei Shang[5*] and Xiaojing Wang[1*]

Abstract

Background: This study aimed to investigate the prevalence and associated factors of malocclusion among children with primary dentition in Xi'an, China.

Methods: A total of 2,974 subjects were selected from local schools in Xi'an city using a stratified cluster sampling method from January to September 2015. After screening samples according to the inclusion criteria, the final sample size comprised 2,235 pre-school children, with a mean age of 4.82 (SD, 1.76; range, 2.63–6.12) years. Malocclusion traits were assessed by trained clinicians followed by the evaluation of associated factors through clinical examination and a precisely designed questionnaire including data regarding gender, birth place, parental education level, monthly familial income, parental attitude toward the problem of malocclusion, feeding methods of the children, feeding postures, pacifier use, and delivery methods. Data were analyzed using the Chi-square test and logistic regression analysis.

Results: The most common type of malocclusion was increased overjet (34.99 %) in the sagittal direction, deep overbite (37.58 %), and midline deviation (25.32 %) in the vertical and transverse directions, respectively. The prevalence of posterior crossbite, anterior crossbite, and anterior open bite was 7.56, 6.80 and 6.98 %, respectively. The prevalence of the anterior edge-to-edge occlusion was the lowest (2.46 %). The variables associated with malocclusion ($P < 0.05$) were birth place (odds ratio [OR] = 1.741 with 95 % CI of 1.384–2.162), insufficient abrasion of primary canines (OR = 1.465; 95 % CI of 1.153–1.894), caries in primary teeth (OR = 2.045; 95 % CI of 1.665–2.539), tongue thrusting (OR = 2.833; 95 % CI of 1.640–3.649), mandibular prognathism (OR = 2.621; 95 % CI of 1.574–3.689), and finger sucking (OR = 1.573 with 95 % CI of 1.098–2.014). The feeding methods (OR = 3.614 with 95 % CI of 3.087–4.596) along with the method of delivery (OR = 1.847 with 95 % CI of 1.323–2.451) have been observed to play an important role in the morbidity of malocclusion ($P < 0.05$).

Conclusions: The prevalence of malocclusion among pre-school children in Xi'an is higher compared to that in other geographical parts of China. Therefore, early attention to the development of occlusion and necessary interventions toward the associated factors are important to reduce its prevalence and further adverse effects.

Keywords: Cross-sectional study, Epidemiology, Malocclusion, Prevalence, Primary dentition

Abbreviations: CI, Confidence interval; ICC, Intraclass correlation coefficient; OR, Odds ratio; WHO, World Health Organization

* Correspondence: shanglei@fmmu.edu.cn; wxjingpd@hotmail.com
[†]Equal contributors
[5]Department of Health Statistics, School of Public Health, Fourth Military Medical University, Xi'an, People's Republic of China
[1]State Key Laboratory of Military Stomatology, National Clinical Research Center for Oral Diseases, Department of Pediatric Dentistry, School of Stomatology, Fourth Military Medical University, Xi'an, People's Republic of China
Full list of author information is available at the end of the article

Background

Malocclusion is a condition characterized by abnormal relationships among the teeth or dentitions. It is one of the most common problems affecting the human oral cavity along with caries, gingivitis, and dental fluorosis [1]. It leads to symptoms such as deficient chewing, speech articulation, undesirable development of the jaw bones [2], etc. The prevalence of malocclusion is usually high among adolescents with permanent or mixed dentition. Kaur et al. reported a high prevalence of malocclusion (87.79 %) among Indian adolescents aged 13–17 years [3]. The prevalence of normal occlusion among Nigerian children (aged 13–20 years) was only 11.8 % in 2014 [4]. The total prevalence of Class I, II, and III types of malocclusion among Iranian children aged 11–14 years old was 77.1 % [5].

Some cohort studies have already indicated that malocclusion in primary dentition is the determinant of malocclusion in permanent dentition [6–8]. Moreover, it would also increase the potential needs of orthodontic treatment in permanent dentition [9]. In addition, malocclusion may lead to low self-esteem in later years, as children with primary dentition undergo a period during which they establish self-identity and early personality [10]. The prevalence of malocclusion in primary dentition is more than 50 % worldwide [11, 12], and whether malocclusion during this period needs early management is debatable [9, 13]. However, scholars have confirmed that the severity of malocclusion in primary dentition would affect permanent dentition; thus, rather than early management, it is more important to identifying the influencing factors of malocclusion in this period and implement some preventive strategies [14, 15], in order to decrease the severity and lower the prevalence of malocclusion in future.

Therefore, proper and timely evaluation of the factors associated with malocclusions in the primary dentition could help in the prevention and better management of occlusion-related problems later in life [16]. Malocclusion is generally considered as a multifactorial condition that is linked to developmental factors (such as nasal obstruction impairing the nasal breathing), habits (such as thumb sucking), genetics, hereditary factors, and ethnicity [13, 17]. To date, very limited information is available regarding the prevalence of malocclusion among children with primary dentition in Chinese populations. Moreover, because of the different criteria and investigated indices, previous studies have reported different results among various ethnic groups [18, 19].

Currently, there is lack of information regarding the prevalence of malocclusion among the residents of Xi'an city. This epidemiological study aimed to investigate the prevalence and associated factors of malocclusion in primary dentition among children in Xi'an.

Methods

Sample selection

Xi'an is a main regional city in Northwest China, with an area of 10,108 square kilometers and a diverse population of more than eight million. A cross-sectional study was conducted in Xi'an city from January to September 2015. A total of 24 kindergarten schools registered with the pre-school education administration institute in the northern, central, and western districts of Xi'an city were randomly selected. From each kindergarten, two classes in each grade were randomly selected. All children of the selected classes ($n = 2{,}974$) were included in this study. Children with fully erupted primary dentition and without any permanent teeth including the first molars or permanent incisors, and those who co-operated well with the examiners were included in the study. Children who had previously undergone orthodontic or occlusal guidance treatment and those with a history of current or previous systemic diseases or craniofacial anomalies were excluded.

Among all children ($n = 2{,}974$), a remarkable proportion ($n = 739$) did not meet the inclusion criteria and were excluded. The remaining children ($n = 2{,}235$, 1,185 [53.02 %] boys and 1,050 [46.98 %] girls) were included in the research for further investigations. The mean age of the participants was 4.82 (SD, 1.76; range, 2.63–6.12) years.

Ethics approval and consent to participate

The parents of the participating children were informed of the objectives of this research, and written informed consent was obtained from all the parents prior to conducting the study. The study was approved by the Ethical Committee of the School of Stomatology, Fourth Military Medical University, Republic of China (committee's reference number: IRB-REV-2014068).

Criteria of different types of malocclusion and associated variables

The clinical examinations for different types of malocclusion and occlusive variables such as fused teeth, insufficient abrasion of the primary canines, primate space, and caries in the primary teeth and premature exfoliation of primary teeth were performed by trained and calibrated clinicians using a mouth mirror, a graduated periodontal probe, and a tongue blade. The diagnosis criteria for each type of malocclusion were adopted from a previous study [20], as shown in Table 1.

The diagnostic criteria for fused teeth were defined as two teeth with fused enamel or dentin with a forking crown. Insufficient abrasion of the primary canines was noted when the canine cusp was significantly higher than the normal occlusal plane, leading to an early occlusal contact with antagonistic teeth. Primate spaces were located mesial to the upper canines and distal to

Table 1 Types of malocclusion and related diagnostic criteria

	Types	Diagnosis criteria
Sagittal anomalies	Anterior crossbite	Recorded when the lower incisors or canines are in front of the corresponding upper teeth
	Edge-to-edge occlusion	Recorded when the maxillary incisors and the corresponding mandibular incisors are occluded in an edge-to-edge status, without overbite or overjet
	Increased overjet	Recorded when the distance from the most labial point of the incisal edge of the maxillary incisors to the most labial surface of the corresponding mandibular incisors is more than 3 mm, measured to the nearest 0.5 mm
Vertical anomalies	Open bite	Recorded when the upper and lower incisors are vertically separated regardless of the extent, without any overbite
	Deep overbite	Recorded when the vertical overlap of the incisors, when the posterior teeth are in contact is more than two thirds covered or when the overlap is more than 3 mm, measured to the nearest 0.5 mm
Transversal anomalies	Posterior crossbite	Recorded when the buccal cusps of the maxillary molars occlude lingually to the buccal cusps of the mandibular antagonists in at least one pair of teeth, uni- or bilaterally. Teeth in an edge-to-edge position were also included
	Midline deviation	Recorded when the position of the mandibular midline had a more than 2-mm discrepancy relative to the maxillary midline, with the posterior teeth in full occlusion

the lower canines. No visible primate space was considered as the absence of the primate space. In this study, both decayed and filled carious primary teeth were defined as carious [21]. Premature exfoliation of primary teeth was defined as loss of a tooth due to diseases or injuries outside the physiological exfoliation period.

Design of questionnaire for parents

A questionnaire was designed focusing on the demographic characteristics of the children such as gender, birth place (urban/rural), parental education level (high school and below/undergraduate/master and above), monthly familial income, and parental attitude toward the problem of malocclusion (positive/not concerned). In addition, the feeding methods of the children (such as breast milk/milk powder/both), feeding postures (sitting/half sitting/flat/unfixed), pacifier use (yes/no), and delivery methods (such as natural labor/cesarean section) were investigated in this questionnaire. Moreover, the dental visit experiences of the children including the visiting frequency, the facility visited, and the visiting experience (pleasant/unpleasant) were assessed. Finally, the parents were asked regarding current or previous improper oral habits of their children, such as regular tongue thrusting, finger sucking, bruxism, mandibular prognathism, lip biting, and mouth breathing. The questionnaires were completed by the parents of the participating children by following the instructions and under the observation of trained examiners. Each of the improper habits was explained by the examiners and any queries raised by the participants were satisfactorily addressed.

Data collection

Six examiners, who were all faculty members at the Department of Pediatric Dentistry, School of Stomatology, Fourth Military Medical University, Republic of China, participated in this study. Prior to the investigation, serial training sessions were arranged to clarify the purpose of this study, creating awareness about the correct methods for examining primary teeth, and guiding parents to fill the questionnaires accurately. In order to test the intra-examiner reproducibility, following four weeks of their initial examination, 30 children were selected for re-examination. The results showed a high intra-examiner agreement for each type of malocclusion (i.e., maximum and minimum Kappa values were 1.00 and 0.73, respectively). The inter-examiner reliability was determined by two observers who independently evaluated 30 children on the same day. All measurements showed a high degree of inter-examiner reliability, with the intra-class correlation coefficients higher than 0.88.

Statistical analysis

Data were recorded and analyzed using the SPSS statistical software version 22.0. For different types of malocclusions, frequencies and percentages were generated; correlations between the selected variables and malocclusion were determined using the Chi-square test. Statistical significance was considered when $P < 0.05$. Statistically significant independent variables in the Chi-square test were further analyzed using binary logistic regression taking malocclusion as a dependent ($P < 0.05$), and odds ratios (ORs) were then obtained in addition to calculating 95 % confidence intervals (CIs).

Results

Prevalence of different types of malocclusion

Normal occlusion was observed in only 753 children (33.69 %), while 1,482 (66.31 %) children had one or more types of anomalies.

Table 2 Prevalence of different types of malocclusion

Type	N	Percentage (%)
Malocclusion in sagittal direction		
Anterior crossbite	152	6.80
Edge to edge occlusion	55	2.46
Increased overjet	782	34.99
Malocclusion in transversal direction		
Posterior crossbite	169	7.56
Midline deviation	566	25.32
Malocclusion in vertical direction		
Deep overbite	840	37.58
Open bite	156	6.98

The general prevalence of malocclusion is presented in Table 2. The most common type of malocclusion in the sagittal direction was the increased overjet (34.99 %), while the most prevalent malocclusions in the vertical and transverse directions were deep overbite (37.58 %) and midline deviation (25.32 %), respectively. Deep overbite was the most common type of malocclusion among children with primary dentition. The prevalence of posterior crossbite, anterior crossbite, and anterior open bite was 7.56, 6.80 and 6.98 %, respectively. The prevalence of the anterior edge-to-edge occlusion was the lowest (2.46 %).

Relationship between different types of malocclusion and demographic characteristics

The prevalence of malocclusion among children with different demographic characteristics is shown in Table 3. It indicated that the prevalence in urban children was significantly lower than that in children residing in rural areas (61.59 % vs. 76.29 %). The highest prevalence (77.91 %, $P <$ 0.001) was observed in the group of children with monthly familial income less than 2,000 yuan. No statistically significant ($P > 0.05$) association was observed between malocclusion and parental education level or gender.

Factors associated with oral examination and malocclusion

The results of Chi-square test indicated that children with insufficient abrasion of the primary canines, those lacking primate spaces, and those with caries in the primary teeth had a higher prevalence of malocclusion ($P < 0.05$, Table 4). No significant difference in malocclusion was detected between groups of children with premature exfoliation of primary teeth or fused teeth ($P > 0.05$, Table 4).

Relationship between improper oral habits and malocclusion

The relationship between improper oral habits and malocclusion was also confirmed by Chi-square test (Table 4). The results showed that children with tongue thrusting and mandibular prognathism had a higher probability of malocclusion ($P < 0.05$) compared to normal children. Moreover, mouth breathing or finger sucking were associated with a higher prevalence of malocclusion in the primary dentition ($P < 0.05$). The data showed that bruxism together with lip biting did not display any statistical significance with malocclusion ($P > 0.05$).

Relationship between feeding/delivery methods and malocclusion

With regard to the feeding methods (Table 4), Chi-square test demonstrated that the majority of the children were fed on both breast milk and milk powder during infancy. The prevalence of malocclusion showed a significant difference between these groups ($P < 0.001$), while breastfed children had the lowest incidence of malocclusion (23.10 %). With regard to the feeding postures, majority of the children were fed in sitting or half-sitting positions compared to flat or unfixed postures. However, there was no statistically significant difference among these groups ($P > 0.05$). Most children with primary dentition had never used a pacifier. However, the prevalence of malocclusion was higher than in those who did not use pacifiers as infants (73.98 % vs. 64.56 %, $P < 0.001$). With regard to the delivery method, children born via natural labor were less likely to experience malocclusion in the primary dentition than children born via cesarean section ($P < 0.05$).

Relationship between dental visit experience and malocclusion

The experience of previous dental visits was also investigated for its association with malocclusion (Table 4). With regard to the visiting frequency, children who never underwent a routine oral examination or never visited dental clinics when necessary had a significantly higher rate of malocclusion ($P < 0.05$) compared to children who visited dental clinics more frequently at regular intervals of three to six months. In terms of the experience of visiting dental clinics, 14.27 % of the children reported unpleasant experiences. Surprisingly, children in this group had a higher prevalence of malocclusion ($P < 0.05$). Majority of the parents (92.45 %) preferred public hospitals for their children, followed by community hospitals (5.75 %) and private practices (1.80 %). The hospital type (public, community, or private) had no remarkable effects on the prevalence of malocclusion among children with primary dentition ($P > 0.05$). Regardless of the education level of the parents and the monthly familial income, proper parental monitoring and understanding of malocclusion were correlated with a lower prevalence of malocclusion in

Table 3 Prevalence of different types of malocclusion based on demographic characteristics

Variables	Prevalence of malocclusion (present/total)	χ^2	P	Prevalence of anterior crossbite (present/total)	Prevalence of edge to edge occlusion (present/total)	Prevalence of increased overjet (present/total)	Prevalence of posterior crossbite (present/total)	Prevalence of midline deviation (present/total)	Prevalence of deep overbite (present/total)	Prevalence of open bite (present/total)
Gender										
Male	65.49 (776/1185)			6.58 (78/1185)	2.36 (28/1185)	33.33 (395/1185)	7.26 (86/1185)	28.10 (333/1185)	42.45 (503/1185)	7.26 (86/1185)
Female	67.24 (706/1050)	0.766	0.382	7.05 (74/1050)	2.57 (27/1050)	36.86 (387/1050)	7.90 (83/1050)	22.19 (233/1050)	32.10 (337/1050)	6.67 (70/1185)
Birth Place										
Urban	61.59 (935/1518)			6.06 (92/1518)	1.84 (28/1518)	36.96 (561/1518)	5.47 (83/1518)	22.86 (347/1518)	39.26 (596/1518)	8.17 (124/1518)
Rural	76.29 (547/717)	47.078	<0.001	8.37 (60/717)	3.77 (27/717)	30.82 (221/717)	11.99 (86/717)	30.54 (219/717)	34.03 (244/717)	4.46 (32/717)
Parental education level										
High school and below	67.81 (394/581)			8.09 (47/581)	2.41 (14/581)	38.55 (224/581)	7.92 (46/581)	29.09 (169/581)	39.93 (232/581)	8.26 (48/581)
Undergraduate	64.95 (921/1418)			5.71 (81/1418)	2.26 (32/1418)	31.88 (452/1418)	6.63 (94/1418)	22.14 (314/1418)	34.56 (490/1418)	5.57 (79/1418)
Graduate and above	70.76 (167/236)	3.856	0.145	10.17 (24/236)	3.81 (9/236)	44.92 (106/236)	12.29 (29/236)	35.17 (83/236)	50.00 (118/236)	12.29 (29/236)
Familial monthly income (Yuan)										
< 2000	77.91 (261/335)			9.85 (33/335)	3.28 (11/335)	47.16 (158/335)	12.84 (43/335)	33.43 (112/335)	52.84 (177/335)	11.64 (39/335)
2000–5000	65.98 (516/782)			6.01 (47/782)	2.17 (17/782)	30.82 (241/782)	6.01 (47/782)	17.77 (139/782)	32.74 (256/782)	6.27 (49/782)
5000–8000	57.97 (389/671)			4.92 (33/671)	1.34 (9/671)	25.93 (174/671)	6.11 (41/671)	22.95 (154/671)	28.02 (188/671)	4.02 (27/671)
> 8000	70.69 (316/447)	44.937	<0.001	8.72 (39/447)	4.03 (18/447)	46.76 (209/447)	8.50 (38/447)	36.02 (161/447)	48.99 (219/447)	9.17 (41/447)

Table 4 Bivariate analysis of factors associated with oral examination, improper oral habits, feeding and delivery methods, dental visit experience, and malocclusion

	Variables	Prevalence of malocclusion (present/total)	χ^2	P
Oral examination	Fused tooth			
	Present	65.18 (73/112)		
	Absent	66.37 (1409/2123)	0.067	0.795
	Insufficient abrasion of primary canines			
	Present	73.28 (181/247)		
	Absent	65.44 (1301/1988)	6.040	0.014
	Primate space			
	Present	48.13 (775/987)		
	Absent	80.69 (707/1248)	117.996	<0.001
	Caries among primary teeth			
	Present	68.08 (1171/1720)		
	Absent	60.39 (311/515)	10.499	0.001
	Premature exfoliation of primary teeth			
	Present	66.36 (73/110)		
	Absent	66.31 (1409/2125)	0.00016	0.990
Improper oral habits	Tongue thrusting			
	Present	84.38 (54/64)		
	Absent	65.78 (1428/2171)	9.626	0.002
	Mouth breathing			
	Present	77.99 (163/209)		
	Absent	66.09 (1319/2026)	14.083	<0.001
	Bruxism			
	Present	64.76 (441/681)		
	Absent	66.99 (1041/1554)	1.055	0.304
	Mandibular prognathism			
	Present	82.86 (29/35)		
	Absent	66.05 (1453/2200)	4.359	0.037
	Lip biting			
	Present	74.04 (77/104)		
	Absent	65.93 (1405/2131)	2.917	0.088
	Finger sucking			
	Present	54.25 (287/400)		
	Absent	48.50 (1195/2835)	6.457	0.011
Feeding and delivery methods	Feeding methods			
	Breast milk	23.10 (131/567)		
	Milk powder	76.78 (443/577)		
	Both	83.23 (908/1091)	641.829	<0.001
	Feeding postures			
	Sitting	66.86 (577/863)		
	Half sitting	64.10 (557/869)		
	Flat	69.51 (285/410)		
	Unfixed	67.74 (63/93)	3.990	0.263

Table 4 Bivariate analysis of factors associated with oral examination, improper oral habits, feeding and delivery methods, dental visit experience, and malocclusion *(Continued)*

	Use of pacifier			
	Yes	73.98 (307/415)		
	No	64.56 (1175/1820)	13.410	<0.001
	Delivery methods			
	Natural labor	62.97 (670/1064)		
	Caesarean	69.34 (812/1171)	10.133	0.001
Dental visiting experience	Frequency of visiting dental clinic			
	Never	80.28 (635/791)		
	Only when needed	62.71 (676/1078)		
	3 months	38.10 (16/42)		
	Half a year	47.24 (137/290)		
	Irregular	52.94 (18/34)	140.227	<0.001
	Facility of the visited dental clinic			
	Public hospital	59.10 (789/1335)		
	Community hospital	57.83 (48/83)		
	Private practice	38.46 (10/26)	4.505	0.105
	Had unpleasant dental visit experience			
	Yes	74.76 (154/206)		
	No	55.98 (693/1238)	25.685	<0.001
	Parental attitude toward the problem of malocclusion			
	Pay positive attention	52.81 (293/409)		
	Not concerned	69.33 (1189/1826)	6.365	0.012

children compared to children whose parents who lacked these behaviors ($P < 0.05$).

Binary logistic regression analysis of associated factors and malocclusion

The results of conditional binary logistic regression analysis (Table 5) indicated that rural children had a 1.741 times higher risk of suffering from malocclusion than urban children ($P < 0.05$, Table 5). There was no significant difference in the prevalence of malocclusion based on the familial economic status ($P > 0.05$). Insufficient abrasion of the primary canines and caries played a critical role in the morbidity of malocclusion ($P < 0.05$, Table 5). Compared to normal children, the risk of malocclusion among those who suffered from insufficient abrasion of the primary canines or caries was higher (OR = 1.465 and 2.045, respectively). Although the prevalence of malocclusion was higher in the group of children who had lost their primate space, further logistic regression analysis signified no statistical significance. Results of improper oral habits confirmed that children with tongue thrusting and mandibular prognathism had OR = 2.833 and 2.621, respectively. Moreover, children with a habit of finger sucking were at a higher risk (1.573 times) of malocclusion ($P < 0.05$, Table 5). The data showed that mouth breathing did not show any statistical significance with malocclusion in primary dentition. Breast feeding and natural labor did have a positive preventive effect toward malocclusion ($P < 0.05$, Table 5). Although children who had used pacifiers showed an incidence of malocclusion, it was not statistically significant ($P > 0.05$). Regression analysis further confirmed that proper parental monitoring and understanding of malocclusion were correlated with its lower prevalence than in children of parents who lacked these behaviors (Table 5, $P < 0.05$).

Discussion

This epidemiological study revealed a high prevalence of malocclusion in children with primary dentition (66.31 %) residing in Xi'an city. Further statistical analysis revealed that factors such as insufficient abrasion of the primary canines and caries in the primary teeth were associated with malocclusion among these children. In addition, improper oral habits such as tongue thrusting, mandible prognathism, and finger sucking contributed to malocclusion. Children born by natural labor and breastfed children had a lower prevalence of malocclusion. A positive attitude of parents toward this problem is likely to reduce the prevalence of malocclusion in the primary dentition.

Table 5 Binary logistic regression analysis of relative factors and malocclusion

Variables	Prevalence of malocclusion (present/total)	β	S.E.	P	Odds ratio (95 % CI)
Birth place					
Urban	61.59 (935/1518)				
Rural	76.29 (547/717)	1.825	0.309	0.027	1.741 (1.384–2.162)
Insufficient abrasion of primary canines					
Present	73.28 (181/247)				
Absent	65.44 (1301/1988)	0.363	0.395	0.037	1.465 (1.153–.894)
Caries among primary teeth					
Present	68.08 (1171/1720)				
Absent	60.39 (311/515)	1.296	0.78	<0.001	2.045 (1.665–2.539)
Tongue thrusting					
Present	84.38 (54/64)				
Absent	65.78 (1428/2171)	0.725	0.114	0.041	2.833 (1.640–3.649)
Mandibular prognathism					
Present	82.86 (29/35)				
Absent	66.05 (1453/2200)	0.855	0.101	0.023	2.621 (1.574–3.689)
Finger sucking					
Present	54.25 (287/400)				
Absent	48.50 (1195/2835)	0.642	0.173	<0.001	1.573 (1.098–2.014)
Feeding methods					
Breast milk	23.10 (131/567)				
Milk powder	76.78 (443/577)				
Both	83.23 (908/1091)	1.090	0.347	0.012	3.614 (3.087–4.596)
Delivery methods					
Natural labor	62.97 (670/1064)				
Caesarean	69.34 (812/1171)	0.596	0.047	0.028	1.847 (1.323–2.451)
Parental attitude toward the problem of malocclusion					
Paid positive attention	52.81 (293/409)				
Not concerned	69.33 (1189/1826)	1.080	0.452	0.039	1.572 (1.201–2.512)

In the primary dentition, the occlusive relationship is influenced by a dynamic set of forming and adjusting forces [22]. The incidence of suffering from one or more types of malocclusion is high during this period, as demonstrated in our study (66.31 %) and previous studies [23, 24]. The prevalence in the current study was much higher than that in the Brazilian population (46.2 %) [23]. The differences between our study and other published articles [18, 19, 23, 24] could be attributed to the use of variable criteria for the classification of malocclusion; however, more attention needs to be paid to the overall problem.

Deep overbite and increased overjet had the highest morbidity among our subjects; however, the cephalocaudal gradient of craniofacial development should also be taken into consideration. In the preliminary stage of occlusal establishment, the lower dental arch is located in a distal position, exhibiting a vertical or distal terminal plane for the primary molars [25], corresponding to Angle's II occlusion for the permanent dentition. Children with primary dentition usually have a higher risk of developing increased overjet. Insufficient distance between the dental arches may result in a deep overbite [26]. With the development of roots and forward movement of the lower dentition, the occlusion noted as deep overbite and increased overjet can gradually normalize. Borzabadi-Farahani et al. [5] performed a similar investigation on malocclusion in permanent dentition and reported a similar prevalence of different types of malocclusion; however, the prevalence of increased overjet and class II division I malocclusion in primary dentition was lower than the prevalence of increased overjet reported by our study. As previously mentioned, change in occlusion in the primary dentition is a dynamic process.

Therefore, dynamic observations are also needed to differentiate between temporary malocclusion and pathological malocclusion in this period.

With regard to parental characteristics, our study showed that education level had no relationship with malocclusion. Regardless of the education level, positive parental attitude toward oral health is important. Monitoring of primary dentition in a regular and timely manner was associated with a lower incidence of malocclusion. This finding was in accordance with the traditional perception that positive parental participation would lead to early prevention and timely treatment of malocclusion. A higher prevalence of malocclusion was observed among children born and living in the rural areas who were less likely to visit pediatric dentists at regular intervals. Our results are in agreement with Guan et al. study, which reported an increased prevalence of dental caries associated with lower socioeconomic classes but not with parental education levels [27].

Children having primary dentition with insufficient abrasion of the primary canines and a high caries risk showed a higher incidence of malocclusion. Our finding that children who suffered from caries had a higher incidence of malocclusion was slightly different from those of previous studies [28, 29]. Feldens et al. [28] confirmed that there was a correlation between caries and handicapping malocclusion, and between maxillary irregularity and abnormal molar relationship in subjects with permanent dentition. However, no statistically significant correlation was observed in malocclusion in the primary dentition. Singh et al. [29] reported similar findings, that only those who had caries in the mixed and young permanent dentition had a higher probability of suffering from malocclusion. Borzabadi-Farahani et al. [30] found a different interrelationship among children in the older age group, but not among those in lower socioeconomic status groups. In contrast, our study reported that socioeconomic status was not an associated factor for malocclusion. Although we considered a different evaluating indicator for socioeconomic status, the relationship between caries experience and malocclusion should be assessed in a wider context of socioeconomic status and background factors. The association of dental caries with malocclusion is controversial. On the one hand, the authors of this study believed that caries would lead to changes in the length or width of the dentition, thereby leading to abnormal alignment of the primary teeth. On the other hand, caries in the primary molars might lead to crown disintegration, subsequently changing the normal chewing habits of children in their primary dentition, which, to a certain degree, could alter the position of the temporomandibular joint, ultimately resulting in malocclusion.

Primary anterior teeth, especially the primary canines, typically have insufficient abrasion that may affect the relationship among the anterior teeth. Consequently, the mandible may not move back to a relatively normal position, leading to a crossbite of the anterior primary teeth. Caries in the primary dentition, especially primary molars, is interrelated to insufficient abrasion of the primary canines. Soft food items consumed by children may contribute to the insufficient abrasion of the primary canines along with caries. Additionally, severe caries could decrease the intermaxillary height, leading to the primary canines being positioned relatively higher corresponding to insufficient abrasion.

Several studies [31–33] have reported a higher incidence of malocclusion among children with improper oral habits compared to normal children. Some of the most common improper oral habits, such as lip biting, finger sucking, and tongue thrusting have been correlated with various types of malocclusions including inclined teeth, dental arch constriction, open bite, and increased interdentium [34]. However, the current study showed slightly different results; it was observed that in children with primary dentition, malocclusion had no statistical significant correlation with bruxism and lip biting. Our results were supported by Hella et al. [35], who first stated that most lip habits would not lead to an occlusion problem unless they attained a certain degree of strength, frequency, and duration. Hence, if lip habits lead to malocclusion, their effects would appear only in the permanent or mixed dentition.

From the parental questionnaires, it was noted that breastfed children in their primary dentition were less likely to suffer from malocclusion. These findings are similar to another Puerto Rican study [36], which reported that an increased duration of breastfeeding was associated with a decline in the proportion of children suffering from malocclusion. Some scholars [37] believed that compared to other feeding patterns, breastfeeding could significantly reduce the risk of caries. Considering our previous finding that caries may be related to the development of malocclusion, breastfeeding could have a significantly positive effect on malocclusion in the primary dentition.

The World Health Organization (WHO) reported that the overall rate of cesarean births in China increased to 46.2 % from October 2007 to May 2008, ranking the country highest in the world for cesarean delivery rate. In some cities, this proportion is as high as 70 % [38], which is significantly higher than the 15 % threshold set by the WHO. Our results showed that natural labor may be associated with a lower incidence of malocclusion in the primary dentition. Previously, Cattaneo et al. [39] investigated 106 adults to further explore the relationship between malocclusion and delivery methods. The results showed that none of the subjects with malocclusion were delivered naturally. This could be attributed to the maxillofacial trauma during non-natural deliveries. Although further studies are warranted, data from this study and those of other articles suggested that natural birth and breastfeeding may reduce the prevalence of malocclusion.

This study had several limitations. Firstly, there was more than one type of malocclusion in the primary dentition (Table 2). Individual variations can further complicate the investigation of various malocclusions. However, in this study, it was not explored whether one factor was associated with a certain type of malocclusion. Thus, the results could only partly illustrate the influencing relationships. Secondly, although the examiners did provide explanations when parents were investigated about the improper oral habits of their children, the results could still be subjective to some extent. In addition, some of the parents might not have been able to distinguish between habits and occasional behavior. In other words, the duration and frequency of improper oral habits were not taken into consideration in this study. Therefore, further analysis of the data might be required. Finally, few of the primary dentition malocclusions such as crowding (one of the most commonly seen malocclusion) among children in older age group [5, 40] were not included in this study; therefore, further investigation in this regard is also warranted.

Compared to permanent dentition, fewer studies have focused on malocclusion in the primary dentition. In addition, most of these studies cannot represent the general prevalence of a particular region because of small sample sizes or investigation indices. In this study, the stratified cluster sampling method was used. Moreover, a suitable sample size representative of the general prevalence in the city of Xi'an was ensured. Besides, as Angle's malocclusion classification uses the molar relationship for permanent dentition, it does not incorporate vertical and transverse abnormalities [41]. Thus, Bjoerk's classification [20] better suits the primary dentition.

Conclusions

The prevalence of malocclusion among pre-school children in Xi'an is higher than that in pre-school children in other geographical parts of China. Therefore, early attention to the development of occlusion and necessary interventions toward its influencing factors are important to reduce its prevalence and further adverse effects. This study provided considerable information regarding the prevalence of malocclusion and its contributing factors in the primary dentition. These theoretical evidences could be taken into account for future studies focused on preventing malocclusion in children.

Acknowledgments

The authors are grateful to Dr. Xianjun Yang for his help with the statistical analysis.

Funding

This study was partly supported by the National Natural Science Foundation of China (Grant No. 81470743). The funding body did not participate in the study design, data collection, analysis, interpretation of data, or in writing the manuscript.

Authors' contributions

ZZ and FL were responsible for construction of the study strategy, data collection, content analysis, and preparation of the manuscript draft. SS and LinS were responsible for the study design, content analysis, critical revision, and final approval of this manuscript. LeiS and XW contributed to the design of the study strategy and interpretation of findings as well as to the overall critical appraisal and advice. All authors have read and approved the final manuscript.

Competing interests

The authors declare that they have no competing interests.

Consent for publication

Not applicable.

Ethics approval and consent to participate

The parents of the participating children were informed of the objectives of this research and written informed consent was obtained from all the parents prior to conducting the study. The study was approved by the Ethical Committee of the School of Stomatology, Fourth Military Medical University, Republic of China (committee's reference number: IRB-REV-2014068).

Author details

[1]State Key Laboratory of Military Stomatology, National Clinical Research Center for Oral Diseases, Department of Pediatric Dentistry, School of Stomatology, Fourth Military Medical University, Xi'an, People's Republic of China. [2]Department of Oral Medicine, Northwest Women's and Children's Hospital, Xi'an, People's Republic of China. [3]Department of Oral Medicine, PLA 261 Hospital, Beijing, People's Republic of China. [4]Department of Pediatric Dentistry, Foshan Stomatological Hospital, Foshan, People's Republic of China. [5]Department of Health Statistics, School of Public Health, Fourth Military Medical University, Xi'an, People's Republic of China.

References

1. Dhar V, Jain A, Van Dyke TE, Kohli A. Prevalence of gingival diseases, malocclusion and fluorosis in school-going children of rural areas in Udaipur district. J Indian Soc Pedod Prev Dent. 2007;25:103–5.
2. English JD, Buschang PH, Throckmorton GS. Does malocclusion affect masticatory performance? Angle Orthod. 2002;72:21–7.
3. Kaur H, Pavithra US, Abraham R. Prevalence of malocclusion among adolescents in South Indian population. J Int Soc Prev Community Dent. 2013;3:97–102.
4. Aikins EA, Onyeaso CO. Prevalence of malocclusion and occlusal traits among adolescents and young adults in Rivers State, Nigeria. Odontostomatol Trop. 2014;37:5–12.
5. Borzabadi-Farahani A, Borzabadi-Farahani A, Eslamipour F. Malocclusion and occlusal traits in an urban Iranian population. An epidemiological study of 11- to 14-year-old children. Eur J Orthod. 2009;31:477–84.
6. Bishara SE, Khadivi P, Jakobsen JR. Changes in tooth size-arch length relationships from the deciduous to the permanent dentition: a longitudinal study. Am J Orthod Dentofacial Orthop. 1995;108:607–13.
7. Legovic M, Mady L. Longitudinal occlusal changes from primary to permanent dentition in children with normal primary occlusion. Angle Orthod. 1999;69:264–6.
8. Onyeaso CO, Isiekwe MC. Occlusal changes from primary to mixed dentitions in Nigerian children. Angle Orthod. 2008;78:64–9.
9. Peres KG, Peres MA, Thomson WM, Broadbent J, Hallal PC, Menezes AB. Deciduous-dentition malocclusion predicts orthodontic treatment needs

later: findings from a population-based birth cohort study. Am J Orthod Dentofacial Orthop. 2015;147:492–8.
10. van der Watt HP, Wait J, van der Walt P. Malocclusion and the personality of children. J Dent Assoc S Afr. 1984;39:609–11.
11. Chevitarese AB, Della Valle D, Moreira TC. Prevalence of malocclusion in 4-6 year old Brazilian children. J Clin Pediatr Dent. 2002;27:81–5.
12. Normando TS, Barroso RF, Normando D. Influence of the socioeconomic status on the prevalence of malocclusion in the primary dentition. Dental Press J Orthod. 2015;20:74–8.
13. Heimer MV, Tornisiello Katz CR, Rosenblatt A. Non-nutritive sucking habits, dental malocclusions, and facial morphology in Brazilian children: a longitudinal study. Eur J Orthod. 2008;30:580–5.
14. Klocke A, Nanda RS, Kahl-Nieke B. Anterior open bite in the deciduous dentition: longitudinal follow-up and craniofacial growth considerations. Am J Orthod Dentofacial Orthop. 2002;122:353–8.
15. Stahl F, Baccetti T, Franchi L, McNamara Jr JA. Longitudinal growth changes in untreated subjects with Class II Division 1 malocclusion. Am J Orthod Dentofacial Orthop. 2008;134:125–37.
16. Petersen PE. The World Oral Health Report 2003: continuous improvement of oral health in the 21st century–the approach of the WHO Global Oral Health Programme. Community Dent Oral Epidemiol. 2003;31 Suppl 1:3–23.
17. Katz CR, Rosenblatt A, Gondim PP. Nonnutritive sucking habits in Brazilian children: effects on deciduous dentition and relationship with facial morphology. Am J Orthod Dentofacial Orthop. 2004;126:53–7.
18. Zhao FM, Zhu YQ, Wang YJ. Epidemiological study of children in primary dentition in the city of Shanghai China. Shi Yong Kou Qiang Yi Xue Za Zhi. 1999;15:313–4 [Chinese].
19. Huang N, Shi ZD, Wang ZH, Qin JC, Chen E, Guo CL, et al. The malocclusion of primary dentition in the suburb of Chengdu: a cross-section survey. Hua Xi Kou Qiang Yi Xue Za Zhi. 2005;23:173–4 [Chinese].
20. Bjoerk A, Krebs A, Solow B. A method for epidemiological registration of malocclusion. Acta Odontol Scand. 1964;22:27–41.
21. World Health Organization. Oral health surveys. Basic methods, 4th edition. Geneva;1997.
22. Lujan-Climent M, Martinez-Gomis J, Palau S, Ayuso-Montero R, Salsench J, Peraire M. Influence of static and dynamic occlusal characteristics and muscle force on masticatory performance in dentate adults. Eur J Oral Sci. 2008;116:229–36.
23. Carvalho AC, Paiva SM, Scarpelli AC, Viegas CM, Ferreira FM, Pordeus IA. Prevalence of malocclusion in primary dentition in a population-based sample of Brazilian preschool children. Eur J Paediatr Dent. 2011;12:107–11.
24. Onyeaso CO, Sote EO. A study of Malocculusion in the primary dentition in a population of Nigerian children. Niger J Clin Pract. 2004;5:52–6.
25. de Castro LA, Modesto A, Vianna R, Soviero VL. Cross-sectional study of the evolution of the primary dentition: shape of dental arches, overjet and overbite. Pesqui Odontol Bras. 2002;16:367–73.
26. Hegde S, Panwar S, Bolar DR, Sanghavi MB. Characteristics of occlusion in primary dentition of preschool children of Udaipur, India. Eur J Dent. 2012;6:51–5.
27. Guan Y, Zeng X, Tai B, Cheng M, Huang R, Bernabe E. Socioeconomic inequalities in dental caries among 5-year-olds in four Chinese provinces. Community Dent Health. 2015;32:185–9.
28. Feldens CA, Dos Santos Dullius AI, Kramer PF, Scapini A, Busato AL, Vargas-Ferreira F. Impact of malocclusion and dentofacial anomalies on the prevalence and severity of dental caries among adolescents. Angle Orthod. 2015;85:1027–34.
29. Singh A, Purohit B, Sequeira P, Acharya S, Bhat M. Malocclusion and orthodontic treatment need measured by the dental aesthetic index and its association with dental caries in Indian schoolchildren. Community Dent Health. 2011;28:313–6.
30. Borzabadi-Farahani A, Eslamipour F, Asgari I. Association between orthodontic treatment need and caries experience. Acta Odontol Scand. 2011;69:2–11.
31. Calisti LJ, Cohen MM, Fales MH. Correlation between malocclusion, oral habits, and socio-economic level of preschool children. J Dent Res. 1960;39: 450–4.
32. Warren JJ, Bishara SE, Steinbock KL, Yonezu T, Nowak AJ. Effects of oral habits' duration on dental characteristics in the primary dentition. J Am Dent Assoc. 2001;132:1685–93.
33. Backlund E. Facial growth, and the significance of oral habits, mouthbreathing and soft tissues for malocclusion. A study on children around the age of 10. Acta Odontol Scand. 1963;21 Suppl 36:9–139.
34. Dos Santos RR, Nayme JG, Garbin AJ, Saliba N, Garbin CA, Moimaz SA. Prevalence of Malocclusion and Related Oral Habits in 5- to 6-year-old Children. Oral Health Prev Dent. 2012;10:311–8.
35. Hella A, Haavikko K. Prevalence of earlier sucking habits revealed by anamnestic data and their consequences for occlusion at the age of eleven. Proc Finn Dent Soc. 1974;70:191–6.
36. Lopez Del Valle LM, Singh GD, Feliciano N, Machuca MC. Associations between a history of breast feeding, malocclusion and parafunctional habits in Puerto Rican children. P R Health Sci J. 2006;25:31–4.
37. Hong L, Levy SM, Warren JJ, Broffitt B. Infant breast-feeding and childhood caries: a nine-year study. Pediatr Dent. 2014;36:342–7.
38. Lumbiganon P, Laopaiboon M, Gülmezoglu AM, Souza JP, Taneepanichskul S, Ruyan P, et al. Method of delivery and pregnancy outcomes in Asia: the WHO global survey on maternal and perinatal health 2007-08. Lancet. 2010;375:490–9.
39. Cattaneo R, Monaco A, Serafino V, Giannoni M. Birth delivery trauma and malocclusion. J Clin Pediatr Dent. 2005;29:185–8.
40. Lux CJ, Ducker B, Pritsch M, Niekusch U, Komposch G. Space conditions and prevalence of anterior spacing and crowding among nine-year-old schoolchildren. J Orthod. 2008;35:33–42.
41. Brin I, Weinberger T, Ben-Choirin E. Classification of occlusion reconsidered. Eur J Orthod. 2000;22:169–74.

4

A plea for the development of an universally accepted modular tooth wear evaluation system

P. Wetselaar*, A. Faris and F. Lobbezoo

Abstract

Background: Tooth wear is considered an increasing oral health problem. Due to its multifactorial nature, recognizing and diagnosing of tooth wear is difficult but nevertheless important. Over the years, a wide variety of evaluation systems has been developed, yet none of them is universally accepted. This has implications for both research and clinical practice.

Discussion: This paper describes an in-depth analysis of four commonly used tooth wear evaluation systems, namely, the Eccles index, the Tooth Wear Index, the Lussi index, and the Basic Erosive Wear Examination. Comparing those systems revealed that despite several similarities, they differ considerably from each other. Notably, all four systems have their specific advantages and disadvantages. However, neither one of them meets all necessary characteristics of a hypothetical, broadly applicable tooth wear evaluation system. In fact, it is not realistic that a single system qualifies for all purposes (for example, diagnosing or monitoring individual patients, performing epidemiological studies, etc.).

Summary: As a potentially feasible solution for this issue, the development of an evaluation system is recommended that consists of multiple, coherent modules, which cover different purposes.

Keywords: Diagnosis, Evaluation system, Index, Modular evaluation system, Tooth wear

Background

Tooth wear is considered an increasingly prevalent oral health problem, which will mainly manifest in the future. It can be divided in the subtypes "mechanical wear" (attrition and abrasion), and "chemical wear" (erosion, or erosive tooth wear) [1]. Since nowadays most people grow old with their own dentition, tooth wear occurs more frequently [1]. Because tooth wear is always a multifactorial process, its diagnosis can be difficult [2]. Within dentistry, several widely accepted diagnostic tools for various pathologies are used (e.g., Decayed Missing Filled Teeth (DMFT) for caries and the periodontal screening index [3] for periodontal diseases). So far, however, no universally accepted diagnostic tool is available for the evaluation of tooth wear [4]. Most likely, this is due to the fact that a broadly applicable tooth wear evaluation system has not been developed yet. Ideally, such system should have the following characteristics: 1. being able to assess all subtypes of tooth wear, viz., mechanical wear and chemical wear; 2. being useful for research purposes (e.g., epidemiological and etiological assessments) as well as for clinical applications (e.g., screening, diagnosing, and monitoring); It is very important to have an evaluation system for tooth wear, that can be used for epidemiological purposes, because in that way, health care providers can estimate the need for dental care regarding tooth wear. Regarding individuals, since tooth wear is an irreversible process, it is important to screen for tooth wear on a regular basis, in order to prevent wear as much as possible and by doing this, to try to preserve dentitions as long as possible in an ageing population. 3. having well-defined, reproducible scoring criteria; and 4. being easy to use. It was this study's first aim to perform an in-depth analysis of the characteristics of four commonly used tooth wear evaluation systems and to determine if, and if so, to what extent these systems show any one or more of the

* Correspondence: p.wetselaar@acta.nl
Department of Oral Kinesiology, Academic Centre for Dentistry Amsterdam (ACTA), University of Amsterdam and VU University Amsterdam, MOVE Research Institute Amsterdam, Gustav Mahlerlaan 3004, 1081 LA Amsterdam, The Netherlands

above-described characteristics of a hypothetical, broadly applicable evaluation system. The following systems will be analyzed: the Eccles index [5], the Tooth Wear Index, TWI [6], the Lussi index [7], and the Basic Erosive Wear Examination, BEWE [8]. The outcome of the analyses of the four systems will provide input for the second aim of this study, namely to formulate recommendations for the development of a broadly applicable tooth wear evaluation system for use in adults. By using the Eccles index, the Lussi index and the BEWE, chemical tooth wear is overestimated, because the two subtypes of tooth wear (chemical wear and mechanical wear) are summated.

Selection of the most widely quoted tooth wear evaluation systems

The selection of the first three evaluation systems (i.e., the Eccles index, the TWI, and the Lussi index) was based on the frequency of them being quoted in the literature of the past four decades. This was based on several PubMed searches, the last one being performed on the 12th of September 2016. The used query was: "(tooth wear OR tooth surface loss OR attritive tooth wear OR abrasive tooth wear OR erosive tooth wear OR tooth attrition OR teeth attrition OR dental attrition OR tooth erosion OR teeth erosion OR dental erosion OR tooth abrasion OR teeth abrasion OR dental abrasion) AND (index OR indices OR scale OR scales OR measurement OR measurements OR grade OR grades OR grading system OR grading systems OR recording system OR recording systems OR evaluation system OR evaluation systems)". The PubMed search yielded 114 different grading systems for the quantification of tooth wear, including adaptations of already existing systems. It was revealed that in research, the TWI is the most frequently used system, followed by the BEWE and the Lussi index respectively. Of importance for our selection was that these three systems were also used by other authors than those who developed the systems, while for the majority of the system, the use was restricted to the developers. Additionally, Margaritis and Nunn [4] described in their article in Table 3 their PubMed search of the most recently cited indices used in the assessment of erosive wear (years 2000–2013). They found a frequency of use of 13 times for the Lussi index, 11 times for the TWI, 6 times for the BEWE, and 5 times for the Eccles index respectively, when the target group was adults. No other indices with adults as the target group were included in their table. Hence, this is in line with our findings. The Eccles index is considered as one of the basic evaluation systems from which many others originate [9]. The TWI and the Lussi index are the two most commonly used tooth wear evaluation systems, and many other systems are developed based on them. The fourth system that was included, the BEWE, was recently introduced by a group of experts and is since then quoted frequently as well. Although the BEWE is a relatively new index and population-based studies are scarce, the amount of studies is increasing with recent reports from around the globe. The characteristics of these four evaluation systems are described below.

Eccles index

The Eccles index [5] consists of three classes, viz., I, II, and III (Table 1). Classes I and II apply to all surfaces, while Class III differentiates between various surfaces, namely facial surfaces as IIIa, lingual and palatal surfaces as IIIb, incisal and occlusal surfaces as IIIc, and severe multi-surface involvement as IIId.

Tooth Wear Index (TWI)

The Tooth Wear Index (TWI) [6] consists of a five-point ordinal scale. The descriptions of the various grades are shown in Table 2. The grading is identical for all teeth, but different criteria are present for the various surfaces, viz., for the buccal/lingual/occlusal, incisal, and cervical surfaces.

Lussi index

The Lussi index [7] consists of two ordinal scales for all teeth, viz., a four-point ordinal scale for the facial surfaces and a three-point ordinal scale for the occlusal/lingual surfaces. The descriptions of both scales are shown in Table 3.

Basic Erosive Wear Examination (BEWE)

The Basic Erosive Wear Examination (BEWE) [8] consists of a single four-point ordinal scale; the descriptions of the various grades are shown in Table 4.

Characteristics of a hypothetical, broadly applicable tooth wear evaluation system

A hypothetical, broadly applicable tooth wear evaluation system should have the following characteristics:

Tooth wear subtypes: being capable to evaluate both mechanical wear (attrition and abrasion) and chemical

Table 1 Eccles index [5]

Class	Description
I	Superficial lesions involving enamel only
II	Localized lesions involving dentin for less than 1/3 of the surface
III	Generalized lesions involving dentin for more than 1/3 of the surface
IIIa	Facial
IIIb	Lingual and palatal
IIIc	Incisal and occlusal
IIId	Severe multisurface involvement

Table 2 Tooth Wear Index (TWI) [6]

Score	Description		
	Buccal/Lingual/Occlusal	Incisal	Cervical
0	No loss of enamel surface characteristics	No loss of enamel surface characteristics	No change in contour
1	Loss of enamel surface characteristics	Loss of enamel surface characteristics	Minimal loss of contour
2	Loss of enamel exposing dentine for less than 1/3 of the surface	Loss of enamel just exposing dentine	Defect <1 mm deep
3	Loss of enamel exposing dentine for more than 1/3 of the surface	Loss of enamel and substantial loss of dentine, but not exposing pulp secondary dentine	Defect 1–2 mm deep
4	Complete loss of enamel, or pulp exposure, or exposure of secondary dentine	Pulp exposure or exposure of secondary dentine	Defect >2 mm deep, or pulp exposure or exposure of secondary dentine

wear (erosion), and not only one subtype, since the subtypes rarely act alone.

Assessment mode: being applicable to all assessment modes, like chair side, dental casts, photographs, and/or scans, and not only for one or a few of them. This gives the clinician the possibility to choose the most appropriate assessment mode under the given clinical conditions.

Purpose: being capable of screening (both in the clinic and/or in epidemiological studies), diagnosing, and monitoring, and not for only one or two of these purposes.

Clusters of teeth: being suitable for both a partial assessment and a full assessment of the dentition. Examples of a partial assessment are grading only some key elements and grading of teeth per sextant. Also here, researchers and clinicians have the possibility to choose the most appropriate assessment mode.

Surfaces: being suitable for all possible (combinations of) surfaces, viz., occlusal, incisal, lingual/palatal/oral, buccal/labial/facial, cervical, occlusal/incisal, and/or non-occlusal/non-incisal surfaces. It should be noted that tooth wear rarely occurs on only one surface.

Determining: providing a good insight in the amount of tooth wear. To that end, the assessed grades should be noted separately. When the grades are added together, the severity can be camouflaged. Therefore, separate scores are to be preferred.

Type of scale: making use of clear scores, and not of descriptions that are open for multiple interpretations. Therefore, an ordinal scale is to be preferred over a nominal one.

Direction of assessment: using a combination of both surface area criteria (horizontal) and depth criteria (vertical, loss of clinical crown height), since early detection of tooth surface loss can better be determined with the former mentioned, while stages of more advanced tooth wear can better be determined with the latter mentioned.

Amount of subscales/descriptions: using as little subscales as possible, in order to make the use as straightforward as possible, and by this, avoiding the easy introduction of mistakes.

Analysis of the four commonly used tooth wear evaluation systems

The characteristics of the four evaluation systems are described below and summarized in Table 5. In this paragraph, the descriptions are literal according to the mentioned authors.

Tooth wear subtypes

As indicated by the authors themselves, the Eccles index, the Lussi index, and the BEWE focus only on chemical

Table 3 Lussi index [7]

Surface	Score	Description
Facial	0	No erosion. Surface with a smooth, silky-glazed appearance and absence of developmental ridges possible.
	1	Loss of surface enamel. Intact enamel found cervical to the erosion and concavity on enamel whose breadth clearly exceeds its depth, thus distinguishing them from tooth abrasion. Undulating borders of the lesions are possible. Dentin is *not* involved.
	2	Involvement of dentin for less than one half of the attacked area of the tooth surface.
	3	Involvement of the dentin for more than one half of the attacked area of the tooth surface.
Occlusal/lingual	0	No erosion. Surface with a smooth, silky-glazed appearance and absence of developmental ridges possible.
	1	Slight erosion. Rounded cusps, edges of restorations rising above the level of adjacent tooth surface, grooves on occlusal aspects. Loss of surface enamel. Dentin is not involved.
	2	Severe erosion, more pronounced signs than in grade 1. Dentin is involved.

Table 4 Basic Erosive Wear Examination (BEWE) [8]

Score	Description
0	No erosive tooth wear (no surface loss)
1	Initial loss of enamel surface texture
2[a]	Distinct defect, hard tissue loss (dentine) <50 % of the surface area
3[a]	Hard tissue loss >50 % of the surface area

[a]in scores 2 and 3, dentine often is involved

wear (erosion) [5, 7, 8]. The TWI is the only index of the four selected evaluation systems that is applicable to all subtypes of tooth wear [6].

Assessment mode

All four evaluation systems (Eccles index, TWI, Lussi index, and BEWE) are suitable for chair side use [5–8]. For the use on dental casts, only the TWI and the BEWE are suitable [6, 8]. For the use on photographs, only the Lussi index is *not* suitable [7]. For none of the four evaluation systems, it is indicated whether they are suitable for the use with scans, but it must be noted that all systems were introduced before scans were broadly introduced.

Purpose

The BEWE is suitable for screening and monitoring [8]. For screening, a quick but not detailed overview of the dentition is needed. The Eccles index, the TWI, and the Lussi index are only suitable for diagnosing [5–7]. All teeth and surfaces are examined and recorded. This corresponds with the purpose of diagnosing, because this requires a detailed overview of the entire dentition.

Clusters of teeth

The Eccles index, the TWI, and the Lussi index examine and record all teeth [5–7]. The BEWE is the only index of the four selected evaluation systems that uses a partial assessment. The BEWE examines all teeth, but only the most severely affected tooth in a sextant is recorded [8].

Surfaces

The Eccles index grades the occlusal/incisal, facial, and lingual/palatal surfaces [5] (Table 1); the TWI the buccal/lingual/occlusal, incisal, and separately the cervical surfaces [6] (Table 2); the Lussi index the facial and occlusal/lingual surfaces [7] (Table 3); and the BEWE the buccal/facial, occlusal, and lingual/palatal surfaces [8] (Table 4).

Determining

The Eccles index [5], the TWI [6], and the Lussi index [7] determine the scores separately. Only the BEWE uses a cumulative score, whereby the six separate scores of each sextant are added to one cumulative score [8].

Type of scale

All four evaluation systems have an ordinal scale [5–8].

Direction of assessment

All four evaluation systems are based on a combination of grading the amount of the surface area that is involved and the depth of the tooth surface loss [5–8].

Amount of subscales/descriptions

The Eccles index can be considered as having four separate 3-point ordinal scales, namely for the facial surfaces (a), for the lingual and palatal surfaces (b), for the incisal and occlusal surfaces (c), and when multiple surfaces are involved at the same time (d). For each ordinal scale, the descriptions are identical, while the surfaces differ [5] (Table 1). The TWI has three separate 5-point ordinal scales, namely for the buccal/lingual/occlusal surfaces, for the incisal surfaces, and for the cervical surfaces. For each ordinal scale, the descriptions differ [6] (Table 2). The Lussi index consists of a 4-point ordinal scale for the facial surfaces and of a 3-point ordinal sale for the occlusal/lingual surfaces. The description of grade 0 is identical for both scales, while for the other grades (1, 2, and 3) the descriptions differ [7] (Table 3). The BEWE has only one 4-point ordinal scale, the descriptions of which are used for all surfaces [8] (Table 4).

Discussion

The analyzed four evaluation systems (viz., Eccles index, TWI, Lussi index, BEWE) have several similarities, but on the other hand, they differ considerably and do not complement each other (Table 5). None of the four systems shows all characteristics of a hypothetical, broadly applicable tooth wear evaluation system (Table 5). Below, those characteristics will be discussed.

Tooth wear subtypes

It is often stated that the subtypes of tooth wear hardly exist separately [2, 10]. Also the developers of the four selected tooth wear evaluation systems mentioned that in their articles. For example, Eccles [5] stated:" *Loss of tooth substance as a result of erosion is frequently made worse by abrasion, so that it may be impossible to make a clear distinction between the two conditions"* and *"Attrition, wear due to opposing teeth, will also exacerbate the effects of erosion."* [7] stated for other than facial surfaces: *"Erosion, attrition and abrasion are difficult to distinguish in their initial stages,"* and *"When erosion is present, abrasion and attrition can cause it to increase."*. While the BEWE was originally developed for the

Table 5 Characteristics of the four selected tooth wear evaluation systems (viz., Eccles index, Tooth Wear Index [TWI], Lussi index, and Basic Erosive Wear Examination [BEWE]), and of the hypothetical, broadly applicable, tooth wear evaluation system (h-TWES)

Characteristics	Evaluation systems				
	Eccles	TWI	Lussi	BEWE	h-TWES
Tooth wear subtypes					
tooth wear		x			x
mechanical					x
chemical	x		x	x	x
Possible overestimating chemical wear	x		x	x	
Assessment mode					
chair-side	x	x	x	x	x
dental casts		x		x	x
photographs	x	x		x	x
scans					x
Purpose					
screening				x	x
diagnosing	x	x	x	x	x
monitoring				x	x
Cluster of teeth					
partial assessment				x	x
full assessment	x	x	x		x
Surfaces					
occlusal	x	x	x	x	x
incisal	x	x	x	x	x
palatal/lingual/oral	x	x	x	x	x
buccal/labial/facial	x	x	x	x	x
cervical		x			
Determining					
cumulative				x	
separate	x	x	x		x
Type of scale					
ordinal	x	x	x	x	x
nominal					
Direction of assessment					
surface area	x	x	x	x	x
depth	x	x	x	x	x
Amount of Subscales and/or descriptions					
1				x	x
2			x		x
3		x			
4	x				

(x = meets the required characteristics)

assessment of erosion [8], the system was later described as "a proposed system for screening tooth wear" [11]. Smith and Knight [6] designed a tool for diagnosing all three subforms of tooth wear and their combinations. They stated: *"Together with the fact that there is often a combined cause, the simple term tooth wear is proposed to embrace all three conditions plus their combination."* [6]. Since it can be concluded that the different subtypes of tooth wear are difficult to differentiate, it can be stated that the Eccles index, the Lussi index, and the

BEWE do measure different types of tooth wear, and not only one of the subtypes.

Assessment mode

All four evaluation systems were designed to assess tooth wear chairside. For three of them, the authors stated that the use of photographs was possible as well [5, 6, 8], while for two of them the authors stated that the use of dental casts was a third option [6, 8]. Lussi and coauthors only mention the chairside use [7]. There is evidence that several evaluation systems can be used both on dental casts and on photographs [12] as well as both clinical and on casts [13]. Although this evidence concerns other evaluation systems than the four described in this article, namely the Visual Erosion Dental Examination (VEDE) [14] and an occlusal and non-occlusal Tooth Wear Grading System [13], it is an interesting finding. In the future, when dentals casts are possibly replaced by intraoral scans, it must be tested if the use of scans is as accurate as assessments performed chairside, on casts, and on photographs.

Purpose

All four evaluation systems were designed, according to the authors, to diagnose (erosive) tooth wear. It goes without saying that only grading (quantifying) the amount of tooth surface loss is nowhere near a proper diagnosis [2]. Also qualification, recognizing the clinical signs of tooth wear [15], a proper oral history [2], and perhaps saliva tests are required [10]. Nevertheless, quantification is necessary, and for an individual patient, a thorough assessment of the present amount of tooth wear must be performed. The four evaluation systems all seem to be appropriate for this purpose. For screening (of individual patients and in epidemiological studies), a simple and short assessment is preferred. For this purpose, a partial assessment is appropriate. The BEWE uses a partial assessment by only writing down the surfaces/teeth with the highest amount of tooth surface loss per sextant [8]. For a more detailed assessment per individual, the BEWE grading could be used to assess all teeth and surfaces. The other way around is perhaps also possible, namely using the Eccles index, the TWI, or the Lussi index to assess the amount of tooth surface loss of all elements and surfaces (as aimed by the developers), but then only writing down the worst affected surfaces/teeth per sextant. It should be tested if the evaluation systems can be used in this manner. Concerning monitoring, it first needs to be clarified what is meant by this term. The authors of the BEWE consider monitoring a management strategy, that follows the effects the preventive measurements after counseling, and a guidance towards other treatment modalities (e.g., restorative treatment) [8]. In general, monitoring is considered a technique to measure progression. The authors of the BEWE mention that their system is not suitable for monitoring, because the distinction between the various levels is too crude [8]. The authors of the other three indices do not mention monitoring in their respective articles [5–7]. It is obvious that these evaluation systems fail twofold in this respect: I. the distinction between the levels is too crude, and II. for more advanced stages of tooth surface loss, there are no grades described. Regarding the too crude distinctions (I.), adaptations for all the four evaluation systems could be the introduction of intermediate steps (for example separating a score 2 into sub-scores 2a, 2b, and 2c). Regarding the more advanced stages of tooth surface loss (II.), for example for the TWI, this was already mentioned and adapted by Donachie & Walls [16]. They extended the TWI with a score 5, so changing the original 5-point ordinal scale into a 6-point ordinal scale [17].

Clusters of teeth

The Eccles index, the TWI and the Lussi index use full assessment, which means, all teeth and all surfaces are graded [5–7]. Only the BEWE uses a partial assessment, by which the authors mean that all teeth and surfaces are assessed, but only the surface/tooth with the highest grade per sextant is recorded [8]. In fact, this is a full assessment as well, but with partial recording. During a real partial assessment, only so called key elements are graded and noted. An example of this way of assessing is the simplified erosion partial recording system (SEPRS) by Hasselkvist and coauthors, using only four permanent surfaces [18]. For screening purposes (on a patient level and/or in epidemiological studies), a partial assessment or a full assessment with a partial recording could be sufficient. For diagnosing, a full assessment is a necessity, while for monitoring (i.e., measuring progression) a full assessment is required.

Surfaces

All four evaluation systems grade all surfaces of the clinical crown [5–8]. Only the TWI also grades the cervical surfaces [6]. Although it is clear that the surface structure of the roots is different from that of crowns, the necessity to grade the cervical surfaces separately can be discussed. The other three evaluation systems grade the cervical areas as part of the non-occlusal/non-incisal surfaces (buccal/lingual/palatal/oral). Since for the cervical areas in the TWI an extra ordinal scale with different description is necessary, this can make the use of the TWI unnecessarily difficult.

Determining

The Eccles index [5], the TWI [6], and the Lussi index [7], determine the scores separately. Only BEWE uses a cumulative score, whereby the six separate scores of the sextants are combined into a single cumulative score [8]. Although it is highly attractive to give a tooth wear patient only one score, this not realistic. When adding up the different scores and calculating a cumulative score, the risk is that higher grades of tooth wear in one of the sextants are masked by lower ones in the other sextants. For example, a patient with severe tooth wear on the palatal surfaces of the second sextant, perhaps needs restorative treatment. When the scores remain separate, the clinician is alert, but when the scores are combined, the clinician can overlook the necessity for restorative treatment.

Type of scale

All four evaluation systems have an ordinal scale (Table 5). A nominal scale is only useful for determining which subtype of tooth wear is present, based on clinical signs [15].

Direction of assessment

All four evaluation systems are based on a combination of grading the amount of the surface area (horizontal) that is involved and the depth of the tooth surface loss (vertical, loss of clinical crown height). For assessing the early stages of tooth wear, grading the surface area is necessary. When the tooth surface loss progresses, grading in depth is necessary.

Amount of subscales/descriptions

For an easy-to-use evaluation system, with well-defined, reproducible scoring criteria, it is useful that the system only has one ordinal scale, like the BEWE [8] has. Nevertheless, the occlusal/incisal surfaces differ that much from the non-occlusal/non-incisal surfaces, that this is not possible when the index is used for monitoring or diagnosing. The most important difference between these two groups of surfaces is the loss of clinical crown height, which is the case on occlusal/incisal surfaces, while on non-occlusal/non-incisal surfaces the clinical crown length is not affected.

Recommendations for the development of a broadly applicable tooth wear evaluation system

After analyzing the four commonly used tooth wear evaluation systems in depth, comparing their characteristics towards an hypothetically broadly applicable tooth wear evaluation system, the following recommendations for the development of a broadly applicable tooth wear evaluation system are raised. It must be concluded that, taking into account all the different characteristics, only one single evaluation systems is not realistic. Therefore, the development of a modular evaluation system seems to be a workable solution. Below, a possible solution is proposed, based on the above described analyses of the four evaluation systems. In a modular evaluation system, the following modules should be included: 1. A screening module (both for epidemiological studies and for screening individual patients in the clinic) (Table 6); and 2. A module for diagnosing or monitoring individual patients, for which both occlusal/incisal and non-occlusal/non-incisal (finer grained) evaluation systems are needed (Table 7). Regarding the management of an individual patient, we think that during every recall appointment, assessment of tooth wear is a necessity. Because a lack of time can be a factor, the screening module is suitable. When the health care provider want to monitor the progress of the tooth wear, the finer grained assessment can be performed during the recall sessions. Also, when a treatment plan for an individual patient is needed, one can assess the tooth wear in detail. One must realize that by the proposed modular evaluation system only quantification is performed and no qualification is done. Concerning the screening module, the proposal is a 4-point ordinal scale as shown in Table 6. One can discuss about the cluster of teeth, as well as about the surfaces. One can assess only some key elements, per sextant, or all elements. One can assess only occlusal/incisal or also non-occlusal/non-incisal. Until agreement is reached, every individual researcher and/or dental clinician can make his/her own decision, based on the specific goal of the assessment. Concerning the diagnosing/monitoring module, the proposals are a 6-point ordinal scale for the occlusal/incisal surfaces, and a 5-point ordinal scale for the non-occlusal/non-incisal surfaces. These ordinal scales are based on the descriptions of the four analyzed tooth wear evaluation systems [5–8], and on the tooth wear evaluation systems as described by Lobbezoo and Naeije [19] and Wetselaar and coworkers [13]. The modular evaluation system consists of three different ordinal scales. The descriptions for these three scales are similar for scores 0 and 1. For score 2, a different description exists; in the screening module the distinction in clinical crown height is ≤1/2, while in the finer

Table 6 Modular evaluation system, module for screening, both occlusal/incisal and non-occlusal/non-incisal [4-point ordinal scale]

Score	Description
0	No (visible) wear
1	Wear within the enamel
2	Wear with dentin exposure - horizontal less than 50 % of the area *or* - loss of clinical crown height ≤1/2
3	Wear with dentin exposure - horizontal more than 50 % of the area *or* - loss of clinical crown height >1/2

Table 7 Modular evaluation system, module for diagnosing/monitoring occlusal/incisal [6-point ordinal scale], and non-occlusal/non-incisal [5-point ordinal scale]

Score	Description -occlusal/incisal	Description -non-occlusal/non-incisal
0	No (visible) wear	No (visible) wear
1	Wear within the enamel	Wear within the enamel
2	Wear with dentin exposure -horizontal less than 50 % of the area *or* -vertical loss of clinical crown height ≤1/3	Wear with dentin exposure -less than 50 % of the area
3	Wear with dentin exposure -horizontal more than 50 % of the area *or* -vertical loss of clinical crown height >1/3 but ≤1/2	Wear with dentin exposure -more than 50 % of the area
4	Wear with dentin exposure -horizontal complete loss of enamel *or* -vertical loss of clinical crown height >1/2 but ≤2/3	Wear with dentin exposure -complete loss of enamel *or* -pulp exposure
5	Wear with dentin exposure -horizontal complete loss of enamel *or* -vertical loss of clinical crown height >2/3	

grained diagnosing/monitoring scale the cutoff point is ≤1/3. The same applies to score 3; in the screening module the distinction in clinical crown height is >1/2, while in the finer grained diagnosing/monitoring scale the cutoff point is >1/3 but <2/3. Score 4 is similar for the occlusal/incisal surfaces and the non-occlusal/non-incisal surfaces. Score 5 only exists for the occlusal/incisal finer grained module. By this, the amount of scales and descriptions are as limited as possible.

Conclusion

Four of the most commonly used evaluation systems have been analyzed in this paper to formulate recommendations for the development of a universally and broadly applicable "ideal" tooth wear evaluation system. The analyses reveal that none of the systems is suitable as a universal evaluation system in its current form. In addition, the study reveals that it is not feasible that a single evaluation qualifies for all purposes as a universal evaluation system should do. As the purpose determines which cluster of teeth and which surfaces should be examined, and since each purpose dictates a different examination, it is not realistic to have a single multi-purpose universal evaluation system for clinical use.

A potentially feasible solution could be a modular evaluation system that consists of multiple modules. It is stated that the modular system must be able to grade all subtypes of tooth wear, be applicable for all mentioned assessment modes, all purposes, all surfaces, and all directions of assessment. The types of scales are ordinal, the scores remain separate. One can choose for partial or full assessment, and the amount of subscales or descriptions must be as limited as possible.

More research is required to explore the feasibility of such a modular evaluation system. The dental community must take its responsibility to reach an agreement upon this topic.

Abbreviations

BEWE: Basic erosive wear examination; DMFT: Decayed missing filled teeth; SEPRS: Simplified erosion partial recording system; TWES: Tooth wear evaluation system; TWI: Tooth wear index; VEDE: Visual erosion dental examination

Acknowledgements

Not applicable.

Funding

This research was carried out without funding, the authors declare no conflicts of interest.

Authors' contributions

PW and AF both made substantial contributions to the conception, design, analysis and interpretation. FL revised the manuscript critically for important intellectual content. All authors read and approved the final manuscript.

Competing interests

The authors declare that they have no competing interests.

Consent for publication

Not applicable.

Ethics approval and consent to participate

Not applicable.

Disclosures

This research was carried out without funding, the authors declare no conflicts of interest.

References

1. Lussi A, Carvalho TS. Erosive tooth wear: a multifactorial condition of growing concern and increasing knowledge. Monogr Oral Sci. 2014;25:1–15. doi:10.1159/000360380. Epub 2014 Jun 26. Review.
2. Ganss C, Lussi A. Diagnosis of erosive tooth wear. Monogr Oral Sci. 2014;25:22–31. doi:10.1159/000359935. Epub 2014 Jun 26. Review.
3. Beckhof G, Kutschmann M, Bardehle D. Methodological considerations concerning the development of oral dental erosion indexes: literature survey, validity and reliability. Clin Oral Invest. 2008;12 Suppl 1:S51–8.
4. Margaritis V, Nunn J. Challenges in assessing erosive tooth wear. Monogr Oral Sci. 2014;25:46–54. doi:10.1159/000359937. Epub 2014 Jun 26. Review.
5. Eccles JD. Dental erosion of nonindustrial origin. A clinical survey and classification. J Prosth Dent. 1979;42:649–53.
6. Smith BGN, Knight JK. An index for measuring the wear of tooth. Br Dent J. 1984;156:435–8.

7. Lussi A, Schaffner M, Hotz P, Suter P. Dental erosion in a population of Swiss adults. Community Dent Oral Epidemiol. 1991;19:286–90.
8. Bartlett D, Ganss C, Lussi A. Basic Erosive Wear Examination (BEWE): a new scoring system for scientific and clinical needs. Clin Oral Invest. 2008;12 suppl 1:S65–8.
9. Bardsley PF. The evolution of tooth wear indices. Clin Oral Invest. 2008;12 Suppl 1:S15–9.
10. Shellis RP, Addy M. The interactions between attrition, abrasion and erosion in tooth wear. Monogr Oral Sci. 2014;25:32–45. doi:10.1159/000359936. Epub 2014 Jun 26. Review.
11. Bartlett D. A proposed system for screening tooth wear. Br Dent J. 2010;208: 207–9. doi:10.1038/sj.bdj.2010.205.
12. Hove LH, Mulic A, Tveit AB, Stenhagen KR, Skaare AB, Espelid I. Registration of dental erosive wear on study models and intra- oral photographs. Eur Arch Paediatr Dent. 2013;14:29–34.
13. Wetselaar P, Lobbezoo F, Koutris M, Visscher CM, Naeije M. Reliability of an occlusal and nonocclusal tooth wear grading system: clinical use versus dental cast assessment. Int J Prosthodont. 2009;22:388–90.
14. Mulic A, Tveit AB, Wang NJ, Hove LH, Espelid I, Skaare AB. Reliability of two clinical scoring systems for dental erosive wear. Caries Res. 2010;44:294–9. doi:10.1159/000314811. Epub 2010 May 27.
15. Gandara BK, Truelove EL. Diagnosis and management of dental erosion. J Contemp Dent Pract. 1999;1:16–23.
16. Donachie MA, Walls AW. Assessment of tooth wear in an ageing population. J Dent. 1995;23:157–64.
17. Donachie MA, Walls AW. The tooth wear index: a flawed epidemiological tool in an ageing population group. Community Dent Oral Epidemiol. 1996; 24:152–8. Review.
18. Hasselkvist A, Johansson A, Johansson AK. Dental erosion and soft drink consumption in Swedish children and adolescents and the development of a simplified erosion partial recording system. Swed Dent J. 2010;34:187–95.
19. Lobbezoo F, Naeije M. A reliability study of clinical tooth wear measurements. J Prosthet Dent. 2001;86:597–602.

5

The differences in healthcare utilization for dental caries based on the implementation of water fluoridation in South Korea

Myung-Soo Cho[1,2†], Kyu-Tae Han[3,4†], Sohee Park[5], Ki Tae Moon[6] and Eun-Cheol Park[4,7*]

Abstract

Background: There were some debates about the water fluoridation program in South Korea, even if the program had generally substantial effectiveness. Because the out-of-pocket expenditures for dental care were higher in South Korea than in other countries, an efficient solution was needed. Therefore, we examined the relationship between the implementation of water fluoridation and the utilization of dental care.

Methods: We used the National Health Insurance Service National Sample Cohort. In this study, data finally included 472,250 patients who were newly diagnosed with dental caries during 2003–2013. We performed survival analysis using cox proportional hazard model, negative binomial-regression, and regression analyses using generalized estimating equation models.

Results: There were 48.49 % outpatient dental care visit during study period. Individuals with water fluoridation had a lower risk of dental care visits (HR = 0.949, 95 % CI = 0.928–0.971). Among the individuals who experienced a dental care visit, those with water fluoridation program had a lower number of dental care visits (β = −0.029), and the period of water fluoridation had an inverse association with the dental care expenditures.

Conclusion: The implementation of water fluoridation programs and these periods are associated with reducing the utilization of dental health care. Considering these positive impacts, healthcare professionals must consider preventive strategies for activating water fluoridation programs, such as changes in public perception and relations, for the effective management of dental care in South Korea.

Keywords: Water fluoridation, Dental caries, Healthcare expenditures, Public program

Background

Dental caries are the most common diseases related to oral health worldwide [1]. The insufficient management of oral health to prevent dental caries could cause several symptoms and large cost burdens associated with the treatment of dental caries. Naturally, many strategies for preventing dental caries were developed, such as the improvement of oral health behaviors, changes in dietary patterns, the brushing of teeth, the use of fluoride toothpaste, flu dental screenings, dental scaling, and water fluoridation programs [2–4]. Recently, the oral health, especially that related to dental caries, of individuals has been generally improved compared with that in the past [5].

Water fluoridation is a program that introduces fluoride at an optimal level into drinking water to improve pubic dental health. It was first introduced in Grand Rapids in 1945 and was considered effective in the prevention of dental caries [6]. A previous report by the World Health Organization (WHO) suggested that the program could positively affect oral health, and the WHO recommended introducing water fluoridation in countries where such programs would be technically and culturally feasible [7]. Hence, many countries began to introduce water fluoridation. In the previous study which was conducted based on systematic review in UK,

* Correspondence: ecpark@yuhs.ac
†Equal contributors
[4]Institute of Health Services Research, Yonsei University College of Medicine, Seoul, Republic of Korea
[7]Department of Preventive Medicine, Yonsei University College of Medicine, Seoul, Republic of Korea
Full list of author information is available at the end of the article

the water fluoridation had positive impact for reducing dental caries about 14 % [8]. This program in New Zealand and Australia also made about positive outcomes in oral health related to dental caries [9, 10]. The result in Japan also showed that positive effect too [11].

Since 1981, South Korea has implemented and gradually expanded a water fluoridation program. In 2002, the 32 regions among the ~250 regions in South Korea had implemented water fluoridation programs [12]. Since the late 1990s, some concerns about adverse effects of water fluoridation have been generally raised through media sources in South Korea. Each local government, with the support of voters, faces choices in its decision making for the implementation of water fluoridation. The expansion of water fluoridation thus faces difficulties, even if the program is effective in aspects of both quality of life and costs. Finally, only 17 regions implemented water fluoridation in 2013. Previous studies suggest, however, that there have been no significant adverse effects of introducing water fluoridation since the beginning of the 21st century [7, 8, 13].

Because of the effectiveness of water fluoridation and the continuous progress against dental caries in South Korea (age-adjusted prevalence rates of dental caries: 39.1 % in 2007, 31.4 % in 2014), we assumed that water fluoridation programs could significantly affect the reduction of dental caries in South Korea [14]. Although some previous studies in South Korea examined the effectiveness of water fluoridation, there were no studies took the perspective of the whole nation in South Korea. Also, the cost burden, including out-of-pocket expenses, for dental care is one of the major causes of medical expenditures (2011: Organization for Economic Co-operation and Development [OECD] average = 55 %, South Korea = 84 %) [15]. Therefore, we examined the relationship between the implementation of water fluoridation and the utilization of dental care using national sample cohort data. Based on our findings, we expect that decision makers could make appropriate strategies for the management of oral health in South Korea.

Methods

Study population

The data used in this study was the National Health Insurance Service National Sample Cohort 2002–2013. It include a random sample of 1,025,340 individuals as about 2.2 % of the overall South Korean in 2002. To represent total medical expenditure per year of South Korean within each of 1,476 strata (defined by age, sex, types of insurance coverage, and income level), this data was made through using probability sampling methods, and the model used proportional allocation. Thus, total medical claims of 1,025,340 individuals during 2002–2013 was included in this data. To examine the association between the implementation of water fluoridation program and the utilization of outpatient care for dental caries, represented by factors such as the frequency of outpatient visits and the medical expenditures by individuals, we only included patients who lived in non-metropolitan areas, because water fluoridation programs were rarely implemented in metropolitan areas (one metropolitan area in 2013). Then, we included only the patients who were newly diagnosed with dental caries (International Classification of Diseases [ICD]-10: K02) through outpatient care after 2003 (589,346 patients). We excluded those who were first diagnosed with dental caries before 2003 to ensure that only newly diagnosed patients were included. These patients were annually followed up. Finally, the data included 472,250 patients in 164 regions during 2003–2013 (average 9.12 years follow up). In addition, we added information about which regions had implemented water fluoridation from the Ministry of Health & Welfare. Regional variables were obtained from the 'e-provincial indicators' which was collected by Statistics Korea. It contained the regional characteristics of about 250 Si-Gun-Gu in South Korea. This data was used in this study for reflecting regional characteristics for each region where the patients with dental caries lived.

Variables

The outcome variables used in this study were based on information about healthcare utilization for dental caries within the study population. The first outcome variable used in this study was whether each patient visited to dental clinic due to dental caries through outpatient care during study period. Next, other outcome variables were used in this study were the frequencies of dental care visits and the cost of outpatient care as indicators of medical expenditures for only the patients who had experienced outpatient care for dental caries in each year.

The major variables of interest were whether or not each community implemented water fluoridation during the study period and how long the period of the program was. Based on 2013, the water fluoridation program was implemented in 13 Si-Gun-Gu among 164 non-metropolitan areas. In this study, the patients who lived in those regions were considered to live in regions where water fluoridation had been implemented. Additionally, to consider the effect of the time since the initial implementation the program, the time since the implementation of water fluoridation was also included in this study. We hypothesized that the implementation of water fluoridation and the time since the implementation in each region would affect the outpatient visits and medical expenditures by the patients.

The patients and regional variables were controlled in analyses for association between water fluoridation and the outcome variables. The patient variables were as follows: age, sex, income, type of insurance coverage, study year, dental care expenditures in the previous year, dental care visits in the previous year, dentofacial anomalies, and disorders of tooth development and eruption. The patients' age was categorized based on 10 years. The income was divided into deciles based on mean household income as follows: ≤10, 11–20, 21–30, 31–40, 41–50, 51–60, 61–70, 71–80, 81–90, and ≥91 %. The types of insurance coverage were categorized based on the NHI criteria as: medical aid, National Health Insurance (NHI) employee insurance, or NHI self-employed insurance. First, medical aid was defined as individuals with income less than poverty level in South Korea or individuals with a physical or mental disability. They could receive the healthcare services as free or low copayment by government funds. And, the other individuals were defined as NHI beneficiaries. The NHI beneficiaries were categorized in employee or self-employed based on job status. If individuals included workers and employers in all workplaces, they were included to NHI employee insurance, and paid a premium of about 7 % in their monthly income as withholding tax.The NHI self-employed insurance defined as individuals who did not fall into the NHI employee insurance group. They paid NHI premium based on their income, property, and living standard. Thus, this category could reflect the socio-economic status of each individual. We also included the number of pre-dental care visits, the pre-dental care cost, dentofacial anomalies (ICD-10: K07), and disorders of tooth development and eruption (ICD-10: K00) to adjust the severity of disease which could affect to the risk in dental caries in each patient. The number of pre-dental care visits was defined as the number of outpatient visits related to dental care during the previous year after the baseline year. The pre-dental care costs were calculated as the sum of the healthcare expenditures for dental care during the previous year after the baseline year. Dentofacial anomalies and disorders of tooth development and eruption were defined based on whether the patient was diagnosed with those symptoms as comorbidities in a specific year. The regional variables were the number of dentists per 1,000 people and the financial independence rate of the local government. The financial independence rate of the local government is an index of the finance utilization capacity of a local government with independent discretionary power. It was calculated as follows: (local taxes + non tax revenue)/budgets of local government × 100.

Statistical analysis

First, we showed the frequencies of categorical variable and averages of continuous variable to examine the distribution of general characteristics at the baseline. We also performed χ^2 tests and Cochran–Mantel–Haenszel tests to investigate the association between each categorical variables and visiting dental care by the implementation of water fluoridation as unit of person-years during study period. Next, we showed the averages and standard deviation of each continuous variable at the baseline and also performed a Mann-Whitney test, a Kruskal-Wallis test, and an analysis of covariance for continuous variable by the water fluoridation program during the study period. We also showed the Kaplan-Meier survival curve to compare the risk for visiting dental care by the water fluoridation. Finally, we performed a survival analysis using cox proportional hazard model to investigate whether patient visited to dental clinic due to dental caries during study period. Then, for the patients who had experienced outpatient care for dental caries during the study period, to examine the associations with the number of dental care visits and the dental care expenditures, we performed a multiple negative binomial regression, and regression analysis using a Generalized Estimating Equation (GEE) model with link logit regarding the overdispersion of outcome variables [16]. Additionally, we performed subgroup analyses according to age group or experience of pre-dental care within each region to examine the difference of association related to water fluoridation. The statistical analyses in used this study were analyzed using SAS statistical software version 9.4.

Results

The data included 472,250 patients at baseline. Appendix 1 shows the general characteristics of the study population at baseline. The patients with water fluoridation were 10.40 % of the total patients at baseline. The average follow-up time was 9.12 years during the study period.

Table 1 shows the associations among the patient and regional characteristics of baseline, the outpatient dental care visits for dental caries, and the presence of water fluoridation during the study period. The average percentage of patients that experienced an outpatient dental visit was 46.98 % in regions with water fluoridation and 48.66 % in regions without water fluoridation, respectively (p-value < .0001). The distributions of the other independent variables based on water fluoridation were similar among the groups. Females more frequently experienced outpatient dental care than males (p-value < .0001). In addition, younger or wealthier groups were generally more likely to make dental visits because of dental caries than other groups (p-value < .0001). Beneficiaries of NHI employee insurance more visited to dental care than individuals with other types of insurance (p-value < .0001).

Table 1 The association between baseline characteristics and dental care visit during study period by water fluoridation program

Variables	Water flouridation										*P*-value
	Yes					No					
	Visit		Non-visit		*P*-value					*P*-value	
	N/Mean	%/SD	N/Mean	%/SD		N/Mean	%/SD	N/Mean	%/SD		
Regional variables											
Period from introduction of water fluoridation	6.40	±4.67	6.64	±4.74	<.0001	–	–	–	–	–	–
Number of dentists per 1,000 residents	0.29	±0.15	0.29	±0.15	<.0001	0.28	±0.12	0.27	±0.12	<.0001	0.0021
Financial independence rate of local government	46.48	±23.11	47.56	±23.36	<.0001	51.77	±24.63	50.36	±24.45	<.0001	<.0001
Individual variables											
Sex											
Male	10,934	44.14	13,837	55.86	<.0001	98,496	45.88	116,178	54.12	<.0001	<.0001
Female	12,142	49.86	12,209	50.14		107,402	51.52	101,052	48.48		
Age (Years)											
-19	8,880	59.43	6,063	40.57	<.0001	78,779	61.62	49,071	38.38	<.0001	<.0001
20–29	3,546	51.14	3,388	48.86		31,139	51.96	28,790	48.04		
30–39	3,663	43.75	4,710	56.25		32,436	45.26	39,233	54.74		
40–49	3,290	43.90	4,205	56.10		29,275	44.93	35,884	55.07		
50–59	1,872	43.30	2,451	56.70		16,961	44.98	20,743	55.02		
60–69	1,366	34.45	2,599	65.55		12,956	37.25	21,824	62.75		
< 70	459	14.86	2,630	85.14		4,352	16.71	21,685	83.29		
Income (percentile)											
-10 % (low)	1,911	35.95	3,405	64.05	<.0001	15,930	35.78	28,588	64.22	<.0001	<.0001
11–20 %	1,404	43.58	1,818	56.42		12,124	44.91	14,874	55.09		
21–30 %	1,705	44.68	2,111	55.32		14,157	46.55	16,253	53.45		
31–40 %	2,014	45.56	2,407	54.44		16,787	46.70	19,163	53.30		
41–50 %	2,289	46.19	2,667	53.81		19,872	48.74	20,899	51.26		
51–60 %	2,518	47.58	2,774	52.42		21,769	49.95	21,811	50.05		
61–70 %	2,818	49.68	2,854	50.32		24,962	50.83	24,148	49.17		
71–80 %	2,988	50.50	2,929	49.50		27,172	52.05	25,032	47.95		
81–90 %	2,840	50.87	2,743	49.13		28,038	52.66	25,206	47.34		
+ 91 % (high)	2,589	52.55	2,338	47.45		25,087	54.13	21,256	45.87		
Types of insurance coverage											
Medical Aid	449	22.90	1,512	77.10	<.0001	3,868	23.24	12,778	76.76	<.0001	<.0001
NHI, self-employed insured	10,619	46.96	11,995	53.04		92,100	48.14	99,217	51.86		
NHI, employee insured	12,008	48.92	12,539	51.08		109,930	51.09	105,235	48.91		
Year of baseline											
2003	20,564	47.40	22,819	52.60	<.0001	180,731	49.01	187,996	50.99	<.0001	<.0001
2004	661	55.22	536	44.78		5,917	58.95	4,120	41.05		
2005	412	61.40	259	38.60		3,783	65.57	1,986	34.43		
2006	346	58.25	248	41.75		3,595	58.85	2,514	41.15		
2007	271	51.82	252	48.18		3,056	57.40	2,268	42.60		
2008	272	47.97	295	52.03		2,897	57.84	2,112	42.16		
2009	221	42.91	294	57.09		2,276	49.04	2,365	50.96		

Table 1 The association between baseline characteristics and dental care visit during study period by water fluoridation program *(Continued)*

2010	170	37.53	283	62.47		1,808	41.23	2,577	58.77		
2011	96	24.55	295	75.45		1,093	26.17	3,083	73.83		
2012	44	10.21	387	89.79		563	12.55	3,924	87.45		
2013	19	4.79	378	95.21		179	4.01	4,285	95.99		
Dentofacial anomalies											
Yes	13	100.00	0	0.00	0.0001	70	100.00	0	0.00	<.0001	<.0001
No	23,063	46.96	26,046	53.04		205,828	48.65	217,230	51.35		
Disorders of toothe development and eruption											
Yes	89	100.00	0	0.00	<.0001	792	100.00	0	0.00	<.0001	<.0001
No	22,987	46.88	26,046	53.12		205,106	48.56	217,230	51.44		
Total	23,07	46.98	26,046	53.02		205,898	48.66	217,230	51.34		<.0001

†The results of a Cochran-Mantel-Haenszel test to investigate the differences of distribution for categorical variables based on water fluoridation

Appendix 2 shows the Kaplan-Meier survival curve for time to first diagnosis of dental caries by the implementation water fluoridation. Individuals in regions with water fluoridation program was less likely to visit dental care than individuals in regions without program (p-value for log-rank test < .0001).

Table 2 shows the distribution based on water fluoridation of the average values and the standard deviation for dental care visits or cost per year among only the patients who made dental visits because of dental caries. The average number of dental care visits and the costs were lower among patients with water fluoridation than among those without the program (p-value < .0001).

Table 3 shows the results of the survival analysis using cox proportional hazard model, negative binomial regression, and regression analysis for dental care expenditures, represented by the number of visits or the costs, among only the patients that experienced a dental visit. Patient with water fluoridation program had higher risk in the dental care visit during study period (Yes = HR: 0.949, 95 % CI: 0.928–0.971, p-value < .0001). Female and younger people was had more tend to dental care visits due to dental caries (p-value < .0001). By the economic status, people with higher income or employee insured NHI had high risk in dental care visits than other groups (p-value < .0001). In addition, people with dental comorbidities was also more visited in dental care (p-value < .0001).

The results of the regression analysis for dental care expenditures showed that patients in regions that implemented a water fluoridation program had a lower number of dental visits or lower costs, although the results about dental care cost was not statistically significant (number of dental visits: $\beta = -0.029$, p-value = 0.0431; dental care costs: $\beta = -0.008$, p-value = 0.7097). In addition, patients in regions with more dentists made less dental visits and spent less on dental care. On the other hand, the financial independence rate in each region had an inverse association with the risk of dental visits (p-value < .05). For the patient characteristics, males had an inverse association with the number of dental visits and costs (p-value < .0001). On the other hand, beneficiaries of Medical Aid or self-employed NHI had a lower number of dental visits and lower costs than beneficiaries of employee NHI (p-value < .05). Expenditures related to pre-dental care or comorbidity had a positive association with the outcome variables (p-value < .001).

We performed subgroup analyses for the survival analysis using cox proportional hazard model, negative binomial regression, and regression analyses using GEE models to investigate the relationship between water fluoridation and the outcome variables based on experience of pre-dental care visits (visit or no visit), income (−50 % and +51 %), and age group (≤19 years, 20–39 years, 40–59 years, ≥60 years). The associations between the presence of a water fluoridation program and the number of dental visits was greater for patients who had not experienced a pre-dental care visit in the previous year than for patients who had experienced a pre-dental care visit in the previous year (with, water fluoridation = β: 0.043, p-value = 0.2901; without, water fluoridation = β: −0.031, p-value = 0.0424). By age group, the inverse associations between water fluoridation and outcome variables were greater in the elderly population than in the younger population. In the younger groups, the inverse associations with dental care expenditures were analyzed based on period from implementation of water fluoridation (Table 4).

Discussion

To effectively manage oral health, and particularly patients with dental caries in South Korea, the South Korean government has introduced water fluoridation

Table 2 The averages and standard deviations of dental care visits and costs for patients who visited dental care through outpatient care†

Variables	Water flouridation						*P*-value	Water flouridation						*P*-value†
	Yes			No				Yes			No			
	Number of dental care visits		*P*-value	Number of dental care visits		*P*-value		Dental care costs (KRW)		*P*-value	Dental care costs (KRW)		*P*-value	
	Mean	SD		Mean	SD			Mean	SD		Mean	SD		
Individual variables														
Sex														
Male	0.28	±0.75	<.0001	0.30	±0.79	<.0001	0.9079	8485.36	±26,233.38	0.0167	8758.21	±27,035.59	<.0001	0.6855
Female	0.29	±0.77		0.30	±0.81			8567.78	±26,234.69		8790.68	±26,725.42		
Age (Years)														
-19	0.38	±0.90	<.0001	0.42	±0.95	<.0001	<.0001	12358.18	±32,803.66	<.0001	12790.26	±33,474.42	<.0001	0.2527
20–29	0.26	±0.72		0.27	±0.76			7478.72	±24,358.22		7636.75	±24,858.38		
30–39	0.22	±0.65		0.23	±0.67			6137.69	±20,783.50		6353.85	±21,809.12		
40–49	0.22	±0.63		0.24	±0.68			6118.31	±20,360.00		6575.26	±22,017.51		
50–59	0.25	±0.69		0.24	±0.68			7203.43	±22,910.40		7305.94	±23,947.33		
60–69	0.26	±0.77		0.27	±0.75			7729.45	±25,167.92		7685.72	±24,254.82		
< 70	0.26	±0.76		0.27	±0.76			7378.33	±23,917.36		7392.36	±23,288.21		
Income (percentile)														
-10 % (low)	0.25	±0.74	0.0003	0.27	±0.81	<.0001	0.2805	7745.45	±25,837.11	0.0003	7969.37	±26,342.94	<.0001	0.0164
11–20 %	0.28	±0.78		0.29	±0.81			8170.88	±26,355.37		8539.98	±26,535.13		
21–30 %	0.28	±0.79		0.29	±0.80			8300.89	±26,029.00		8530.71	±26,384.56		
31–40 %	0.26	±0.70		0.29	±0.80			7579.31	±24,080.07		8585.70	±27,179.61		
41–50 %	0.28	±0.76		0.30	±0.80			8685.57	±27,015.42		8710.41	±26,762.40		
51–60 %	0.29	±0.77		0.30	±0.80			8869.81	±27,295.76		8910.14	±27,358.22		
61–70 %	0.30	±0.78		0.31	±0.81			8887.83	±26,420.46		9195.21	±27,617.53		
71–80 %	0.29	±0.77		0.32	±0.81			8868.81	±26,543.89		9330.15	±27,794.34		
81–90 %	0.30	±0.79		0.32	±0.80			9128.50	±27,290.42		9128.64	±27,025.66		
+ 91 % (high)	0.28	±0.72		0.30	±0.76			8348.43	±24,746.39		8392.44	±25,500.98		
Types of insurance coverage														
Medical Aid	0.17	±0.65	<.0001	0.19	±0.73	<.0001	0.9777	5463.02	±24,295.15	<.0001	5569.94	±23,732.00	<.0001	0.6780
NHI, self-employed insured	0.27	±0.75		0.29	±0.79			8349.77	±25,975.77		8657.48	±26,710.94		
NHI, employee insured	0.29	±0.77		0.31	±0.81			8768.09	±26,464.81		8971.88	±27,079.50		

Table 2 The averages and standard deviations of dental care visits and costs for patients who visited dental care through outpatient care† *(Continued)*

Index year														
2003	0.25	±0.61	<.0001	0.25	±0.63	<.0001	<.0001	8034.83	±24,159.19	<.0001	8080.83	±24,641.98	<.0001	0.0003
2004	0.25	±0.63		0.25	±0.62			8382.93	±26,010.94		8009.35	±24,967.53		
2005	0.25	±0.61		0.25	±0.63			8297.59	±25,261.94		8270.24	±25,774.14		
2006	0.25	±0.63		0.25	±0.63			8283.21	±25,874.99		8310.02	±26,017.55		
2007	0.29	±0.78		0.30	±0.82			8302.10	±25,361.18		8447.74	±25,742.34		
2008	0.33	±0.90		0.34	±0.93			8527.55	±25,215.56		8613.98	±25,737.46		
2009	0.32	±0.87		0.34	±0.91			8484.86	±25,234.96		8797.15	±26,417.00		
2010	0.30	±0.83		0.32	±0.88			8363.59	±26,338.25		8692.93	±26,825.06		
2011	0.31	±0.84		0.34	±0.90			8821.34	±27,704.86		9519.33	±28,487.64		
2012	0.30	±0.83		0.33	±0.88			9062.00	±28,211.94		9642.10	±29,482.37		
2013	0.29	±0.79		0.33	±0.87			9443.44	±29,389.48		10376.20	±31,264.12		
Dentofacial anomalies														
Yes	1.75	±1.32	<.0001	1.91	±1.42	<.0001	0.0774	60991.70	±60,760.65	<.0001	68584.30	±65,057.42	<.0001	0.0088
No	0.28	±0.76		0.30	±0.80			8503.58	±26,182.17		8742.72	±26,802.56		
Disorders of toothe development and eruption														
Yes	1.89	±1.43	<.0001	1.95	±1.39	<.0001	0.1953	70958.60	±56,207.42	<.0001	71028.40	±54,669.15	<.0001	0.8636
No	0.28	±0.75		0.29	±0.79			8287.70	±25,760.74		8526.49	±26,412.60		
Total	0.28	±0.76		0.30	±0.80		<.0001	8528.51	±26,234.03		8775.16	±26,874.15		<.0001

† The results of analysis of covariance to investigate the differences of distribution for continuous variables based on water fluoridation

Table 3 The results of survival analysis, negative binomial regression, and regression for dental care visits and expenditures including both patient and regional characteristics

Variables	Dental care visits[a]				Only patient with dental care visit					
					Number of dental care visits[b]			Dental care costs (KRW)[c]		
	HR	95 % CI		*P*-value	β	SE	*P*-value	β	SE	*P*-value
Regional variables										
Water fluoridation										
Yes	0.949	0.928	0.971	<.0001	−0.029	0.014	0.0431	0.008	0.021	0.7097
No	1.000	–	–	–	Ref	–	–	Ref	–	–
Period from implementation of water fluoridation	0.998	0.995	1.001	0.2302	−0.003	0.001	0.0177	−0.006	0.002	0.0024
Number of dentists per 1,000 residents	1.007	0.975	1.041	0.6700	−0.045	0.016	0.0068	−0.026	0.024	0.2812
Financial independence rate of local government	0.999	0.999	0.999	<.0001	−0.003	0.000	<.0001	−0.003	0.000	<.0001
Individual variables										
Sex										
Male	0.795	0.788	0.801	<.0001	−0.051	0.004	<.0001	−0.071	0.005	<.0001
Female	1.000	–	–	–	Ref	–	–	Ref	–	–
Age (Years)										
-19	4.835	4.695	4.979	<.0001	0.408	0.010	<.0001	0.662	0.013	<.0001
20–29	3.069	2.977	3.163	<.0001	0.064	0.011	<.0001	0.020	0.014	0.1451
30–39	2.466	2.392	2.542	<.0001	−0.073	0.011	<.0001	−0.134	0.014	<.0001
40–49	2.502	2.427	2.579	<.0001	−0.069	0.011	<.0001	−0.101	0.013	<.0001
50–59	2.531	2.452	2.613	<.0001	−0.022	0.011	0.0487	−0.030	0.014	0.0316
60–69	2.044	1.978	2.112	<.0001	0.033	0.012	0.0045	0.055	0.016	0.0004
< 70	1.000	–	–	–	Ref	–	–	Ref	–	–
Income (percentile)										
-10 % (low)	0.751	0.736	0.767	<.0001	0.003	0.009	0.7721	−0.085	0.013	<.0001
11–20 %	0.751	0.736	0.767	<.0001	−0.004	0.009	0.6797	−0.094	0.013	<.0001
21–30 %	0.762	0.747	0.777	<.0001	−0.004	0.009	0.6740	−0.099	0.013	<.0001
31–40 %	0.770	0.756	0.784	<.0001	−0.026	0.008	0.0018	−0.121	0.012	<.0001
41–50 %	0.805	0.790	0.819	<.0001	0.006	0.008	0.4173	−0.069	0.012	<.0001
51–60 %	0.835	0.821	0.850	<.0001	0.011	0.008	0.1536	−0.045	0.012	0.0001
61–70 %	0.880	0.866	0.895	<.0001	0.028	0.007	0.0002	−0.007	0.011	0.5510
71–80 %	0.916	0.901	0.931	<.0001	0.030	0.007	<.0001	0.025	0.011	0.0267
81–90 %	0.943	0.928	0.959	<.0001	0.023	0.007	0.0007	0.025	0.011	0.0190
+ 91 % (high)	1.000	–	–	–	Ref	–	–	Ref	–	–
Types of insurance coverage										
Medical Aid	0.410	0.396	0.425	<.0001	−0.573	0.018	<.0001	−0.956	0.017	<.0001
NHI, self-employed insured	0.872	0.865	0.879	<.0001	−0.033	0.004	<.0001	−0.097	0.006	<.0001
NHI, employee insured	1.000	–	–	–	Ref	–	–	Ref	–	–
Year of baseline/Index year										
2003	1.000	–	–	–	Ref	–	–	Ref	–	–
2004	1.052	1.026	1.079	<.0001	−0.015	0.003	<.0001	−0.126	0.013	<.0001
2005	1.126	1.092	1.162	<.0001	−0.018	0.003	<.0001	−0.102	0.013	<.0001
2006	1.124	1.089	1.160	<.0001	−0.017	0.003	<.0001	−0.108	0.013	<.0001
2007	1.143	1.104	1.183	<.0001	0.128	0.004	<.0001	−0.037	0.013	0.0037

Table 3 The results of survival analysis, negative binomial regression, and regression for dental care visits and expenditures including both patient and regional characteristics *(Continued)*

2008	1.104	1.065	1.144	<.0001	0.209	0.004	<.0001	0.016	0.013	0.2238
2009	1.038	0.997	1.080	0.0710	0.192	0.004	<.0001	0.000	0.013	0.9752
2010	0.974	0.931	1.018	0.2418	0.176	0.004	<.0001	−0.073	0.013	<.0001
2011	0.736	0.695	0.779	<.0001	0.163	0.004	<.0001	0.079	0.013	<.0001
2012	0.483	0.445	0.523	<.0001	0.157	0.004	<.0001	0.045	0.013	0.0007
2013	0.304	0.265	0.350	<.0001	0.149	0.004	<.0001	0.091	0.014	<.0001
Pre-dental care costs (per 1,000 KRW)					0.001	0.000	<.0001	0.004	0.000	<.0001
Number of pre-dental care					0.183	0.004	<.0001	0.309	0.009	<.0001
Dentofacial anomalies										
Yes	21.614	17.417	26.821	<.0001	1.925	0.022	<.0001	8.832	0.037	<.0001
No	1.000	–	–	–	Ref	–	–	Ref	–	–
Disorders of toothe development and eruption										
Yes	16.465	15.392	17.614	<.0001	1.563	0.008	<.0001	8.348	0.012	<.0001
No	1.000	–	–	–	Ref	–	–	Ref	–	–

[a]The survival analysis using cox proportional hazard models was applied to investigate the association with risk of dental care visits during study period
[b]The negative binomial regression using GEE models was performed for patients who had experienced a dental care visit at least once per year to investigate the associations with dental care visits
[c]The regression using GEE models was performed for patients who had experienced a dental care visit at least once per year to investigate the associations with dental care cost

programs since 1981 [12]. Previous studies of the water fluoridation programs showed that the programs had a positive role in preventing dental caries and improving oral health [10, 17, 18]. Based on those results, the water fluoridation programs seemed to gradually expand on the whole in South Korea. However, in the late 20th century, some concerns related to negative effects of water fluoridation, such as fluoride toxicity, were raised and proliferated. After that, the activation of the programs faced difficulties such as a negative public awareness. However, the previous studies of the adverse effects of water fluoridation found no significant adverse effects related to fluoride [7, 8, 13]. There was a need to change the public perception and provide evidence supporting the activation of water fluoridation programs for effective public health. Therefore, we examined the relationship between the implementation of water fluoridation and dental care utilization by South Koreans using a national sample cohort during 2003–2013.

Our findings showed that the implementation of the water fluoridation program in each region had a preventive role, decreasing dental care utilizations such as dental visits and expenditures. In the regions with water fluoridation programs, the duration of the program had an inverse association with the number of dental visits per year. Those findings were similar to the findings of previous studies including results in the other countries [8–11]. Water fluoridation programs as a prevention strategy could positively affect the improvement of oral health, and individuals who lived in regions with water fluoridation had less need to access dental care because of their improved oral health. The out-of-pocket expenditures for dental care in South Korea were remarkably higher than those in other OECD countries; introducing such prevention strategies had a quite positive affect on the reduction of the disease burden in South Korea [15]. Therefore, the implementation of water fluoridation improved oral health in South Korea, and a national recommendation for the activation of this program would be worthwhile based on our findings.

In addition, our study suggests some interesting results related to other covariates. The results for the financial independence rate of the local government as an indirect indicator of regional wealth revealed some inequalities in oral health among regions based on wealth, even if some community oral health programs were already implemented [19]. Hence, governments need to consider public health programs, such as regular dental screening programs, which could reduce inequalities. Also, the patients with a lower economic level, represented by income or type of insurance coverage, had a lower risk of dental visits and expenditures. Such results might be caused by the accessibility of health care. The wealthier individuals made more dental visits in the early stages of their clinical symptoms, and they used regular screening or consultation as part of primary and secondary prevention. On the other hand, individuals with low economic status could not make dental visits in the early stages of their symptoms and could not engage in prevention behaviors because of the cost burden [20, 21]. Therefore, the makers of health policy such as Korea

Table 4 The results of subgroup analysis for survival analysis, negative binomial regression, and regression by pre-dental care and patient age

Sub group		Variables	Dental visits[a]				Only patient with dental care visit					
							Number of dental care visits[b]			Dental care costs (KRW)[c]		
			HR	95 % CI		*P*-value	β	SE	*P*-value	β	SE	*P*-value
Experience of pre-dental care in previous year	With	Water fluoridation					0.043	0.041	0.2901	0.064	0.047	0.1712
		Period from implementation of water fluoridation					−0.007	0.004	0.0689	−0.003	0.004	0.4521
	Without	Water fluoridation					**−0.031**	**0.015**	**0.0424**	−0.009	0.018	0.6180
		Period from implementation of water fluoridation					−0.002	0.001	0.3959	**−0.004**	**0.002**	**0.0115**
Income (percentile)	−50 %	Water fluoridation	**0.934**	**0.900**	**0.968**	**0.0002**	**−0.0532**	**0.0247**	**0.0315**	−0.0106	0.0288	0.7131
		Period from implementation of water fluoridation	1.001	0.996	1.006	0.6484	−0.0004	0.0022	0.8424	−0.0026	0.0025	0.2927
	51 %	Water fluoridation	**0.957**	**0.930**	**0.985**	**0.0032**	−0.0083	0.0178	0.6422	0.0173	0.0212	0.4162
		Period from implementation of water fluoridation	0.997	0.993	1.000	0.0792	**−0.0050**	**0.0016**	**0.0014**	**−0.0056**	**0.0018**	**0.0020**
	−19	Water fluoridation	**0.941**	**0.906**	**0.976**	**0.0013**	−0.0086	0.0232	0.7117	0.0048	0.0276	0.8617
		Period from implementation of water fluoridation	0.996	0.992	1.001	0.1132	**−0.0070**	**0.0021**	**0.0007**	**−0.0054**	**0.0025**	**0.0270**
Age group	20–39	Water fluoridation	**0.959**	**0.922**	**0.998**	**0.0408**	−0.0113	0.0263	0.6675	0.0274	0.0309	0.3755
		Period from implementation of water fluoridation	1.001	0.996	1.006	0.8145	−0.0034	0.0023	0.1495	**−0.0068**	**0.0027**	**0.0104**
	40–59	Water fluoridation	**0.952**	**0.908**	**0.999**	**0.0461**	−0.0568	0.0301	0.0595	−0.0211	0.0352	0.5493
		Period from implementation of water fluoridation	1.000	0.994	1.006	0.9847	−0.0001	0.0026	0.9676	−0.0025	0.0029	0.3957
	60+	Water fluoridation	**0.912**	**0.840**	**0.991**	**0.0297**	−0.0518	0.0465	0.2648	0.0010	0.0568	0.9864
		Period from implementation of water fluoridation	0.998	0.987	1.010	0.7551	0.0022	0.0039	0.5666	0.0008	0.0048	0.8707

The reference level of water fluoridation was that of regions without a program, and the period since the implementation of water fluoridation was a continuous variable
The bold face indicates statistically significant results
These were results of sub group analyses for survival analysis and negative binomial regression analyses
[a]The survival analysis using cox proportional hazard models was applied to investigate the association with the risk of dental care visits
[b]The negative binomial regression using GEE model was performed for patients who had experienced a dental care visit at least once per year to investigate the associations with dental care visits.
[c]The regression using GEE model was performed for patients who had experienced a dental care visit at least once per year to investigate the associations with dental care costs

Health Promotion Foundation must consider some interventions to reduce economic barriers for those with low economic status to reduce health inequalities caused by economic issues. Finally, there were results showing that younger patients or patients with comorbidities utilized more dental care. Those results were similar to previous results about dental care. That is because younger patients are at a period of change from primary teeth to permanent teeth, whereas the elderly had fewer teeth because of deformation [22, 23]. Also, the patients with comorbid conditions such as dentofacial anomalies or disorders of tooth development and eruption made more dental visits than patients without those problems [24, 25]. Such patients need to activate preventive healthcare to reduce preventable expenditures.

The reduction of dental care utilization by the introduction of water fluoridation showed some differences in the subgroup analyses. The results showed that such associations were greater among patients that had not experienced dental care. It was suggested that the water fluoridation program had a major role in the reduction of the incidence of dental caries as a primary prevention rather than a secondary prevention. The implementation of such programs would be effective for individuals who managed their dental care well without clinical symptoms. Therefore, healthcare professionals need to recommend the importance of managing oral health even for individuals without any symptoms [26].

Our study has some strengths compared with previous studies. First, we used national health insurance national sampling cohort data to analyze the relationship between the implementation of water fluoridation programs and dental visits or expenditures. Therefore, the data used in our study are especially helpful for establishing evidence-based health policy for dental care. Second, to our best knowledge, this study is the first attempt to investigate the impact of water fluoridation programs on the whole nation of South Korea. So far, several previous studies of water fluoridation have been conducted, but most of those only investigated the impact of the programs at the community level [27–29]. Therefore, our findings would be effective evidence for establishing public health programs or policies. Third, we included the dental visits and expenditures as outcome variables. Therefore, our results could reflect overall dental care utilization by each patient. Finally, we adjusted the data for pre-dental care and other comorbid conditions to provide a more detailed study. Thus, we could reflect the severity of the dental caries experienced by the patients in our analyses.

Our study had also some limitations. Based on previous studies of dental caries or oral health, various factors including lifestyles, types of tooth paste, and frequencies of tooth brushing could affect the health outcome [1, 30]. The impact of water fluoridation program could be different by cultural factors which affect to heathy behaviors in each countries. Also, the outcome variables in previous studies were used with other clinical indicators including the Patient Hygiene Performance index [31]. However, the relevant details were not included in the data, as the data used in our study had the characteristics of health insurance claim data. Therefore, we were unable to consider other variables that could affect dental caries. Next, we could not consider the fluoride level in the water or the actual consumption volume for each individual because of limitations of the data [32, 33]. In addition, we excluded the regions that quit the program during the study period, because we could not clearly identify the period effect after the introduction of water fluoridation. Therefore, more detailed studies are needed. Third, in the characteristics of dental care, there were many non-payment items related to dental care in South Korea. However, because of the characteristics of the NHI claim data, we could not consider those items. Thus, it is possible that the measurement of the dental care expenditures could have been underestimated. Finally, regarding some studies of water fluoridation programs that suggested that the programs had an adverse effect, there was a need to evaluate adverse effects. However, we only analyzed the dental care utilization and did not include any adverse effects.

Despite those limitations, our findings suggest that the implementation of water fluoridation programs had a positive role in improving oral health, and especially dental caries. Regarding the negative public perception of water fluoridation programs and the high out-of-pocket expenditures for dental care in South Korea, those findings could be helpful in the management of dental care expenditures from the perspective of health policy and public health. Although further detailed studies using clinical factors will be needed in the near future, makers of health policy and professionals in the area of dental care must consider efficient strategies for activating water fluoridation programs.

Conclusions

The implementation of water fluoridation programs is inversely associated with the risk of dental visits and expenditures related to dental caries. Considering that association, makers of health policy and decision makers such as Korea Health Promotion Foundation have to consider preventive strategies for activating water fluoridation programs, such as changes in public perception and relations, in order to effectively manage dental care in South Korea.

Appendix 1

Table 5 Characteristics of study population at baseline

Variables	N/Mean	%/SD
Regional variables		
Water fluoridation		
Yes ($n = 13$)	49,122	10.40
No ($n = 151$)	423,128	89.60
Period from implementation of water fluoridation	0.68	2.51
Number of dentists per 1,000 residents	0.28	0.12
Financial independence rate of local government	50.63	24.45
Individual variables		
Sex		
Male	239,445	50.70
Female	232,805	49.30
Age (Years)		
-19	142,793	30.24
20–29	66,863	14.16
30–39	80,042	16.95
40–49	72,654	15.38
50–59	42,027	8.90
60–69	38,745	8.20
> 70	29,126	6.17
Income (percentile)		
-10 % (low)	49,834	10.55
11–20 %	30,220	6.40
21–30 %	34,226	7.25
31–40 %	40,371	8.55
41–50 %	45,727	9.68
51–60 %	48,872	10.35
61–70 %	54,782	11.60
71–80 %	58,121	12.31
81–90 %	58,827	12.46
+ 91 % (high)	51,270	10.86
Types of insurance coverage		
Medical Aid	18,607	3.94
NHI, self-employed insured	213,931	45.30
NHI, employee insured	239,712	50.76
Year of baseline		
2003	412,110	87.27
2004	11,234	2.38
2005	6,440	1.36
2006	6,703	1.42
2007	5,847	1.24
2008	5,576	1.18
2009	5,156	1.09
2010	4,838	1.02
2011	4,567	0.97
2012	4,918	1.04
2013	4,861	1.03
Dentofacial anomalies		
Yes	83	0.02
No	472,167	99.98
Disorders of toothe development and eruption		
Yes	881	0.19
No	471,369	99.81
Follow up time (year)	9.12	2.80
Total	472,250	100.00

Appendix 2

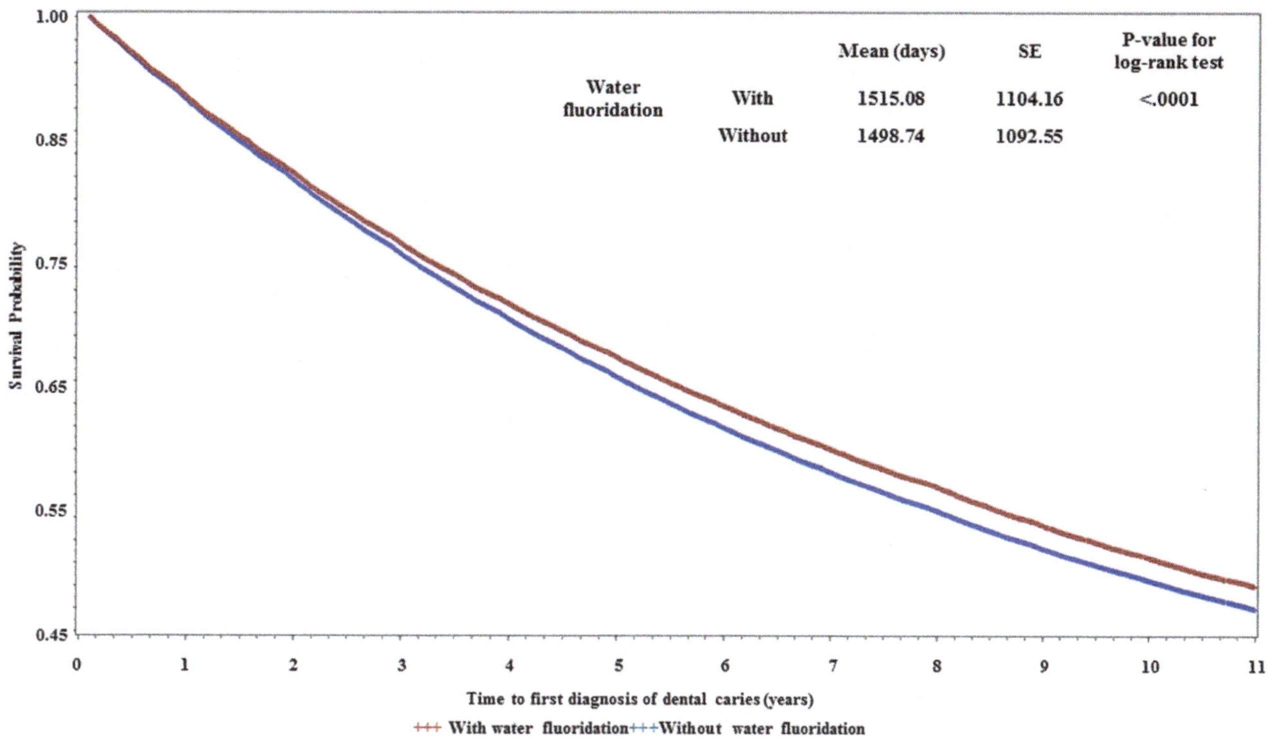

Fig. 1 The Kaplan-Meier Survival curve for time to first diagnosis of dental caries by the implementation water fluoridation

Abbreviations

CI: Confidence interval; GEE: Generalized estimating equation; HR: Hazard ratio; ICD: International classification of diseases; KNHIS: Korean National Health Insurance Service; NHI: National Health Insurance; OECD: Organization for Economic Co-operation and Development; SE: Standard error; WHO: World Health Organization

Acknowledgement

No specific funding supported this study.

Authors' contributions

MSC and KTH designed the study, performed the research and statistical analyses, and wrote the manuscript. SHP, KTM, and ECP contributed to the discussion and reviewed and edited the manuscript. ECP is the guarantor of this work and as such has full access to all the data in the study and takes responsibility for the integrity of the data and the accuracy of the data analysis. The English in this document has been checked by at least two professional editors, both native English speakers. All authors read and approved the final manuscript.

Competing interests

The authors declare that they have no competing interests.

Consent for publication

Not applicable.

Ethics approval and consent to participate

The data used in this study included the information about dental care utilization of patients, and it was not included informed consents of each patient. This is because that the data was anonymized and not identified prior to analysis. This study was approved by the Institutional Review Board, Yonsei University Graduate School of Public Health (2014-239).

Author details

[1]Department of Health Policy and Management, Graduate School of Public Health, Yonsei University, Seoul, Republic of Korea. [2]Division of Management & Planning, Korea Health Promotion Foundation, Seoul, Republic of Korea. [3]Department of Public Health, Graduate School, Yonsei University, Seoul, Republic of Korea. [4]Institute of Health Services Research, Yonsei University College of Medicine, Seoul, Republic of Korea. [5]Department of Biostatistics, Graduate School of Public Health, Yonsei University, Seoul, Republic of Korea. [6]National Evidence-Based Healthcare Collaborating Agency, Seoul, Republic of Korea. [7]Department of Preventive Medicine, Yonsei University College of Medicine, Seoul, Republic of Korea.

References

1. Selwitz RH, Ismail AI, Pitts NB. Dental caries. Lancet. 2007;369(9555):51–9.
2. Marinho VC, Higgins J, Logan S, Sheiham A. Fluoride toothpastes for preventing dental caries in children and adolescents. The Cochrane Libr. 2003.
3. Tinanoff N, Palmer CA. Dietary determinants of dental caries and dietary recommendations for preschool children. J Public Health Dent. 2000;60(3): 197–206.
4. Axelsson P, Lindhe J, Nyström B. On the prevention of caries and periodontal disease. J Clin Periodontol. 1991;18(3):182–9.

5. Lee HJ, Han DH: Exploring the determinants of secular decreases in dental caries among Korean children. Community Dent Oral Epidemiol. 2015;43(4):357–65.
6. Arnold Jr FA, Dean HT, Jay P, Knutson JW. Effect of fluoridated public water supplies on dental caries prevalence: tenth year of the Grand Rapids-Muskegon study. Public Health Rep. 1956;71(7):652.
7. Petersen PE, Lennon MA. Effective use of fluorides for the prevention of dental caries in the 21st century: the WHO approach. Community Dent Oral Epidemiol. 2004;32(5):319–21.
8. McDonagh MS, Whiting PF, Wilson PM, Sutton AJ, Chestnutt I, Cooper J, Misso K, Bradley M, Treasure E, Kleijnen J. Systematic review of water fluoridation. BMJ. 2000;321(7265):855–9.
9. Lee M, Dennison PJ. Water fluoridation and dental caries in 5-and 12-year-old children from Canterbury and Wellington. N Z Dent J. 2004;100(1):10–5.
10. Armfield JM. Community effectiveness of public water fluoridation in reducing children's dental disease. Washington, DC: Public Health Reports; 2010:655–64.
11. Kobayashi S, Kawasaki K, Takagi O, Nakamura M, Fujii N, Shinzato M, Maki Y, Takaesu Y. Caries experience in subjects18–22 years of age after 13 years' discontinued water fluoridation in Okinawa. Community Dent Oral Epidemiol. 1992;20(2):81–3.
12. DI P, Hs M, Horowitz AM, Gift HC, KI J, Ss S. Knowledge of and practices related to caries prevention among Koreans. J Public Health Dent. 1994; 54(4):205–10.
13. Parnell C, Whelton H, O'Mullane D. Water fluoridation. Eur Arch Paediatr Dent. 2009;10(3):141–8.
14. Prevalence of dental caries. http://kosis.kr/statHtml/statHtml.do?orgId=117&tblId=DT_11702_N116&conn_path=I2. Accessed 18 July 2016.
15. Organization for Economic Cooperation and Development. Health at a Glance 2013: OECD Indicators. 2013.
16. Zorn CJ: Generalized estimating equation models for correlated data. A review with applications. Am J Pol Sci. 2001;45(2):470–90.
17. Armfield JM, Spencer AJ, Roberts-Thomson KF, Plastow K. Water fluoridation and the association of sugar-sweetened beverage consumption and dental caries in Australian children. Am J Public Health. 2013;103(3):494–500.
18. Cobiac LJ, Vos T. Cost-effectiveness of extending the coverage of water supply fluoridation for the prevention of dental caries in Australia. Community Dent Oral Epidemiol. 2012;40(4):369–76.
19. Hobdell M, Petersen PE, Clarkson J, Johnson N. Global goals for oral health 2020. Int Dent J. 2003;53(5):285–8.
20. Jeon JE, Chung WG, Kim NH. The reason of unmet dental need related socioeconomic status in Korea: Using the 4th Korea National Health and Nutritional Examination Survey. J Korean Acad Oral Health. 2012;36(1):73–81.
21. Swank ME, Vernon SW, Lairson DR. Patterns of preventive dental behavior. Public Health Rep. 1986;101(2):175.
22. Fure S, Zickert I. Incidence of tooth loss and dental caries in 60-, 70- and 80-year-old Swedish individuals. Community Dent Oral Epidemiol. 1997;25(2):137–42.
23. Harris R, Nicoll AD, Adair PM, Pine CM. Risk factors for dental caries in young children: a systematic review of the literature. Community Dent Health. 2004;21(1):71–85.
24. Solorzano I, Salas M, Chavarría P, Beltrán-Aguilar E, Horowitz H. Prevalence and severity of dental caries in Costa Rican schoolchildren: results of the 1999 national survey. Int Dent J. 2005;55(1):24–30.
25. Barmes DE. Epidemiology of dental disease. J Clin Periodontol. 1977;4(5):80–93.
26. Wilkins EM. McCullough PA. Clinical practice of the dental hygienist. Philadelphia: Lea & Febiger; 1983.
27. Cho HJ, Lee HS, Paik DI, Bae KH. Association of dental caries with socioeconomic status in relation to different water fluoridation levels. Community Dent Oral Epidemiol. 2014;42(6):536–42.
28. Kim M-K, Jung J-I, Kim M-J, Jun E-J, Kim H-N, Kim S-Y, Han D-H, Jeong S-H, Kim J-B. Cost-benefit analysis of a water fluoridation program for 11 years in Jinju, Korea. J Korean Acad Oral Health. 2014;38(2):118–28.
29. Cho HJ, Jin BH, Park DY, Jung SH, Lee HS, Paik DI, Bae KH. Systemic effect of water fluoridation on dental caries prevalence. Community Dent Oral Epidemiol. 2014;42(4):341–8.
30. Petersen PE. Sociobehavioural risk factors in dental caries–international perspectives. Community Dent Oral Epidemiol. 2005;33(4):274–9.
31. Ismail AI, Sohn W, Tellez M, Willem JM, Betz J, Lepkowski J. Risk indicators for dental caries using the International Caries Detection and Assessment System (ICDAS). Community Dent Oral Epidemiol. 2008;36(1):55–68.
32. Bassin EB, Wypij D, Davis RB, Mittleman MA. Age-specific fluoride exposure in drinking water and osteosarcoma (United States). Cancer Causes Control. 2006;17(4):421–8.
33. Pizzo G, Piscopo MR, Pizzo I, Giuliana G. Community water fluoridation and caries prevention: a critical review. Clin Oral Investig. 2007;11(3):189–93.

6

Should oral anticoagulant therapy be continued during dental extraction?

Shuo Yang[1], Quan Shi[1], Jinglong Liu[1], Jinru Li[2] and Juan Xu[1*]

Abstract

Background: Oral anticoagulation therapy is widely used to reduce the risks of thromboembolism. However, the therapy increases the risk of hemorrhage during the surgical procedures. The aim of this meta-analysis was to evaluate the bleeding risk of patients continuing or discontinuing oral anticoagulant therapy while undergoing dental extractions.

Methods: Six electronic databases, including PubMed, Embase, Cochrane library, Web of Science, China Biology Medicine disc (CBM), and China National Knowledge Infrastructure (CNKI), were searched in March, 2016. Relevant articles were screened by two independent reviewers under our inclusion criteria. Quality was evaluated using the Cochrane Collaboration risk of bias tool. Meta-analyses were conducted with fixed and random effects models as appropriate.

Results: Six studies (with a total of 591 patients) were included in our meta-analysis. Our results showed that there was no significant difference in the bleeding risk between patients continuing or discontinuing oral anticoagulant therapy while undergoing dental extractions (risk ratio, 1.31; 95 % CI, 0.79, 2.14; $P > 0.05$). There was also no significant difference in bleeding risk 1 day (risk ratio, 0.91; 95 % CI, 0.35, 2.37; $P > 0.05$) and 7 days (risk ratio, 1.47; 95 % CI, 0.83, 2.59; $P > 0.05$) after the dental extraction.

Conclusion: Under current studies and evidence, it appears that patients continuing oral anticoagulant therapy do not have an increased risk of bleeding after dental extractions compared to patients who discontinue oral anticoagulant therapy.

Keywords: Oral anticoagulant therapy, Dental extraction, Bleeding, Meta-analysis

Abbreviations: NOACs, New oral anticoagulants; OAT, Oral anticoagulant therapy

Background

With the living standard gradually increasing and diet habits continuously changing, cardiovascular diseases, such as mechanical heart valve, atrial fibrillation and venous thromboembolism, have become more and more common. Millions of people receive oral anticoagulant therapy (OAT). Used to reduce thrombosis, oral anticoagulation therapy is one of the most effective prophylactic medications for preventing life-threatening events [1, 2]. Oral anticoagulant drugs mainly include heparin, warfarin and new oral anticoagulants (NOACs) [3]. Heparin should be administered intravenously, and its action is to interfere with thrombin-antithrombin pathways and reduce fibrin formation. Warfarin, which is derived from 4-hydroxycoumarin, is a competitive inhibitor of vitamin K. It is widely used all over the world [4]. New oral anticoagulants (NOACs) include factor Xa inhibitors, such as rivaroxaban, apixaban, and edoxaban, which mainly inhibit the factor Xa activity of the prothrombinase complex in the propagation phase, and factor IIa inhibitors such as dabigatran. Although their advantages included a rapid onset and a short half-life, NOACs are still not ready to completely replace conventional anticoagulants [3].

* Correspondence: newxj@hotmail.com
[1]Department of Stomatology, Chinese People's Liberation Army General Hospital, 28 Fuxing Road, Beijing 100853, China
Full list of author information is available at the end of the article

However, with the wide use of oral anticoagulant therapy (OAT), a major disadvantage of OAT that should receive more attention, is the increased risk of hemorrhage during surgical procedures. OATs are frequently prescribed to elder patients, who also have a higher demand for dental extraction caused by caries, periodontitis or other dental diseases. So, the problem of postoperative bleeding becomes a major concern for the dentist. Whether to continue or discontinue OAT has become a strong controversy. If OAT is continued, there is a high risk of bleeding, and if OAT is discontinued, the thromboembolic complications are potentially deadly.

Discontinuing OAT 2 or 3 days before oral surgery has been a widely used strategy for managing patients on warfarin [5, 6]. However,the risk of postoperative bleeding apparently does not decrease, and the thromboembolic risk increases [7]. There have been documented incidences of thromboembolic events when warfarin was stopped prior to a dental procedure or a minor oral surgery [8, 9]. Garcia et al. [10] published the first important prospective study on the risk of thromboembolism with a short-term interruption of OAT by reporting that the incidence of thromboembolism within a 30-day follow-up period was 0.5 %. Though the incidence of thromboembolism is low, the consequence may be deadly. These thromboembolic events can have devastating clinical consequences, such as an embolic stroke, which can result in major disability or death, or myocardial ischaemia, which can increase risk of death two to four fold [11]. To solve this problem, some strategies have been developed in the last few decades. These strategies include reducing the dose of the anticoagulant drugs [12, 13] or bridging it with heparin [14, 15]. These two methods, however, do not completely eliminate the risk of thromboembolic events, such as stroke [9]. Currently, there are a lot of publications suggest that dental extractions may be carried out with no OAT interruption if local hemostasis is adequately maintained in the OAT patients [14, 16–20]. Nevertheless, there is still a lack of public recognition of the treatment guidelines for treating these patients. To address this controversy and to provide evidence-based recommendations, we have completed a meta-analysis. Articles on randomized controlled trials (RCTs) or controlled clinical trials (CCTs), including patients under OAT who undergo dental extractions were collected, and the postoperative bleeding was compared between patients who continued OAT and patients who discontinued OAT.

Methods

The methods for this review were based on the Cochrane Handbook for Systematic Reviews of Interventions. Throughout the whole process, the studies were assessed by 2 observers independently, and any disagreement was resolved by discussion.

Database search

A comprehensive search of the PubMed, EMBASE, Web of Science, Cochrane Library, China Biology Medicine disc (CBM), and China National Knowledge Infrastructure(CNKI) databases was conducted in March 2016. The search strategies for PubMed, EMBASE, Web of Science and Cochrane Library are shown in Table 1.

Study selection

Two reviewers independently evaluated all of the search results, and the inclusion criteria were as follows:

1. Study design—studies were designed as randomized controlled trials (RCTs) or controlled clinical trials (CCTs)
2. Participants—patients were receiving OAT and required dental extractions
3. Comparators—the postoperative bleeding between patients who continue or discontinue OAT.
4. Outcomes—postoperative bleeding (spontaneous bleeding, induced bleeding and minor bleeding)

The exclusion criteria were as follows:

1. In vitro study (laboratory studies or animal studies), case reports or letters.
2. Studies on antiplatelet medications.
3. Study outcomes were not clearly reported or the data could not be used for our meta-analysis.

Data extraction

The following parameters were extracted from each of the selected studies: the first author, country, year of publication, design type, patient characteristics, intervention method, and bleeding outcomes. The information is recorded in the table.

Because there is no accepted standardized definition of bleeding outcomes for patients undergoing surgical procedures, we aimed to use the postoperative bleeding to

Table 1 The key words, database and search result

Database	Key words	Result
Pubmed	(oral anticoagulant therapy OR OAT OR anticoagulant*) AND (dental surgery OR dental extraction* OR tooth extraction*)	879
Embase	(oral anticoagulant therapy OR OAT OR anticoagulant*) AND (dental surgery OR dental extraction* OR tooth extraction*)	634
Cochrane Library	(oral anticoagulant therapy OR OAT OR anticoagulant*) AND (dental surgery OR dental extraction* OR tooth extraction*)	2
Web of Science	(dental surgery OR dental extraction* OR tooth extraction*) AND (oral anticoagulant therapy OR OAT OR anticoagulant*)	664
Total		2179

summarize the bleeding outcome after thoroughly reading the included articles. The bleeding outcomes can be defined as two processes during the follow-up days. One is the patient's own perceived bleeding, such as spontaneous bleeding that continues for more than 20 min [21] and oozing from the extraction site [7]. The other bleeding outcome is examined by doctors during the appointment, and the presence of a solid clot covering the extraction socket was considered as no bleeding, while the presence of a fresh clot that shed easily or oozing blood was considered to be positive bleeding [4].

Risk of bias evaluation

The following seven items were taken into consideration:

(1) allocation concealment, (2) random sequence generation, (3) blinding of participants and personnel, (4) blinding of outcome assessment, (5) incomplete outcome data, (6) selective reporting, and (7) other bias. The risk of bias for each item was judged as low risk, high risk, or unclear risk. The overall risk of bias for each study was evaluated by the following criteria: If the risk of bias was low for all the items, the study was of low risk. If one (or more than one) of the risk factors for bias was high for key items, the study was of high risk. If one (or more than one) of the risk factors for bias was unclear, the study had an unclear risk.

Statistical analysis

The bleeding outcomes of the included studies were combined, and a meta-analysis was performed using RevMan software (version 5.3). Subgroup analyses were performed once the included studies had the same evaluation intervals. The risk of bleeding for continuing or discontinuing OAT was expressed as a relative risk (RR) with an associated 95 % CI. In addition, a chi-square and I^2 test were used to estimate the degree of heterogeneity, with values of 25, 50, and 75 % corresponding to the low, moderate, and high heterogeneity, respectively. Substantial heterogeneity was defined as a P value <0.05 and $I^2 >50$ %. The fixed-effects model was applied when $I^2 <50$ %, and the random-effects model was applied when $I^2 >50$ %.

Results

Literature search

The search process is shown in Fig. 1. There were 968 relevant studies identified during the database search, and after the exclusion of duplication as well as titles, abstracts, and full-text screening, finally, we included six

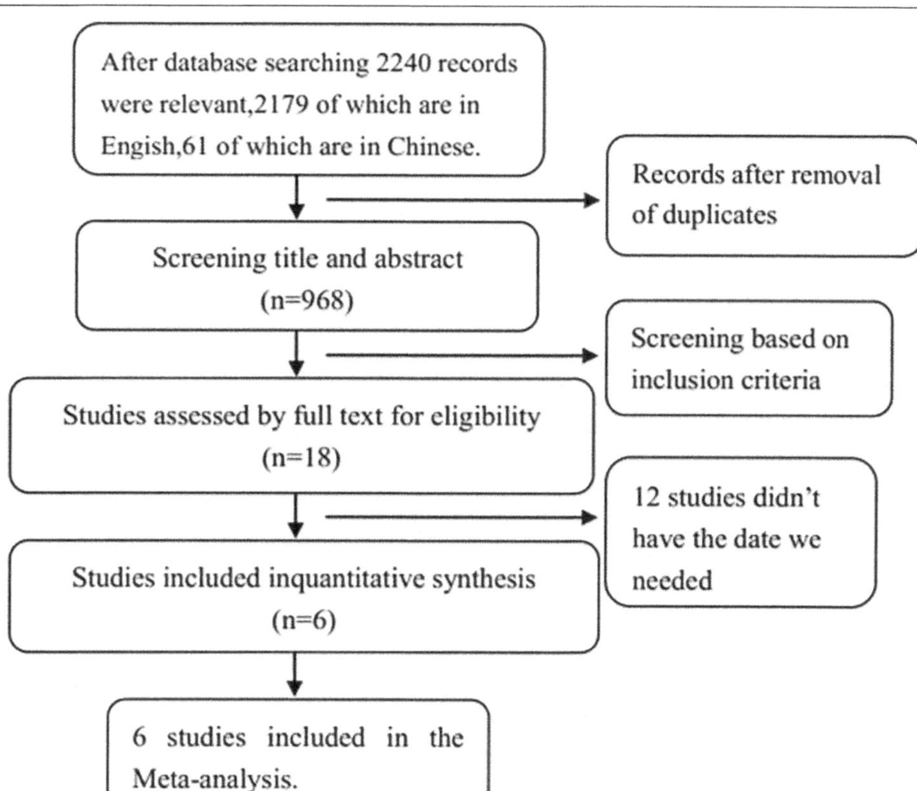

Fig. 1 Study flow diagram

studies [4, 7, 16, 21–23] in our meta-analysis. Five of the studies are in English, and the other one [22] is in Chinese.

Data extraction

The characteristics of the selected six studies are summarized in Tables 2 and 3. The studies were published between 1993 and 2010. Four of the six studies were RCT, and the other two were CCT. The total number of patients under OAT who received dental extractions was 581. The patients were divided into the following two groups: an OAT continued group and an OAT discontinued group. In the OAT continued group, patients did not stop their anticoagulant therapy when they needed dental extractions. In the OAT discontinued group, patients stopped their anticoagulant therapy 2 or 3 days before the dental extraction procedure and usually resumed the therapy on the same day. Four of the studies used warfarin as the anticoagulant drug, one used a vitamin K inhibitor and one had not report the anticoagulant. The details of the bleeding outcomes are shown in Table 3. The follow-up ranged from 1 to 7 days. The bleeding outcomes during patients' review visits were recorded if the article mentioned.

Risk of bias evaluation

The risk of bias summary is shown in Fig. 2. Of the six included studies, one [21] was judged to have a low risk of bias because all of the items had a low risk of bias. Five [4, 7, 16, 22, 23] of the studies were judged to have a high risk of bias because all of the studies failed to blind participants and personnel, and three [4, 22, 23] studies failed to describe the method of randomization and had no report of the allocation concealment.

Meta-analysis

According to the postoperative bleeding outcomes, we performed a meta-analysis to compare the bleeding risk of the OAT continued and OAT discontinued groups. Six studies were included, with 314 subjects in the treated group and 277 in the control group.

The incidence of postoperative bleeding was 10.8 % (34/314) in the OAT continued group and 8.30 % (23/277) in the OAT discontinued group. A fixed-effects model was applied because of the low heterogeneity across the studies. There was no significant difference in bleeding risk between the OAT continued group and OAT discontinued group ($P = 0.29$). The risk ratio was 1.31 and 95 % CI (0.79, 2.14) (Fig. 3).

Subgroup analyses were performed when three or more studies recorded the bleeding incidence using the same evaluation intervals. Two time points (1 and 7 days after the operation) fit the criteria. Three studies [7, 21, 22], with 115 subjects in the treated group and 96 in the control group were included in the 1 day subgroup. The bleeding occurred in 8 of 115 (6.9 %) patients in the treated group and in 7 of 96 (7.2 %) in the control group. A fixed-effects model was applied, and there was no significant difference between the two groups ($P = 0.85$). The risk ratio was 0.91 and 95 % CI (0.35, 2.37) (Fig. 4).

Four studies [4, 16, 21, 23], with 214 subjects in the treated group and 196 in the control group were included in the 7 day subgroup. The bleeding occurred in 27 of 214 (12.6 %) patients in the treated group and in 17 of 196 (8.7 %) in the control group. A fixed-effects model was applied and there was no significant difference between the two groups (P = 0.19). The risk ratio was 1.47 and 95 % CI (0.83, 2.59) (Fig. 5).

Discussion

Numerous studies have reported that OAT reduces the risks of thromboembolism significantly [24, 25]. Other studies have documented that serious embolic complications, including death, are three times more likely to occur in patients whose anticoagulant therapy was interrupted, compared to patients with bleeding complications associated with anticoagulation [26]. For oral surgery procedures, no case of lethal postoperative bleeding in patients who continued OAT has been reported [16, 26], whereas several fatal thromboembolic events after stopping OAT for dental extractions have

Table 2 Characteristics of included studies

Study	Country	No.(T/C)[a]	Design	Anticoagulants	Average age (mean ± SD or mean (range))
Borea (1993) [21]	Italy	30(15/15)	RCT	NR[b]	T: 62.7 ± 6.1 C: 61.1 ± 10
Gaspar (1997) [23]	Israel	47(32/15)	CCT	Vitamin K inhibitor	T: 61.1(34–85) C: 53.4(35–72)
Devani (1998) [7]	UK	65(33/32)	CCT	Warfarin	T: 62.3(30–82) C: 61.3(32–81)
Evans (2002) [16]	UK	109(57/52)	RCT	Warfarin	T: 67(36–92) C: 66 (30–93)
Al-Mubarak (2007) [4]	Saudi Arabia	214(110/114)	RCT	Warfarin	T: 51.7 ± 14.7 53.1 ± 13.7
					C: 52.3 ± 14.3 48.7 ± 13.1
Duan XQ (2010) [22]	China	116(67/49)	RCT	warfarin	T: 59.5 ± 12.6 C: 61.5 ± 11.3

[a] *T* treatment group, continue oral anticoagulant therapy group, *C* control group, discontinue oral anticoagulant therapy group
[b] *NR* not report

Table 3 Characteristics of included studies

Study	Group	INR (mean/range)	Intervention method	Number of extraction	Follow up	Bleeding outcomes
Borea (1993) [21]	T: continued OAT. C: discontinued OAT.	T: 3–4.5 C: 1.5–2.5	T: Sutures and TA irrigation at surgery and MS for 7 day. C: Sutures and physiologic irrigation at surgery and MS for 7 days.	Single dental	7 days	Day 1: Spontaneous bleedings T: 1/15 C:2/15 Induced bleedings T:1/15 C:0/15 Day 2 to day 7: none
Evans (2002) [16]	T: continued OAT. C: discontinued OAT 2 days before extractions and resumed on the same day.	T: 2.5(1.2–4.7) C: 1.6(1.2–2.3)	All groups: Oxycellulose dressing and sutures for all patients.	T: 2(1–7) C: 3(1–9)	7 days	Postoperative bleeding T:15/57 C:7/52
Devani (1998) [7]	T: continued OAT. C: discontinued OAT 2 days before extractions.	T: 2.7(2.2–3.9) C: 1.6(1.2–2.1)	All groups: Placing haemostatic pack and sutures.	T: 2.1(1–9) C: 2(1–9)	5 days	Minor bleeding: Day 1 T:0/33 C:0/32 Day 2 T:0/33 C:1/32 Day 3 T:1/33 C:0/32 Day 4 to day 5:none
Gaspar (1997) [23]	T: continued OAT C: discontinued OAT 3 days before and resumed the same day	T: 2.5(1.9–3.5) C: 1.4(1.3–1.9)	All groups: Sutures and TA irrigation at surgery and MS for 2 min.MS for 7 days postoperativedays	NR	7 days	Postoperative bleeding T:2/32 C:1/15
Al-Mubarak (2007) [4]	T: continued OAT (group2 no sutures,group4 sutures). C: discontinued OAT 2 days before and resumed 12 h after dental extractions (group1 no sutures, group 3 sutures).	T: 1.85(1.4–2.3) C:2.55(1.9–3.1)	Local pressure (all) and sutures (group 3 and 4).	All patients range 1–5, single extraction (63.3) two teeth (25 %), three teeth (7.5 %) four teeth (3.3 %) and five teeth (0.8 %).	7 days	Postoperative bleeding T:8/110 C:7/114
Duan XQ (2010) [22]	T: continued OAT. C: discontinued OAT 3 days before and resumed the next day.	ALL: 1.80–2.67	All groups: Local pressure and sutures.	T:1.5(1–5) C:1.3(1–5)	1 day	Postoperative bleeding T:6/67 C:5/49

OAT oral anticoagulant therapy, *T* treatment group, *C* control group, *INR* international normalized ratio, *MW* mouthwash, *TA* tranexamic acid, *NR* not report

occurred [8, 27]. Nevertheless, there is still a lack of consensus regarding preoperative alteration of the anticoagulant regimen to prepare OAT patients for dental extractions.

Summary of results

The results of our meta-analysis revealed that patients continuing oral anticoagulant therapy do not have an increased risk of bleeding after dental extraction compared to patients who discontinue oral anticoagulant therapy. However, the follow-up dates were not the same between these studies. One of the studies [22] only reported the first day bleeding outcome, and one study [7] followed-up for 5 days with a detailed record of everyday situations. The other four studies [4, 16, 21, 23] followed up for 7 days after the dental extraction, but three studies only mentioned the total number of bleeding events and the remaining one recorded everyday situations. Subgroup analyses were performed since three of the included studies [7, 21, 22] recorded the bleeding outcome 1 day after surgery, and four included studies [4, 16, 21, 23] collected measurements for 7 days after the surgery. The results were consistent with the previous results. There was no significant difference in bleeding risk between the OAT continued group and the OAT discontinued group 1 and 7 days after the surgery. Of all the studies, none of these patients suffered serious bleeding, and the bleeding was easily controlled by patients at home or controlled with local measures during their visit to the hospital. No thromboembolic event was reported in these studies, whether OAT was continued or not. However, this outcome could be a result of the short follow-up period of these studies (from 1 to 7 days), which made it difficult assess the thromboembolism risk in patients who discontinued OAT.

All of the 6 included studies came to the conclusion that OAT patients who do not discontinue the anticoagulant medication do not have a significantly higher risk of postoperative bleeding than OAT patients who stop the therapy. Some of the studies mentioned the importance of international normalized ratio (INR) and hemostatic procedures. INR has been used as a

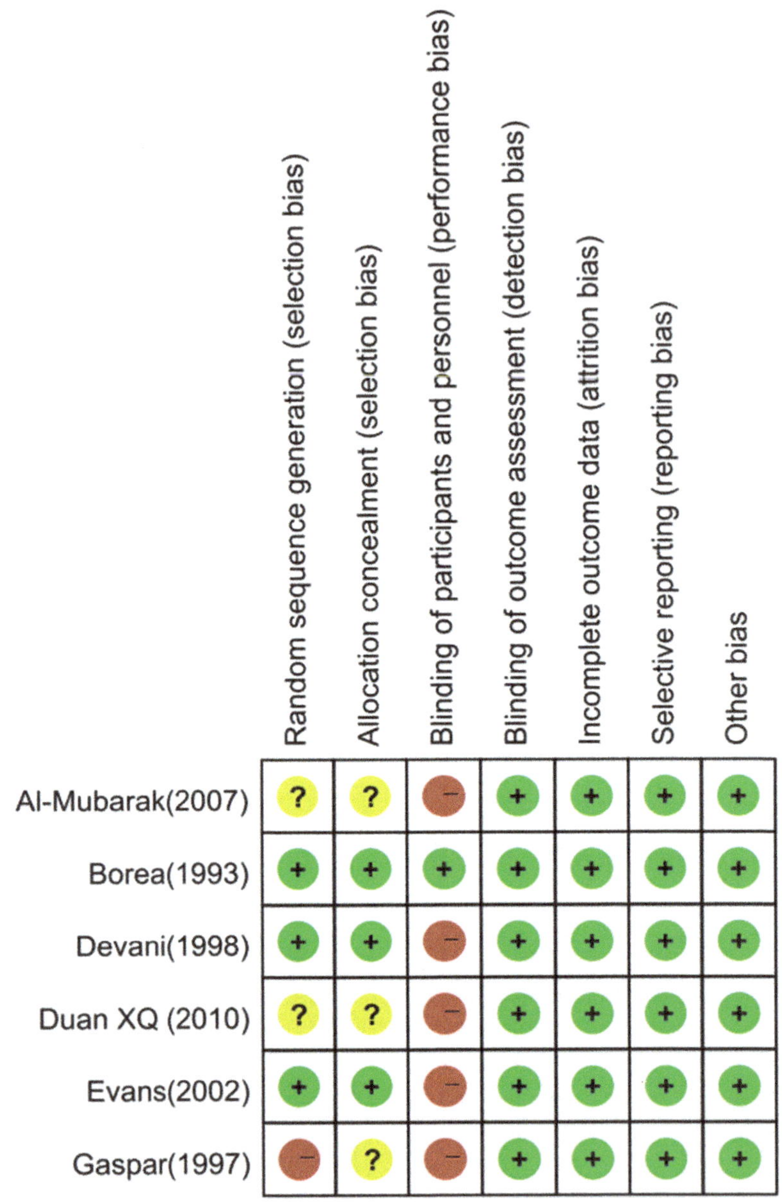

Fig. 2 Risk of bias of the studies. Summary of risk of bias for included studies. Green indicates a low risk of bias, yellow indicates an unclear risk of bias, and red indicates a high risk of bias

	continued OAT		discontinued OAT			Risk Ratio
Study or Subgroup	Events	Total	Events	Total	Weight	M-H, Fixed, 95% CI
Al-Mubarak(2007)	8	110	7	114	28.2%	1.18 [0.44, 3.16]
Borea(1993)	2	15	2	15	8.2%	1.00 [0.16, 6.20]
Devani(1998)	1	33	1	32	4.2%	0.97 [0.06, 14.85]
Duan XQ (2010)	6	67	5	49	23.7%	0.88 [0.28, 2.71]
Evans(2002)	15	57	7	52	30.1%	1.95 [0.87, 4.41]
Gaspar(1997)	2	32	1	15	5.6%	0.94 [0.09, 9.55]
Total (95% CI)		**314**		**277**	**100.0%**	**1.31 [0.79, 2.14]**
Total events	34		23			

Heterogeneity: $Chi^2 = 1.66$, df = 5 (P = 0.89); $I^2 = 0\%$
Test for overall effect: Z = 1.05 (P = 0.29)

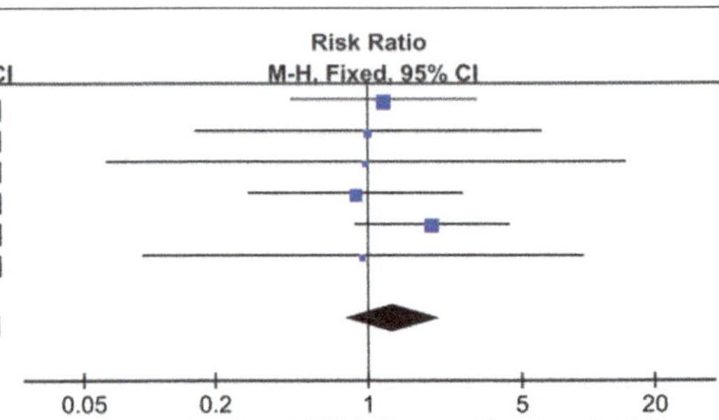

Fig. 3 Forest plot of the difference of postoperative bleeding between OAT continued or discontinued group

Study or Subgroup	continued OAT Events	continued OAT Total	discontinued OAT Events	discontinued OAT Total	Weight	Risk Ratio M-H, Fixed, 95% CI
Borea(1993)	2	15	2	15	25.7%	1.00 [0.16, 6.20]
Devani(1998)	0	33	0	32		Not estimable
Duan XQ (2010)	6	67	5	49	74.3%	0.88 [0.28, 2.71]
Total (95% CI)		**115**		**96**	**100.0%**	**0.91 [0.35, 2.37]**
Total events	8		7			

Heterogeneity: Chi² = 0.01, df = 1 (P = 0.91); I² = 0%
Test for overall effect: Z = 0.19 (P = 0.85)

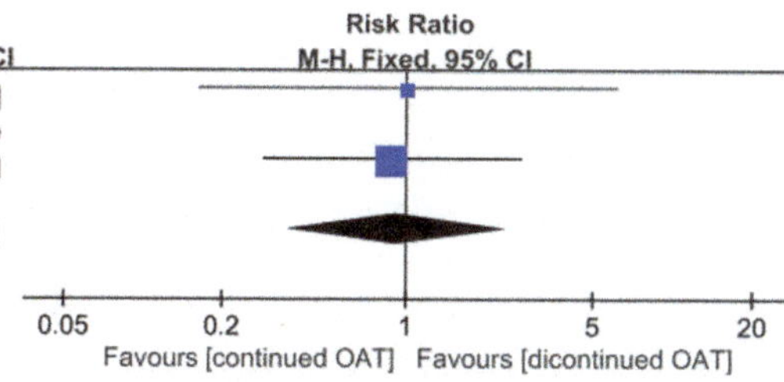

Fig. 4 Forest plot of the difference of postoperative bleeding between OAT continued or discontinued group 1 day after the surgery

recommendation for monitoring patients' oral anticoagulant therapy. For stroke prevention in atrial fibrillation patients, oral anticoagulation therapy that is dose adjusted to maintain an INR range of 2.0 to 3.0 is associated with a 64 % reduction in the risk of stroke compared to placebo [28]. And in patients suffering an acute venous thromboembolism (either deep vein thrombosis or pulmonary embolism), adjusted-dose OAT use significantly reduces the risk of recurrence of thrombotic events with a target INR range of 2.0–3.0. [29]. According to meta-analyses of atrial fibrillation or mixed populations assessing INR control and associated events [30], more than half of all thromboembolic events occurred when patients have an INR <2.0. Besides, the INR has a safe range before surgical procedures. This "safe range" is controversial because some experts recommended an INR of ≤3 [17, 31], whereas others suggest an INR of ≤4 [32, 33] as safe for dental extractions. An INR above 5 has been shown to be an unacceptable risk for postoperative bleeding [34]. However, none of the included patients had an INR of more than 5. Most of the patients had an INR no higher than 4, as shown in Table 3. Next to monitoring the INR, it is recommended to take a special care of patients with renal dysfunction. Given the renal excretion of drugs, renal dysfunction may result in a higher incidence of bleeding associated with oral anticoagulation [35, 36]. A variety of local hemostatic measures are used in oral surgeries, including sutures, local compression, adjuvants (such as fibrin and histoacryl glue), local antifibrinolytic solutions, collagen fleeces, acrylic splints, gelatin sponges and so on [37, 38]. Placing hemostatic, physiological or tranexamic acid irrigation and mouthwash were used in our included studies. However, one of the included studies [4] showed that suturing played no significant role in bleeding status. In their study, patients with sutures showed a higher incidence of bleeding than patients without sutures. This outcome might be caused by the mode of suturing that further traumatizes the soft tissue. Four of the included studies [7, 16, 21, 23] used local hemostatic measures, except for local compression and sutures. The effectiveness of these measures was worth studying.

Limitations

There were some limitations in the included studies. Only one of the six included studies was judged to have a low risk of bias, and the absence of randomization may predispose the analysis to a risk of selection bias and possible confounding effects [39]. Some studies were carried out with limited patient numbers [21, 23] and, as with all meta-analyses, there may be studies published in other languages or unpublished studies that we were not able to access. Additionally, the INR differed between different studies which influenced the bleeding outcomes. Patients with a low INR were less likely to suffer bleeding than patients with a higher INR. Other factors, such as gingival health, numbers and the complexity of the tooth extractions, the surgical skills, anesthesia type, material and suture technique, local hemostatic measures, and the use of anticoagulants differed from one study to another or were not reported. This heterogeneity limited the scientific evidence that could be obtained for this review.

Study or Subgroup	continued OAT Events	continued OAT Total	discontinued OAT Events	discontinued OAT Total	Weight	Risk Ratio M-H, Fixed, 95% CI
Al-Mubarak(2007)	8	110	7	114	39.2%	1.18 [0.44, 3.16]
Borea(1993)	2	15	2	15	11.4%	1.00 [0.16, 6.20]
Evans(2002)	15	57	7	52	41.7%	1.95 [0.87, 4.41]
Gaspar(1997)	2	32	1	15	7.8%	0.94 [0.09, 9.55]
Total (95% CI)		**214**		**196**	**100.0%**	**1.47 [0.83, 2.59]**
Total events	27		17			

Heterogeneity: Chi² = 0.97, df = 3 (P = 0.81); I² = 0%
Test for overall effect: Z = 1.32 (P = 0.19)

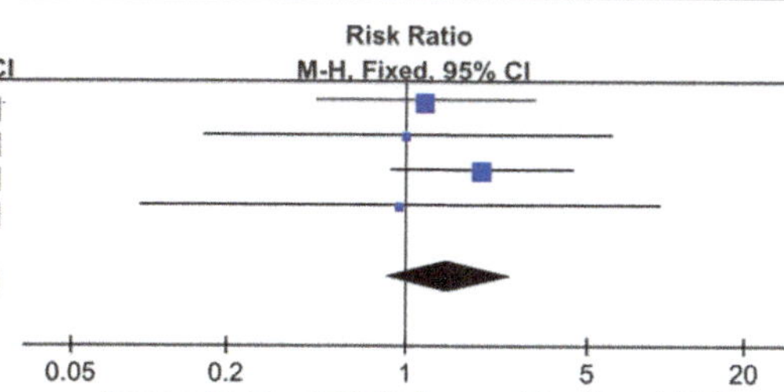

Fig. 5 Forest plot of the difference of postoperative bleeding between OAT continued or discontinued group 7 days after the surgery

Conclusion

Under current studies and evidence, the results of our meta-analysis revealed that patients continuing oral anticoagulant therapy do not increase the risk of bleeding after dental extractions compared to patients who discontinue oral anticoagulant therapy. However, with the limited number of included studies and the risk of bias, well-designed RCTs should be included with a larger sample size as well as specific inclusion and exclusion criteria. Moreover, it would be better if the bleeding outcomes had a reporting standard. This standardization would enhance the comparability of studies based on identical outcome measurements, which would help to establish guidelines for dentists who treat these patients with complex medical needs.

Acknowledgements

This work was supported by a grant from the National Natural Science Foundation of China emergency management project (No. 81541111) and Clinical scientific research fund (No.320.6750.15029) from Wu Jieping Medical Foundation.

Authors' contributions

YS carried out the literature research and drafted the manuscript. YS, SQ, LJL and LJR gathered the information and performed the statistical analysis. XJ is the Corresponding author and she designed this meta-analysis, and helped to draft the manuscript. All authors read and approved the final manuscript.

Competing interests

The authors declare that they have no competing interests.

Consent for publication

Not applicable.

Ethics approval and consent to participate

Not applicable.

Author details

[1]Department of Stomatology, Chinese People's Liberation Army General Hospital, 28 Fuxing Road, Beijing 100853, China. [2]Department of Stomatology, Chinese People's Liberation Army 322 Hospital, 2 Yunzhong Road, Datong 037000, China.

References

1. Mok CK, Boey J, Wang R, Chan TK, Cheung KL, Lee PK, Chow J, Ng RP, Tse TF. Warfarin versus dipyridamole-aspirin and pentoxifylline-aspirin for the prevention of prosthetic heart valve thromboembolism: a prospective randomized clinical trial. Circulation. 1985;72:1059–63.
2. Stein PD, Collins JJ, Kantrowitz A. Antithrombotic therapy in mechanical and biological prosthetic heart valves and saphenous vein bypass grafts. Chest. 1986;89:46S–53.
3. CADTH Therapeutic Reviews. Recommendations for antithrombotic agents for the prevention of stroke and systemic embolism in patients with atrial fibrillation. Ottawa: Canadian Agency for Drugs and Technologies in Health; 2013.
4. Al-Mubarak S, Al-Ali N, Abou-Rass M, Al-Sohail A, Robert A, Al-Zoman K, Al-Suwyed A, Ciancio S. Evaluation of dental extractions, suturing and INR on postoperative bleeding of patients maintained on oral anticoagulant therapy. Br Dent J. 2007;203:E15. 410-411.
5. Mulligan R, Weitzel KG. Pretreatment management of the patient receiving anticoagulant drugs. J Am Dent Assoc. 1988;117:479–83.
6. Wahl MJ. Demystifying medical complexities. J Calif Dent Assoc. 2000;28:510–8.
7. Devani P, Lavery KM, Howell CJ. Dental extractions in patients on warfarin: is alteration of anticoagulant regime necessary? Br J Oral Maxillofac Surg. 1998;36:107–11.
8. Wahl MJ. Dental surgery in anticoagulated patients. Arch Intern Med. 1998; 158:1610–6.
9. Dunn AS, Turpie AG. Perioperative management of patients receiving oral anticoagulants: a systematic review. Arch Intern Med. 2003;163:901–8.
10. Garcia DA, Regan S, Henault LE, Upadhyay A, Baker J, Othman M, Hylek EM. Risk of thromboembolism with short-term interruption of warfarin therapy. Arch Intern Med. 2008;168:63–9.
11. Kaplan RC, Tirschwell DL, Longstreth WJ, Manolio TA, Heckbert SR, Lefkowitz D, El-Saed A, Psaty BM. Vascular events, mortality, and preventive therapy following ischemic stroke in the elderly. Neurology. 2005;65(6):835–42.
12. Johnson WT, Leary JM. Management of dental patients with bleeding disorders: review and update. Oral Surg Oral Med Oral Pathol. 1988;66:297–303.
13. DeClerck D, Vinckier F, Vermylen J. Influence of anticoagulation on blood loss following dental extractions. J Dent Res. 1992;71:387–90.
14. Souto JC, Oliver A, Zuazu-Jausoro I, Vives A, Fontcuberta J. Oral surgery in anticoagulated patients without reducing the dose of oral anticoagulant: a prospective randomized study. J Oral Maxillofac Surg. 1996;54:27–32. 323.
15. Johnson-Leong C, Rada RE. The use of low-molecular-weight heparins in outpatient oral surgery for patients receiving anticoagulation therapy. J Am Dent Assoc. 2002;133:1083–7.
16 Evans IL, Sayers MS, Gibbons AJ, Price G, Snooks H, Sugar AW. Can warfarin be continued during dental extraction? Results of a randomized controlled trial. Br J Oral Maxillofac Surg. 2002;40:248–52.
17 Blinder D, Manor Y, Martinowitz U, Taicher S, Hashomer T. Dental extractions in patients maintained on continued oral anticoagulant: comparison of local hemostatic modalities. Oral Surg Oral Med Oral Pathol Oral Radiol Endod. 1999;88:137–40.
18 Blinder D, Manor Y, Martinowitz U, Taicher S. Dental extractions in patients maintained on oral anticoagulant therapy: comparison of INR value with occurrence of postoperative bleeding. Int J Oral Maxillofac Surg. 2001;30:518–21.
19 Al-Belasy FA, Amer MZ. Hemostatic effect of n-butyl-2-cyanoacrylate (histoacryl) glue in warfarin-treated patients undergoing oral surgery. J Oral Maxillofac Surg. 2003;61:1405–9.
20 Carter G, Goss A, Lloyd J, Tocchetti R. Tranexamic acid mouthwash versus autologous fibrin glue in patients taking warfarin undergoing dental extractions: a randomized prospective clinical study. J Oral Maxillofac Surg. 2003;61:1432–5.
21 Borea G, Montebugnoli L, Capuzzi P, Magelli C. Tranexamic acid as a mouthwash in anticoagulant-treated patients undergoing oral surgery. An alternative method to discontinuing anticoagulant therapy. Oral Surg Oral Med Oral Pathol. 1993;75:29–31.
22 Duan XQ, Lv YL, Zuo J, Gong LN, Wang J, Meng X. Clinical studies in patients with artificial heart valve replacement surgery tooth extraction. Beijing J Stomatol. 2010;18:332–4.
23 Gaspar R, Brenner B, Ardekian L, Peled M, Laufer D. Use of tranexamic acid mouthwash to prevent postoperative bleeding in oral surgery patients on oral anticoagulant medication. Quintessence Int. 1997;28:375–9.
24 Doraiswamy VA, Slepian MJ, Gesheff MG, Tantry US, Gurbel PA. Potential role of oral anticoagulants in the treatment of patients with coronary artery disease: focus on dabigatran. Expert Rev Cardiovasc Ther. 2013;11:1259–67.
25 Agnelli G, Becattini C. Risk assessment for recurrence and optimal agents for extended treatment of venous thromboembolism. Hematology Am Soc Hematol Educ Program. 2013;2013:471–7.
26 Wahl MJ. Myths of dental surgery in patients receiving anticoagulant therapy. J Am Dent Assoc. 2000;131:77–81.
27 Yasaka M, Naritomi H, Minematsu K. Ischemic stroke associated with brief cessation of warfarin. Thromb Res. 2006;118:290–3.
28 Hart RG, Pearce LA, Aguilar MI. Meta-analysis: antithrombotic therapy to prevent stroke in patients who have nonvalvular atrial fibrillation. Ann Intern Med. 2007;146(12):857–67.
29 Kearon C, Akl EA, Ornelas J, Blaivas A, Jimenez D, Bounameaux H, Huisman M, King CS, Morris TA, Sood N, et al. Antithrombotic Therapy for VTE Disease: CHEST Guideline and Expert Panel Report. Chest. 2016;149(2):315–52.

30 Erkens PM, Ten CH, Buller HR, Prins MH. Benchmark for time in therapeutic range in venous thromboembolism: a systematic review and meta-analysis. Plos One. 2012;7(9):e42269.
31 Campbell JH, Alvarado F, Murray RA. Anticoagulation and minor oral surgery: should the anticoagulation regimen be altered? J Oral Maxillofac Surg. 2000;58:131–5. 135-136.
32 Cieslik-Bielewska A, Pelc R, Cieslik T. Oral surgery procedures in patients on anticoagulants. Preliminary report. Kardiol Pol. 2005;63:137–40. 141.
33 Lippert S, Gutschik E. Views of cardiac-valve prosthesis patients and their dentists on anticoagulation therapy. Scand J Dent Res. 1994;102(3):168–71.
34 Beirne OR, Koehler JR. Surgical management of patients on warfarin sodium. J Oral Maxillofac Surg. 1996;54:1115–8.
35 Piccini JP, Stevens SR, Chang Y, Singer DE, Lokhnygina Y, Go AS, Patel MR, Mahaffey KW, Halperin JL, Breithardt G, et al. Renal dysfunction as a predictor of stroke and systemic embolism in patients with nonvalvular atrial fibrillation: validation of the R(2)CHADS(2) index in the ROCKET AF (Rivaroxaban Once-daily, oral, direct factor Xa inhibition Compared with vitamin K antagonism for prevention of stroke and Embolism Trial in Atrial Fibrillation) and ATRIA (AnTicoagulation and Risk factors In Atrial fibrillation) study cohorts. Circulation. 2013;127(2):224–32.
36 Hart RG, Eikelboom JW, Ingram AJ, Herzog CA. Anticoagulants in atrial fibrillation patients with chronic kidney disease. Nat Rev Nephrol. 2012;8(10):569–78.
37 Rakocz M, Mazar A, Varon D, Spierer S, Blinder D, Martinowitz U. Dental extractions in patients with bleeding disorders. The use of fibrin glue. Oral Surg Oral Med Oral Pathol. 1993;75:280–2.
38 Bajkin BV, Popovic SL, Selakovic SD. Randomized, prospective trial comparing bridging therapy using low-molecular-weight heparin with maintenance of oral anticoagulation during extraction of teeth. J Oral Maxillofac Surg. 2009;67:990–5.
39 Fleming PS, Lynch CD, Pandis N. Randomized controlled trials in dentistry: common pitfalls and how to avoid them. J Dent. 2014;42:908–14.

7

An *in vitro* screening assay for dental stain cleaning

Changxiang Wang[1*], Robert Lucas[2], Anthony J. Smith[1] and Paul R. Cooper[1]

Abstract

Background: The present study aimed to develop an *in vitro* model for stain removal from natural enamel for the assessment and comparison of oral hygiene products.

Methods: Bovine teeth ($n = 8$ per group) were ground/polished to provide flat enamel specimens and ferric-tannate deposits were precipitated onto the enamel surfaces. The ferric-tannate stained enamel specimens were brushed using an *in vitro* tooth-brushing simulator with slurries containing commercially available toothpaste products, dental abrasive particles, and sodium tripolyphosphate (STP) solutions of different concentrations. The colour of the enamel surfaces was measured using a spectrophotometer before and after stain application as well as after the brushing treatments.

Results: Differences in stain removal efficacy were found between the toothpastes categorised as whitening and non-whitening comprising of different types of dental abrasives (hydrated silica and alumina). A mean value of 27% for stain removal was detected for the three non-whitening toothpastes and 59% of stain removal was detected for the three whitening toothpastes after 1000 strokes. Compared with the slurry with Zeodent 113 abrasive alone, the addition of STP provided better performance for stain removal under the same brushing conditions (mean value of 62% for Zeodent 113 abrasive alone and 72% with the addition of 5% (w/w) STP after 1000 strokes). No difference was evident between the STP concentration of 5% (w/w) and 10% (w/w).

Conclusions: The ferric-tannate/bovine enamel model reported here provides good stain retention, is rapidly and easily prepared, and is shown to be progressively and reproducibly sensitive to toothbrushing using different toothpastes and surfactant/chelating agent solutions. Importantly, it provides good discrimination between various oral hygiene products.
The stain removal assay reported here has considerable potential to enable comparative assessments of different toothpaste types in terms of their cleaning capabilities.

Keywords: Enamel, Stain removal efficacy, Tooth whitening, Aesthetics, Toothpaste, Tooth colour, Surface roughness

Background

The natural colour of permanent teeth is largely determined by dentine and modified by the thickness and translucency of the overlying enamel [1]. The appearance of the teeth, particularly whiteness, is aesthetically important to individuals and tooth discolouration is a common dental patient complaint. Personal dissatisfaction with the appearance of the dentition has been reported to range from 17.9 to 52.6% [2–6] and the causes of tooth discolouration are multifactorial and are classified as extrinsic, intrinsic and internalised discolouration [7]. Intrinsic and internalised discolouration arise generally during tooth development or during disease and the more extensive localisation deep within the dental tissues constrains its reversal. Extrinsic staining of the tooth can arise from a variety of sources, such as smoking, red wine consumption, and the intake of cationic compounds, such as chlorhexidine or stannous salts [7–10]. Stain removal can be challenging as staining compounds can be bound to dental plaque and the acquired pellicle, as well as directly to the enamel surface [11]. Thus, oral hygiene strategies need to address both the removal of dental plaque and the extrinsic stain bound in these different ways.

* Correspondence: c.wang@bham.ac.uk
[1]Oral Biology, School of Dentistry, University of Birmingham, 5 Mill Pool Way, Edgbaston, Birmingham B5 7EG, UK
Full list of author information is available at the end of the article

While a variety of stain removal and tooth whitening procedures are used professionally in the clinic [12–15], they are relatively costly and labour intensive [16]. Furthermore, there is considerable demand for 'over-the-counter' (OTC) tooth-whitening products that can be integrated into a normal oral hygiene regime, and whitening toothpastes are commonly used for this [17]. In general, tooth-whitening toothpastes function by abrasive removal of extrinsic stain associated with the dental plaque, the acquired pellicle and the enamel surface together with the chemical cleaning action of constituents, such as sodium tripolyphosphate (STP), sodium pyrophosphate, sodium hexametaphosphate, hydrogen peroxide, as well as by the activity of the enzymes papain and bromelain [4].

Although randomised controlled trials (RCTs) can provide a high degree of evidence for cleaning efficacy, development of a robust laboratory model to evaluate the mechanisms of action and screen efficacy of whitening products or bleaching agents would be of significant benefit [18]. *In vitro* models allow rapid screening of a range of potential products; the most effective can subsequently be clinically assessed in RCTs. Various approaches have been used to investigate extrinsic stain removal by oral care products using a wide range of substrates such as polymethylmethacrylate, hydroxyapatite and enamel (human or bovine). Model stains, including tea, coffee, gastric mucin, soy broth, bacteria, chlorhexidine, saliva, tea with orange II Rhodamine, blood, cola, wine, tobacco and ferric-tannate, have all been used [19–24]. One of the most commonly applied *in vitro* approaches uses cut, polished and acid etched bovine enamel specimens stained with a solution containing a combination of coffee/tea/gastric mucin/Sarcina lutea turtox [19]. The stained specimens are then repeatedly brushed for a period of time using an automated approach with toothpaste slurries. Furthermore, a recent model has utilised a ferric-tannate coating deposited onto highly polished sintered hydroxyapatite discs and was reported to mimic the daily control of pellicle growth, maturation and staining [24].

A significant limitation of current protocols is the weak bonding between the stain and substrate constraining discrimination between different cleaning products and regimes. A further issue is the need for a staining time of several days necessary to achieve sufficient stain build-up for high-throughput analysis and discrimination of cleaning regimes. There is also a need to better model stain interactions with natural enamel to provide good clinical relevance. Subsequently, the aim of this study was to establish a relatively rapid and reproducible staining protocol with appropriate bonding to enamel, which would allow high-throughput assessment of the cleaning ability, and discrimination between oral care products, following brushing.

Methods

Specimen preparation

Previously, a model has been reported to simulate up-to-24 h pellicle formation generated by precipitating an iron (III) complex with tannic acid from aqueous solution directly onto polished hydroxyapatite discs [24]. In the present study, this model was modified to investigate the use of natural enamel specimens and to study the influence of specimen surface finish, which can influence stain retention.

Bovine teeth were collected and stored in 0.1% (w/w) thymol (Sigma-Aldrich, UK) solution at 4 °C prior to use. Bovine enamel specimens (approximate 18 mm × 12 mm) were prepared from tooth crowns by dissection using a diamond-edged saw and embedded in blocks of epoxy resin (Ø25 mm) (Buehler, UK). To investigate the effects of surface roughness on the retention and removal of the stain, eight bovine enamel specimens per treatment group were prepared to either: **a)** 600-grit SiC and 3 μm diamond finish (Polished surface group), **b)** 400-grit SiC ground finish (Partially roughened surface group), or **c)** 280-grit SiC ground finish (Roughened surface group) with 5 min ultrasonication in water following each treatment for removal of any residual grinding/polishing materials. A Phoenix Beta Grinder/Polisher (Buehler, UK) was used with SiC abrasive discs (Buehler, UK) for sample preparation. Samples were then surface profiled using a Talysurf Series 2 inductive gauge profilometer (Taylor-Hobson, UK), which has a 1 mm range in the z-axis and a resolution of 16 nm. The inductive gauge profilometer uses a conical probe with 2 μm diamond tip to accurately measure surfaces at the sub-micron level. Linear line profiles (2D) were measured on the surfaces at a measurement speed of 0.5 mm/s and with points spacing of 0.25 μm, and the arithmetic mean surface roughness (Ra) values were calculated (μltra version 5.1.14, Taylor-Hobson, UK) prior to staining.

Tooth stain development

Freshly combined solutions (0.1% (w/w) of diammonium iron (II) sulphate 6-hydrate (Sigma-Aldrich) and 0.1% (w/w) tannic acid (ACS reagent, Sigma-Aldrich) are initially colourless, but form a dark colloidal iron (III) tannic acid complex ("ferric-tannate") on contact with air, which resembles a dietary tannin staining. The fresh mixture was applied as successive layers on the enamel specimens, with each layer being dried at 40 °C in an oven (D-63450 Hanau, Heraeus Instrument (now Kendro Laboratory Products Ltd), Germany) for 10 mins before application of the subsequent layer. For the first layer, a 40 μl aliquot of the solution was pipetted onto each specimen and allowed to spread evenly over the specimen surface before drying. For the subsequent layers (up to a maximum of 9), 10 μl aliquots of the solutions were applied before drying. A total of 1, 3, 5, 7 and 10 cycles of successive stain deposition layering were investigated to study *in vitro* stain removal efficacy. To mimic the presence of an acquired pellicle layer, one of four different acidic polymers of Carbopol (Lubrizol Advanced Materials, Inc., USA), Carrageenan (Cargill, Incorporated, USA), Gantrez (Ashland, USA) and Xanthan (Cargill, Incorporated, USA) was incorporated and applied to assess stain accumulation and removal. Polymers were incorporated by either: **a)** applying a 40 μl aliquot of 0.1% (w/w) solution of the polymer followed by application of the ferric-tannate stain, or **b)** by reducing the amount of tannic acid in the stain by 50% and replacing it with an equivalent amount of one of the four acidic polymers as described above for the application of the stain.

Stain removal

The stained enamel specimens were mounted in two brushing channels of an *in vitro* brushing simulator, as previously reported [25]. Oral B P35 medium toothbrushes were used for the brushing. Specimens were double brushed at a brushing speed of 120 rpm and a temperature of 20 °C was maintained throughout the entire brushing procedure. 150 g toothpaste/abrasive slurry was used in each channel and a brushing load of 150 g was applied. Specimens were double brushed sequentially for up to 5000 strokes. After brushing for the requisite number of strokes, specimens were thoroughly rinsed with water prior to colour evaluation (as described below). The abrasive slurries examined in the present study included **a)** a range of toothpaste slurries (see Table 1 for a list of products used) prepared with 25 g toothpaste in 40 ml water, **b)** 15% (w/w) of Zeodent 113 (Huber Corporation, USA) silica abrasive in 0.5% (w/w) Hercules 7 MF Carboxymethyl Cellulose (CMC) (Hercules Incorporated, USA) containing 10% (w/w) Glycerol (VWR International BVBA, Belgium), with or without the addition of 5% (w/w) and 10% (w/w) sodium tripolyphosphate (STP) (Sigma-Aldrich), **c)** 10% (w/w) aqueous STP, and **d)** water as a control. Zeodent 113 is a precipitated silica, which has commonly been employed as a toothpaste abrasive [25], with a 15 μm mean particle size (Mastersizer 2000, Malvern Instruments Ltd, United Kingdom).

The cleaning ability of eight dentifrices to remove stain pellicle was determined in parallel by a laboratory testing method (PCR) commonly used within the oral hygiene industry [19]. The results were compared with the stain removal of the same dentifrices using the current stain removal methodology.

Images of the enamel surfaces before staining and post-stain removal with 5000 brush strokes were also captured by using a camera (Nikon D7000, Nikon Corporation) to demonstrate stain removal effects.

Colour evaluation

The colour of each tooth specimen (L^*, a^*, b^*) was measured using a calibrated spectrophotometer (Minolta CM-2600d) before staining (=initial), after up to 10 cycles of stain application and after the brushing treatments. All surfaces were consistently dried by carefully wiping with a soft tissue prior to colour measurements. The L^* value represents the value of 'brightness/darkness' of a colour, such that a perfect black body has an L^* value of zero and the perfect reflecting diffuser has an L^* values of 100. The a^* and b^* represent two colour axes, with a^* the red-green axis and b^* the yellow-blue axis [25].

Removal of the stain was assessed using the following equation:

$$\%Removal = \frac{L*(Brushed) - L*(Stained)}{L*(Initial) - L*(Stained)} \times 100$$

Where L^* (Initial) is the brightness before staining; L^* (Stained) is the brightness after 10 cycles of stain

Table 1 Toothpastes studied

Group	Toothpaste	Type/relevant ingredients	Manufacturer
A	Aquafresh Multi-Action Whitening	Whitening/hydrated silica, pentasodium triphosphate	GlaxoSmithKline Consumer Healthcare, Brentford, UK
B	Arm and Hammer Advanced Whitening	Whitening/hydrated silica, sodium bicarbonate	Church & Dwight UK Ltd., Kent, UK
C	Colgate Cavity Protection	Non-whitening/dicalcium phosphate dihydrate, tetrasodium pyrophosphate	Colgate-Palmolive, Guildford, UK
D	Colgate MaxWhite	Whitening/hydrated silica, white micro crystals, tetrasodium pyrophosphate	Colgate-Palmolive, Guildford, UK
E	Crest Cavity Protection	Non-whitening/hydrated silica, trisodium phosphate	Procter & Gamble UK, Weybridge, UK
F	Crest Whitening Expressions	Whitening/hydrated silica	Procter & Gamble, Cincinnati, USA
G	Pearl Drops Daily Whitening Toothpolish	Whitening/hydrated silica, alumina, tetrapotassium pyrophosphate	Church & Dwight UK Ltd., Kent, UK
H	Signal White Now	Whitening/hydrated silica, trisodium phosphate	Unilever Deutschland, Hamburg, Germany

application and L* (Brushed) is the brightness after toothbrushing for the requisite number of strokes with water or toothpaste/abrasive slurry.

Pellicle cleaning ratio (PCR)

The pellicle cleaning ratio (PCR) for the same batch of toothpastes was undertaken and the details of the methodology have been previously reported elsewhere by Stookey et al. [19]. The PCR data were compared with those from the present methodology.

Statistical analyses of the data

Data were analysed by single factor ANOVA with a significance level of $p \leq 0.05$ applied. Pearson correlation coefficient was used to determine the linear relationship between two variables, and is denoted by r. Given a value between +1 and −1 inclusive, where one is perfect positive correlation, 0 is no correlation, and −1 is perfect negative correlation.

Results

Effects of enamel surface finish on stain removal

Enamel specimens of mean surface roughness values of approximately 0.4 μm (280-grit ground), 0.15 μm (400-grit ground) and 0.02 μm (diamond polished) were compared with respect to their susceptibility to stain removal after brushing with either water or commercial toothpastes (Fig. 1). Brushing with water resulted in minimal stain removal even after 5000 brush strokes with values of less than 1%, 5% and 10% for the 280-grit ground, 400-grit ground and diamond polished enamel surfaces, respectively. Stain removal was considerably enhanced after brushing with the commercial toothpastes with an inverse relationship between stain removal and specimen surface roughness. Statistically significant differences ($p < 0.05$) were found in the *in vitro* stain removal efficacy for the majority of data between 280-grit ground and 400-grit ground, and 280-grit ground and polished enamel specimens. However no significant differences ($p > 0.05$) were found in the *in vitro* stain removal efficacy between 400-grit ground and polished enamel specimens except for brushing with Colgate MaxWhite toothpaste. The numbers of brush strokes required to remove virtually all of the stain were 3000 or more for the 280-grit ground enamel specimens, 1000 or fewer for the 400-grit ground enamel specimens and 500 strokes or fewer for the diamond polished enamel specimens, respectively. There was a trend for greater stain removal with the whitening toothpastes using the same number of brush strokes. Due to the superior stain retention and greater ability to discriminate between individual commercial toothpastes, the 280-grit ground finish was used for all subsequent studies.

The brightness differences for the 280-grit ground bovine enamel surfaces between the pre- and post-brushing are presented in Fig. 2. Due to the number of brush strokes (800 for PCR methodology [19], 500 and 1000 strokes for present methodology), an average difference for the 500 and 1000 brush stroke procedures (denoted as 750 strokes in Fig. 2) was used for the comparisons between the two methods. No statistically significant differences were detected between the two test methods when brushed with Arm & Hammer Advanced Whitening, Crest Whitening Expressions, Colgate MaxWhite, Pearl Drops Daily Whitening Toothpolish, and Signal White Now toothpastes. Statistically significant differences were however identified when brushed with Crest Cavity, Colgate Cavity, and Aquafresh Multi-Action Whitening, with more stain being removed by using the PCR method, indicating that better retention of stain was achieved using the present methodology. Pearson correlation coefficient result ($r = 0.82$) showed a strong positive linear relationship between these two methods.

Figure 3 shows the images of enamel surfaces before staining and post-stain removal with 5000 brush strokes. Upon inspection it is apparent that relatively little stain remained on the roughened enamel surface group after brushing with the three non-whitening toothpastes, and no stain remained after brushing with the three whitening toothpastes. Relatively little stain remained on the partially roughened enamel surface group only after brushing with the Colgate Cavity Protection toothpaste, but no stain was apparent after brushing with the other tested toothpastes. No stain was apparent on the polished enamel surface group after brushing with all the tested toothpastes.

Effects of successive layers of stain deposition

There was a linear decrease in surface brightness of specimens with deposition of up to 10 successive layers of stain ($r = 0.98$). The effects of the number of layers of stain deposition on stain removal after brushing were assessed by brushing with a typical toothpaste precipitated silica abrasive slurry (15% w/w Zeodent 113) (Fig. 4). Significant differences ($p < 0.05$) in stain removal efficacy were detected between the first and successive cycles of stain deposition after more than 100 brushing strokes, no significant differences ($p > 0.05$) were detected between the staining cycles of 3, 5, 7 and 10. However, inter-sample variation tended to decrease with increasing number of layers of stain deposition.

Modelling the presence of acquired pellicle by application of acidic polymers

The application of an acquired pellicle prior to stain deposition (10 layers) was modelled on 280-grit ground

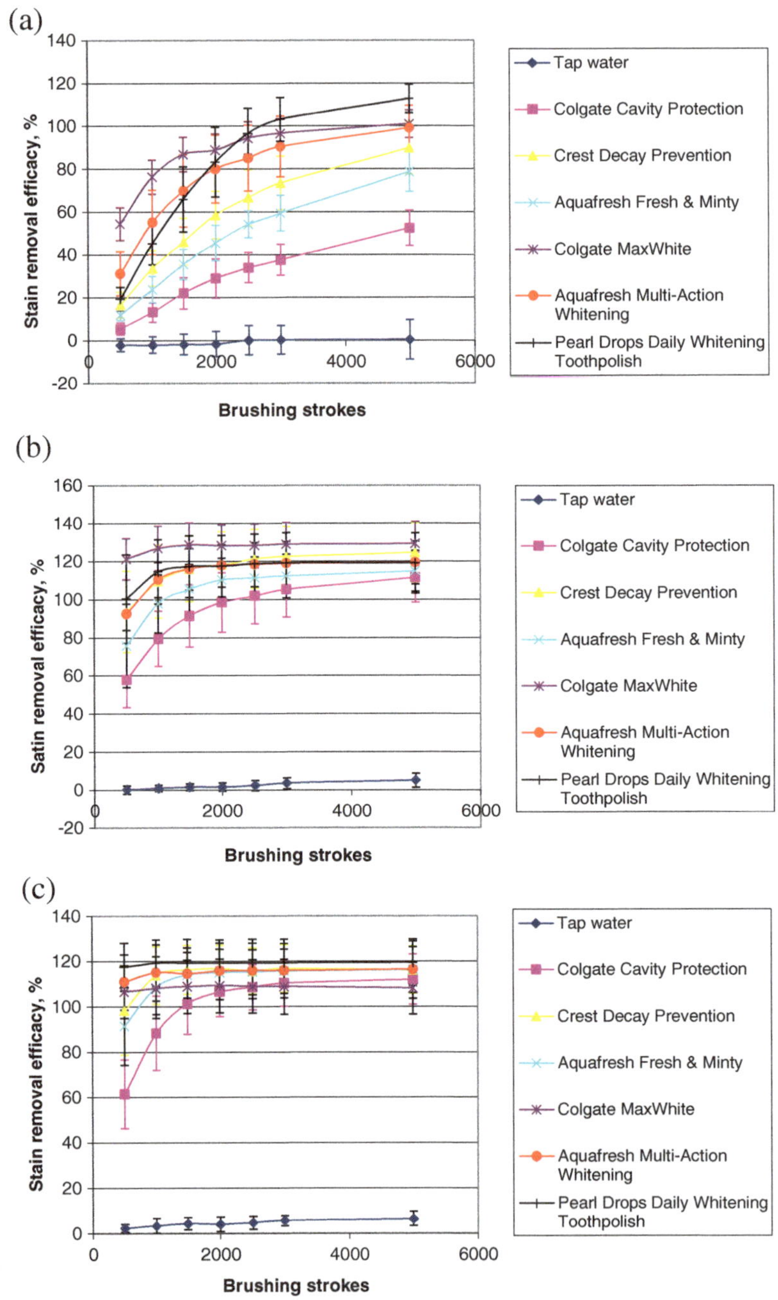

Fig. 1 Effects of initial surface roughness of bovine enamel specimen surfaces on the stain removal efficacy after brushing with the tested toothpaste slurries and water for up to 5000 brush strokes, $n = 8$, mean ± standard deviation. **a** Roughened enamel surface group; **b** Partially roughened enamel surface group; **c** Polished enamel surface group

finish enamel specimens using a variety of acidic polymers. Their effects on stain removal efficacy were subsequently assessed after brushing with a precipitated silica (typically present in commercial toothpastes) abrasive slurry (15% (w/w) Zeodent 113) (Fig. 5a). Significant differences ($p < 0.05$) in stain removal efficacy were observed between the polymers applied with a ranking order of stain retention of Carbopol and Gantrez as the best, then no polymer incorporation followed by Carrageenan and Xanthan being the poorest for stain retention. Treatment with the polymers Gantrez and Carbopol prior to stain deposition resulted in small decreases in stain removal efficacy after brushing, while Carrageenan and Xanthan negatively impacted on stain retention with greater stain removal observed. Application of the polymer by replacing 50% of the Tannic acid

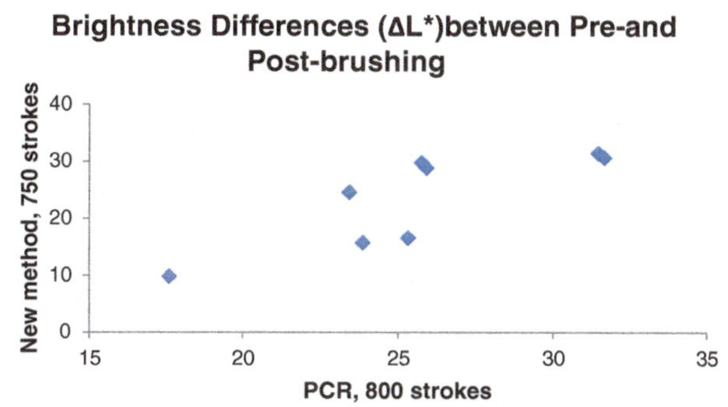

Fig. 2 Comparisons between the PCR [19] and the present methodologies for the brightness changes between pre- and post-brushing after brushing with the toothpastes slurries, $n = 8$, mean value

with the four acidic polymers during stain deposition generally decreased stain retention following brushing compared with the control (Fig. 5b). There were significant differences in stain removal efficacy between the presence of the four polymers versus no polymer inclusion (100% tannic acid) in the stain ($p < 0.05$). Following brushing with 15% (w/w) Zeodent 113, the rank order of stain retention was Gantrez and no polymer as the best, then Carbopol and Carrageenan and Xanthan representing the worst. Only Gantrez increased stain retention after brushing for 100, 500 or 1000 strokes, although such differences were not apparent at 3000 brush strokes. The application of the other polymers provided lower or equal levels of stain retention compared with the control after the various numbers of brush strokes.

STP effect on stain removal

STP is commonly used in oral hygiene products to facilitate stain removal [2]. Brushing of stained enamel specimens with STP both in the absence and presence of silica abrasive (15% (w/w) Zeodent 113) enhanced stain removal (Fig. 6). Brushing with 10% (w/w) STP alone removed approximately 35% of the stain after 5000 strokes and addition of Zeodent 113 abrasive further increased stain removal.

Statistically significant differences in stain removal efficacy were detected between the stained samples brushed with water (Fig. 1a) and 10% (w/w) STP. There were significant differences ($p < 0.05$) in stain removal when the stained enamel specimens were brushed with the three slurries comprising 15% (w/w) Zeodent 113 abrasive particles (+/− STP), while no significant differences were observed between the slurries comprising either 15% (w/w) Zeodent 113 abrasive plus 5% (w/w) or 10% (w/w) STP ($p > 0.05$). The three slurries with 15% (w/w) Zeodent 113 abrasive particles (+/− STP) exhibited the most effective stain removal as measured by brush strokes and linear responses for stain removal were observed during the first 500–1500 brush strokes ($r > 0.98$). The 10% (w/w) STP solution alone (without abrasive particles) showed a reasonably linear response for stain removal throughout the entire range of 500–5000 brush strokes ($r = 0.97$).

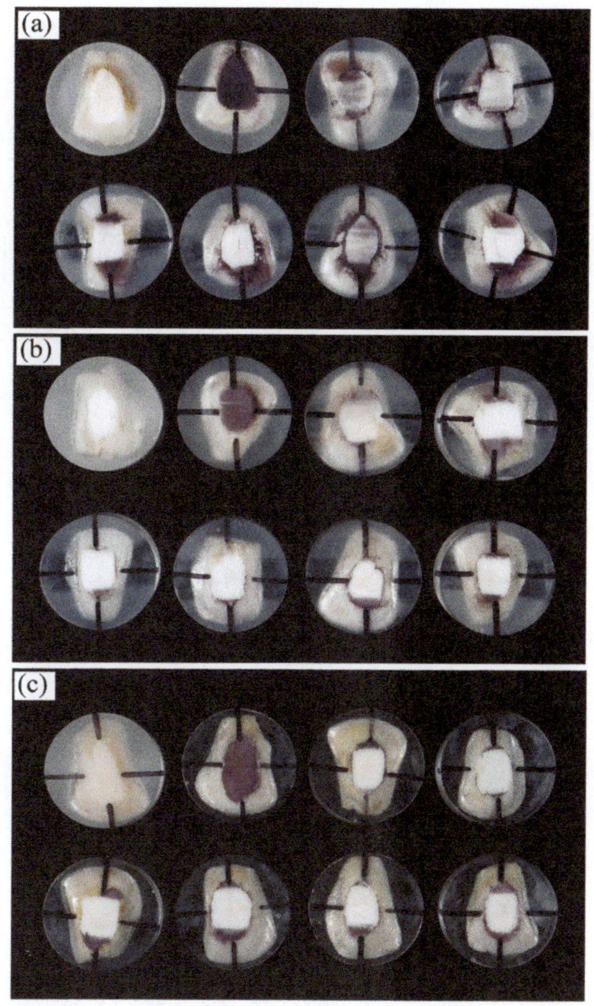

Fig. 3 Images of enamel surfaces before staining, after staining and post-stain removal with 5000 brush strokes. **a** Roughened enamel surface group; **b** Partially roughened enamel surface group; **c** Polished enamel surface group. *Upper row* (left to right): before stain; stain brushing with water; stain brushing with Colgate cavity Protection toothpaste; stain brushing with Crest Decay Prevention toothpaste; *Lower row* (left to right): stain brushing with Colgate MaxWhite toothpaste; stain brushing with Aquafresh Multi-Action Whitening toothpaste; stain brushing with Aquafresh Fresh & Minty toothpaste; stain brushing with Pearl Drops Daily Whitening Toothpolish toothpaste

Discussion

The *in vitro* stain methodology developed in this study provides a relatively inexpensive, easily performed, rapid and reproducible staining protocol which allows examination of stain bound to a natural enamel substrate. Of the many laboratory methods used to evaluate the cleaning potential of toothpaste and toothpaste ingredients, that developed by Stookey et al. [19] (PCR methodology)

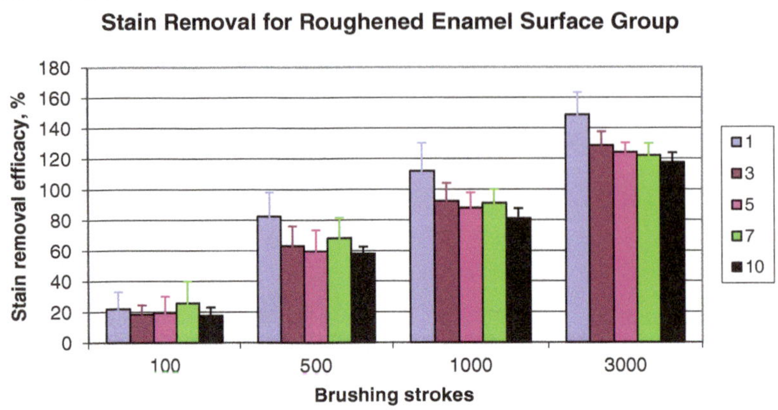

Fig. 4 Stain removal efficacy for 280-grit ground enamel specimens with varying numbers of stain layers after brushing with 15% w/w Zeodent 113 precipitated silica abrasive slurry for up to 3000 brush strokes, $n = 8$, mean ± standard deviation

is commonly used by the oral care industry. However it requires a time consuming stain deposition protocol with opportunities for reproducibility issues when used at different test sites. The data presented here demonstrate good agreement between our stain methodology and the PCR methodology in terms of brightness changes after brushing using the same batches of toothpastes. The current study has also demonstrated the retention of the stain after toothbrushing in the presence of either standard toothpastes or whitening toothpastes

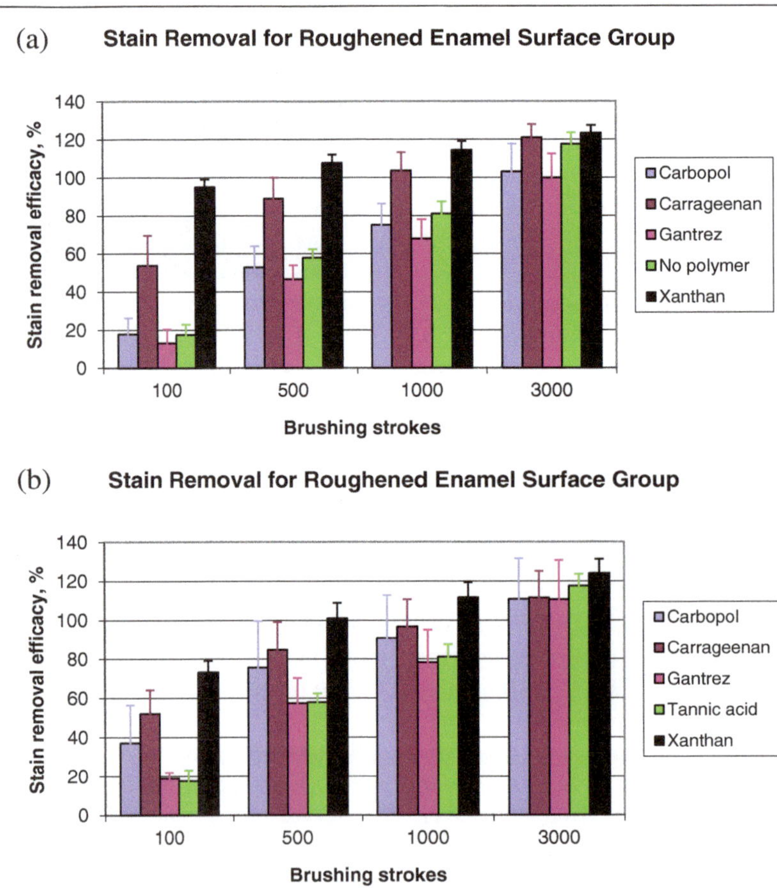

Fig. 5 Modelling the application of an acquired pellicle prior to stain deposition on 280-grit ground finish enamel specimens using a variety of acidic polymers, $n = 8$, mean ± standard deviation. **a** by application of one layer of acidic polymers followed with 10 layers of tannate stain; **b** by replacing half of the tannic acid stain component with acidic polymers for the precipitation of 10 layers of stain

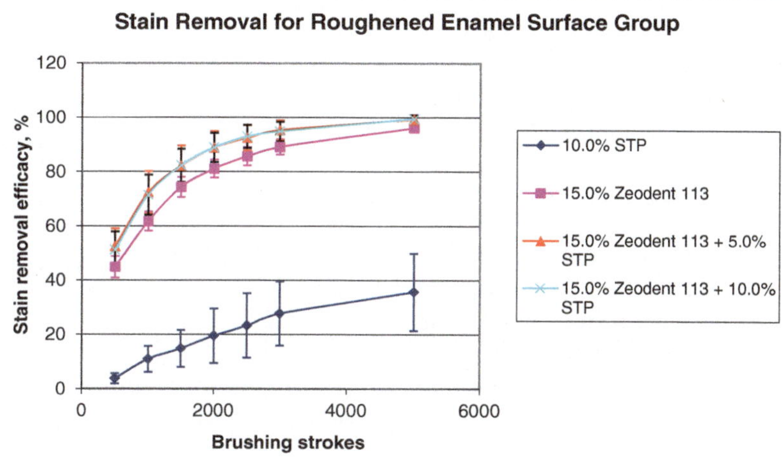

Fig. 6 Stain removal efficacy for stained bovine enamel specimens after brushing for up to 5000 brush strokes with 10.0% (w/w) STP alone, 15.0% (w/w) Zeodent 113 alone, and 15.0% (w/w) Zeodent 113 with 5.0% (w/w) STP and 10.0% (w/w) STP, $n = 8$, mean ± standard deviation

as well as the most common chemically active compound in whitening toothpastes, STP. Furthermore it demonstrates the ability of the methodology to discriminate between these various oral hygiene products.

Model stains have been previously described [19–23] for simulation of the extrinsic staining of the teeth. However, one of the main disadvantages of these staining approaches has been that the stain properties could not be directly compared due to the differences in materials used, i.e., different brand/supplier of reagents used in different studies. However this ferric-tannate stain now provides a reliable standardised model for stain removal purposes in which the stain properties can be controlled due to the chemically defined nature of the stain deposits.

In the previously reported PCR methodology [19], acid etching of polished enamel surfaces has been used to expedite stain accumulation and adherence, although the reproducibility of the etching process can be difficult to accurately reproduce. In the present study, stain could be most readily removed from the diamond polished bovine enamel surfaces, followed by the 400-grit ground enamel bovine surfaces while the stain on the 280-grit ground bovine enamel surfaces was retained to the greatest extent. The surface roughness of enamel specimens can be reproducibly achieved with grinding/polishing protocols contributing to the reproducibility of the presently reported methodology. The surface roughness of the tooth is also of clinical importance, particularly in respect to bacterial retention. A threshold surface roughness for bacterial retention of 0.2 μm has been reported [26]. Indeed, the mean surface roughness values for 400-grit ground bovine enamel were approximately 0.15 μm, which is below the threshold roughness of 0.2 μm and the stain was more readily removed from the 400-grit ground surfaces than from the 280-grit ground bovine enamel surfaces, the latter of which had a mean surface roughness of approximately 0.4 μm. The polished bovine enamel surfaces had mean surface roughness values of approximately 0.02 μm, which is ten-fold less than the threshold roughness for bacterial retention and the stain on these polished surfaces was removed much more readily than that from the 400-grit ground and 280-grit ground bovine enamel surfaces.

The acquired enamel pellicle (AEP) which occurs in vivo results from rapid binding of salivary constituents after saliva contacts a newly exposed enamel surface and reportedly contributes to enamel protection [11]. It is generally understood that the AEP reduces friction between teeth and between teeth and the oral mucosa. It has also been reported that the pellicle enables the initial attachment of bacteria to the tooth surface, which is the first step in plaque formation [11]. In the present study, four acidic polymers were used to mimic an AEP layer on the 280-grit ground bovine enamel surfaces, by either direct application of a thin layer of the acidic polymer prior to application of the ferric-tannate stain or by partly replacing tannic acid with acidic polymers for the stain formation. Appreciable differences in stain removal efficacy were found between the four acidic polymers with a rank order of stain retention of Gantrez > Carbopol > Carrageenan > Xanthan. Gantrez on both occasions showed a very similar pattern of stain removal, indicating its potential to mimic an AEP layer prior to the stain deposits.

STP, a sodium salt of triphosphoric acid with surfactant and chelating properties, has been used in whitening toothpastes for stain removal. *In vitro* studies with crystalline hydroxyapatite (HA) powder showed that STP was effective in removing existing stain and impeding stain formation through inhibition of the adsorption of salivary proteins or tea stain and the desorption of existing protein and stain from HA surfaces [16, 27]. In vivo trials have also reported significant extrinsic stain removal efficacy for a STP containing dentifrice versus the control [28] as well as a reduction in staining by a chewing gum which contained STP [29]. In the present study, the effects of STP on *in vitro* stain removal efficacy were examined both in combination with abrasive particles and alone using 280-grit ground finish bovine surfaces. Approximately 35% of the stain was removed when brushing with 10.0% (w/w) STP alone after 5000 strokes, while a control of water resulted in minimal stain removal (less than 1%). The addition of 5.0 (w/w)% or 10.0 (w/w)% STP to a slurry of 15.0 (w/w)% Zeodent 113 abrasive improved stain removal compared with a 15.0 w/w% Zeodent 113 abrasive slurry alone for the same number of brush strokes. These data also highlight the efficacy of STP in contributing to stain removal during oral hygiene measures. However, no differences were observed between the STP concentration of 5.0 (w/w)% and 10.0 (w/w)%. Interestingly, a lack of influence of STP concentration on stain desorption from HA has also been reported elsewhere [27]. Compared with the 10.0 (w/w)% STP solution alone (without abrasive particles), the slurries with 15.0 w/w% Zeodent 113 abrasive particles (+/− STP) showed significantly higher stain removal efficacy, demonstrating that the abrasive was mainly responsible for the removal of extrinsic stain. Similar results have been reported by others when testing different types of whitening toothpaste products [30].

The present ferric-tannate/bovine enamel (280-grit ground finish) methodology provides an easily performed and reproducible model, which can be readily established in laboratories. The chemically defined nature of the stain contributes to reproducibility of the methodology as does the enamel sample preparation protocol. The rapid stain deposition (about 2 h for 10 cycles) facilitates the use of the methodology for rapid screening of large numbers of oral care products to target those products most suitable for testing under clinical conditions. Importantly, it allows good discrimination between various oral care products, including those used for tooth whitening purposes.

With the growth in the desire for whiter teeth by consumers and patients, toothpaste manufacturers aim to maximise the cleanability of enamel extrinsic staining whilst minimising possible damage (wear) to dental hard tissues. Therefore, it is important to investigate the wear and roughness in parallel to stain removal when using the present methodology.

Conclusion

We conclude that this *in vitro* ferric-tannate stain removal assay provides an easily performed and reproducible screening assay for a variety of oral care products, which can be established in most laboratory settings. Acidic polymers can be applied for the AEP simulation prior to stain formulations.

Abbreviations

AEP: Acquired enamel pellicle; HA: Hydroxyapatite; OTC: Over-the-counter; PCR: Pellicle cleaning ratio; RCTs: Randomised controlled trials; STP: Sodium tripolyphosphate

Acknowledgements

The authors are grateful to Dr Jenny Gordon for helpful discussions and advice during the course of this study.

Funding

This research was financially supported by GSK Consumer Healthcare. RL is an employee of GSK, contributed to the design, analysis and interpretation of the data from this study and contributed to writing of the manuscript.

Authors' contributions

RL, AJS, PRC contributed to the design, analysis and interpretation of the data from this study and contributed to writing of the manuscript. CW contributed to the design, analysis and interpretation of the data from this study as well as conducting the laboratory procedures and contributed to writing of the manuscript. All authors read and approved the final manuscript.

Competing interests

AJS, PRC and CW have no competing interests. RL is an employee of GSK, the sponsor of the study.

Consent for publication

Not applicable.

Ethics approval

The research was performed using food industry animal carcass waste and that ethical approval is not required for waste tissues.

Author details

[1]Oral Biology, School of Dentistry, University of Birmingham, 5 Mill Pool Way, Edgbaston, Birmingham B5 7EG, UK. [2]GlaxoSmithKline Consumer Healthcare, St. George's Avenue, Weybridge, Surrey KT13 ODE, UK.

References

1. Sharif N, MacDonald E, Hughes J, Newcombe RG, Addy M. The chemical stain removal properties of 'whitening' toothpaste products: studies *in vitro*. Br Dent J. 2000;188:620–4.
2. Joiner A. Whitening toothpastes: a review of the literature. J Dent. 2010;38S: e17–24.
3. Alkhatib MN, Holt R, Bedi R. Prevalence of self-assessed tooth discolouration ion the United Kingdom. J Dent. 2004;32:561–6.
4. Alkhatib MN, Holt R, Bedi R. Age and perception of dental appearance and tooth colour. Gerodontology. 2005;22:32–6.
5. Xiao J, Zhou XD, Zhu WC, Zhang B, Li JY, Xu X. The prevalence of tooth discolouration and the self-satisfaction with tooth colour in a Chinese urban population. J Oral Rehabil. 2007;34:351–60.
6. Odioso LL, Gibb RD, Gerlach RW. Impact of demographic, behavioural, and dental care utilization parameters on tooth colour and personal satisfaction. Compend Contin Educ Dent. 2000;21:S35–41.
7. Watts A, Addy M. Tooth discolouration and staining: a review of the literature. Br Dent J. 2001;190:309–16.
8. Joiner A. Review of the extrinsic stain removal and enamel/dentine abrasion by a calcium carbonate and perlite containing whitening toothpaste. Int Dent J. 2006;56:175–80.
9. Ten Bosch JJ, Coops JC. Tooth colour and reflectance as related to light scattering and enamel hardness. J Dent Res. 1995;74:374–80.
10. Nathoo S. The chemistry and mechanisms of extrinsic and intrinsic discolouration. J Am Dent Assoc. 1997;128:S6–S10.
11. Lendenmann U, Grogan J, Oppenheim FG. Saliva and dental pellicle—A review. Adv Dent Res. 2000;14:22–8.

12. Joiner A. The bleaching of teeth: a review of the literature. J Dent. 2006;34: 412–9.
13. Griffiths CE, Bailey JR, Jarad FD, Youngson CC. An investigation into most effective method of treating stained teeth: an *in vitro* study. J Dent. 2008;36: 54–62.
14. Sarrett DC. Tooth whitening today. J Am Dent Assoc. 2002;133:1535–8.
15. Lynch CD, McConnell RJ. The use of microabrasion to remove discoloured enamel: a clinical report. J Prosthet Dent. 2003;90:417–9.
16. Walsh TF, Rawlinson A, Wildgoose D, Marlow I, Haywood J, Ward JM. Clinical evaluation of the stain removal ability of a whitening dentifrice and stain controlling system. J Dent. 2005;33:413–8.
17. Langford J, Pavey KD, Olliff CJ, Cragg PJ, Hanlon GW, Paul F, Rees GD. Real-time monitoring of stain formation and removal on calcium hydroxyapatite surfaces using quartz crystal sensor technology. Analyst. 2002;127:360–7.
18. Sulieman M, Addy M, Rees JS. Development and evaluation of a method in vitro to study the effectiveness of tooth bleaching. J Dent. 2003;31:415–22.
19. Stookey GK, Burkhard TA, Schemehorn BR. *In vitro* removal of stain with dentifrices. J Dent Res. 1982;61:126–9.
20. Addy M, Goodfield S. The use of acrylic to compare the abrasivity and stain removal properties of toothpastes. Clin Mater. 1991;7:219–25.
21. Lee BS, Huang SH, Chiang YC, Chien YS, Mou CY, Lin CP. Development of in vitro tooth staining model and usage of catalysts to elevate the effectiveness of tooth bleaching. Dent Mater. 2008;24:57–66.
22. Freccia WF, Peters DD. A technique for staining extracted teeth: a research and teaching aid for bleaching. J Endod. 1982;82:67–9.
23. Wetter NU, Barroso MC, Pelino JEP. Dental bleaching efficacy with diode laser and LED irradiation: an in vitro study. Lasers Surg Med. 2004;35:254–8.
24. Dawson PL, Walsh JE, Morrison T, Grigor J. Dental stain prevention by abrasive toothpastes: a new in vitro test and its correlation with clinical observations. J Cosmet Sci. 1998;49:275–83.
25. Parry J, Harrington E, Rees GD, McNab R, Smith AJ. Control of brushing variables for the *in vitro* assessment of toothpaste abrasivity using s novel laboratory model. J Dent. 2008;36:117–24.
26. Bollen CML, Lambrechts P, Quirynen M. Comparison of surface roughness of oral hard materials to the threshold surface roughness for bacterial plaque retention: a review of the literature. Dent Mater. 1997;13:258–69.
27. Shellis RP, Addy M, Rees GD. *In vitro* studies on the effect of sodium tripolyphosphate on the interactions of stain and salivary protein with hydroxyapatite. J Dent. 2005;33:313–24.
28. Hughes N, Maggio B, Sufi F, Mason S, Kleber CJ. A comparative clinical study evaluating stain removal efficacy of a new sensitivity whitening dentifrice compared to commercially available whitening dentifrice. J Clin Dent. 2009;20:218–22.
29. Porciani PF, Perra C, Grandini S. Effect on dental occurrence by chewing gum containing sodium tripolyphosphate—a double-blind six-week trial. J Clin Dent. 2010;21:4–7.
30. Alshara S, Lippert F, Eckert GJ, Hara AT. Effectiveness and mode of action of whitening dentifrices on enamel extrinsic stains. Clin Oral Investig. 2013. doi: 10.1007/s00784-013-0981-8.

8

National dental policies and socio-demographic factors affecting changes in the incidence of periodontal treatments in Korean: A nationwide population-based retrospective cohort study from 2002–2013

Jae-Hong Lee[1], Jung-Seok Lee[2], Jung-Kyu Choi[3], Hye-In Kweon[4], Young-Taek Kim[4*†] and Seong-Ho Choi[2*†]

Abstract

Background: Dental insurance coverage has recently expanded in Korea. The number of patients diagnosed with periodontal disease (PD), and the actual number of periodontally compromised patients has increased. However, few studies have investigated the relationships between the prevalence of periodontal disease and the incidence of PD treatment, dental insurance policies, and socio-demographic factors. To determine the incidence of periodontal treatments required, the comprehensive longitudinal data of the National Health Insurance Service were used. This study evaluated changes in the incidence of periodontal treatments, using data from the Korean National Health Insurance Cohort Database.

Methods: A random stratified sample of 1,025,340 Korean patients was selected from National Health Insurance database, using 1,476 multistage samplings (of sex, age, and income level) for 12 years from 2002 to 2013. Chi-square analysis, and univariate, and multivariate logistic regression were used to evaluate the association of socio-demographic factors with the prevalence of PD and the incidence of periodontal treatment.

Results: The incidence of periodontal treatment steadily and significantly increased, in both male and female participants, from 2002 to 2013. The increase was associated with socio-demographic factors and changes in national dental insurance policies. The incidence of periodontal treatment evaluated by age is influenced by the changes in national dental policies. These results suggest that the increase in patients diagnosed with PD reflects changes in dental policies and insurance benefits.

Conclusions: This study confirms that national dental policies and socio-demographic factors are related to the incidence of periodontal treatments. The incidence of periodontal treatment is significantly related to the expansion of insurance coverage in South Korea.

Keywords: Cohort analysis, Dental insurance, Health insurance, Health services accessibility, Periodontal disease

* Correspondence: youngtaek77@naver.com; shchoi726@yuhs.ac

†Equal contributors

[4]Department of Periodontology, Ilsan Hospital, National Health Insurance Service, 100 Ilsan-ro Ilsan-donggu, Goyang 10444, South Korea

[2]Department of Periodontology, Research Institute for Periodontal Regeneration, Yonsei University College of Dentistry, 50 Yonsei-ro, Seodaemun-gu, Seoul 03722, South Korea

Full list of author information is available at the end of the article

Background

The demands for medical care in modern societies are increasing. These demands result from increases in the aging population, household income, and education levels, and changes in health policies and the medical care systems [1]. Recently, the importance of oral-health-related quality of life has been recognized [2, 3]. Periodontal disease (PD) is a disease of the oral cavity, and a major cause of tooth loss in adults [4]. More than half of all adults are affected by some degree of PD, and 11 % of adults suffer from severe and advanced periodontitis [5]. In 2014, in South Korea, 12.9 million people (26 % of the current population) received treatment for PD. Periodontal disease is a highly prevalent disease, and is the second most common outpatient disease, after acute bronchitis [6].

Recent expansion of insurance coverage for dental treatment has resulted in an increase in the number of patients diagnosed with PD, and an increase in the identification of periodontally compromised patients [6]. The incidence of periodontal treatments is closely and consistently related to socio-demographic factors, including age, sex, race, household income, insurance, and health status, and living area [7, 8]. The severity of disease, and the incidence of periodontal treatments, is higher among those in disadvantaged groups, including, individuals who are older, poorer, less educated, and those living in rural areas [9, 10]. In addition, although there is no clear evidence, both public health policy and insurance availability are considered to have an impact on PD treatment efficacy and outcome [11–14].

Universal health care was implemented in Korean in 1989. By 2013, 97.1 % of the Korean population (51.34 million people) was covered by the mandatory social National Health Insurance Service (NHIS) [15]. Insurance for 49.99 million people is provided by NHIS, and the Medical Aid Program (MAP) insures an additional 1.46 million people. The dental health-care service was implemented after the medical-care service and it continues to expand. Major dental insurance policies presently cover the costs of sealant (first and second molars, from May 2013), full complete dentures (from July 2012), removable partial dentures (from July 2013), and dental implant treatment (from July 2014) for individuals aged 75 years and above. They also cover the cost of periodontal scaling (for individuals 20 years and above, from July 2013) [15]. Dental insurance coverage continues to expand and coverage for full and partial dentures, and dental implants is expected to be available by 2015 for individuals aged 70 years and above.

Several studies, such as the National Health and Nutrition Examination Survey (NHANES) from the United States, and the Adult Dental Health Survey from the United Kingdom, have investigated the epidemiology of PD [11, 16]. These reports are useful for assessing the prevalence of PD, and planning national dental services. However, these studies are based on cross-sectional surveys. This method not only limits the ability to assess changes in the incidence of periodontal treatments over time, but also cannot be used to identify the impact of dental insurance coverage on periodontal treatments. When compared with cross-sectional surveys, a longitudinal study can be used to assess changes in the incidence of periodontal treatments over time and to identify the impact of dental insurance coverage on periodontal treatments [17]. In South Korea, several cross-sectional studies, have investigated the association between PD, national dental policies, and socio-demographic factors. However, an observational cohort study has not been conducted [3, 18]. The Korean National Health Insurance Cohort Database (KNHICD) includes 12 years of accumulated individual socio-demographic factors, and is useful for evaluating changes in the incidence of periodontal treatments. Therefore, the aim of our study was to identify national dental policies, and socio-demographic factors, influencing the incidence of periodontal treatments. To accomplish this aim, we used the comprehensive data, accumulated from 2002 to 2013, in the KNHICD.

Methods

Study design and data source

Mandatory national health insurance in South Korea results in a database (DB) of more than one trillion individual cases, involving the entire Korean population of 50 million individuals, and includes data from the start-up of mandatory enforcement of insurance payment benefit in 1977. This DB includes information on qualifications, insurance, medical and dental records, checkups, rare incurable diseases, cancer, and long-term-care insurance services.

The NHIS made the KNHICD available for research purposes in 2013. This nationwide, population-based retrospective cohort study evaluated the association between treatments for PD, national dental policies, and socio-demographic factors of the South Korean population. A random stratified sample of one million Koreans was selected from the DB by the NHIS Big Data Steering Department, using 1,476-stage sampling (of sex, age, and household income level), for the 12 years from 2002 to 2013.

Effective from 2003, records that no longer existed, because of death or emigration, were replaced with records from newborns born in the same year. To protect privacy, the identification number of each patient was anonymized. All personal information is managed solely by NHIS and the request for raw data is offered only with given random identification codes.

Ethics, consent, and permissions

The project was approved by the NHIS Ilsan Hospital, Goyang, Korea. An ethical approval was also obtained by the NHIS Ilsan Hospital (approval #2016-03-019).

Study population clinical characteristics

The KCD-6 (Korean Classification of Disease; modified version of ICD-10 [International Classification of Disease]) guidelines were used to diagnose PD (acute periodontitis [K052]; chronic periodontitis [K053]; periodontosis [K054)]; other PD [K055], and unspecified PD [K056]) according to criteria proposed by the American Academy of Periodontology [19].

The study population was defined as patients who were diagnosed with PD, and treated with periodontal surgery, by a general dentist or a specialized dentist (e.g., periodontist), in 2003. Treatment was defined according to the following NHIS prescription codes: U1051/1052, periodontal flap operation (simple/complicated); U1071/1072, bone graft for alveolar bone defects (allogenic, xenogenic, or substitute bone graft/autogenous bone graft); or U1081–1083, guided tissue regeneration (without bone graft/allogenic, xenogenic, or substitute bone graft/autogenous bone graft).

Definition of socio-demographic factors

Socio-demographic factors were identified from the KNHICD and categorized into the following five groups: sex, age, monthly income, health status, and living area. The groups were further divided (using random stratified analysis by the NHIS Big Data Steering Department) into smaller sub-groups. The factor sex had two groups (male and female participants). Age was divided into eight groups; those < 69 years were divided into 10-year interval groups and those > 70 years formed one group. Monthly household income was divided into 41 groups based on the monthly household income of the participants. It was classified into quintiles, with medical aid beneficiaries in the first-quintile group. Based on health status of the participants, three groups were formed as healthy, minor disability, and major disability (using the Handicapped Welfare Law). Finally, the factor living was divided into two groups on the basis of its population; < 50,000 residents was classified as rural and ≥ 50,000 residents classified as urban.

Statistical analysis

Chi-square analysis, and univariate and multivariate logistic regression were used to evaluate the association between socio-demographic factors and the prevalence of PD. Odds ratios (ORs) and 95 % confidence intervals (CIs) were calculated in all assessments, and a P value of < 0.05 was considered indicative of statistical significance. Statistical analyses were performed using Statistical Analysis System (version 9.2, SAS Institute, Cary, NC, USA) by the Department of Health Insurance Research, Ilsan Hospital, NHIS.

Results

Characteristics of the study population

The baseline characteristics of the cohort are presented in Table 1. Of the 1,025,340 individuals included in the study, male (513,258) and female (512,082) patients were equally represented. Patients aged 20–49 years (526,891) accounted for 51.4 % of the population. Additionally, 97.0 % (994,627) of patients were in the NHIS (employees and self-employed); 97.3 % (998,030) were classified as

Table 1 Baseline characteristics of the study cohort

	Males		Females		Total
	n	%	*n*	%	
Total	513258	50.1 %	512082	49.9 %	1025340
Age group (years)					
≤ 9	71921	14.0 %	64661	12.6 %	136582
10–19	74447	14.5 %	67495	13.2 %	141942
20–29	86355	16.8 %	84492	16.5 %	170847
30–39	95929	18.7 %	91788	17.9 %	187717
40–49	85646	16.7 %	82681	16.1 %	168327
50–59	48254	9.4 %	48862	9.5 %	97116
60–69	34353	6.7 %	41169	8.0 %	75522
≥ 70	16353	3.2 %	30934	6.0 %	47287
Household income[a]					
First quintile	70088	13.7 %	84513	16.5 %	154601
Second quintile	79071	15.4 %	78685	15.4 %	157756
Third quintile	103744	20.2 %	97450	19.0 %	201194
Fourth quintile	123727	24.1 %	118422	23.1 %	242149
Fifth quintile	136628	26.6 %	133012	26.0 %	269640
Insurance status					
MAP	13049	3.2 %	17664	3.4 %	30713
NHIS, employees	248048	48.3 %	248549	48.5 %	496597
NHIS, self-employed	252161	49.1 %	245869	48.0 %	498030
Health status[b]					
Healthy	494934	96.4 %	503096	98.2 %	998030
Major disability	5828	1.1 %	3633	0.7 %	9461
Minor disability	12496	2.4 %	5353	1.0 %	17849
Living area[c]					
Urban	460837	89.8 %	459751	89.8 %	920588
Rural	52421	10.2 %	52331	10.2 %	104752

NHIS National health insurance service, *MAP* Medical aid program
[a]Total of 41 groups classified into quintiles (with MAP beneficiaries in the first quintile)
[b]Classification based on the Handicapped Welfare Law in South Korea
[c]Classification based on rural (<50,000 residents) or urban (≥50,000 residents) living

having good health status; and 89.8 % (920,588) lived in urban areas.

Incidence of periodontal treatments

Of the patients diagnosed with PD, 30.8 % (158,303) were male and 31.8 % (162,800) female. The incidence of periodontal treatments increased significantly from 2002 (n = 71,917; 7.0 %) to 2013 (n = 183,312; 18.1 %). In 2013, the incidence was higher in female patients (n = 91,856; 18.1 %), when compared to male patients (n = 91,456; 18.0 %). The incidence of periodontal treatments increased in all groups in 2013, except in patients 60–69 years of age. The 1-year incidence rate of PD among those aged 10–19 years increased from 2011 (n = 5,529; 4.1 %) to 2013 (n = 22,566; 18.2 %; Fig. 1a). From 2002 to 2013, the accumulated incidence of periodontal treatments peaked among patients 40–49 years of age, for both male (n = 40,426; 47.2 %) and female (n = 39.205; 47.4 %) patients. Among those 30–39 years of age and over 70 years of age, the accumulated incidence was higher in male patients than female patients. The accumulated incidence was higher in female patients for all other age groups (Fig. 1b).

The incidence of periodontal treatments increased from 2002 to 2013; this increase was unrelated to household income level. The increase was greatest in the first quintile, from 5.9 % (n = 9,056) in 2002, to 17.9 % (n = 30,388) in 2013 (Fig. 2a). The accumulated incidence of periodontal treatments in the first quintile, which includes the MAP group (n = 42,102; 27.2 %), increased, and was similar to that in the fifth quintile (n = 96,393; 35.7 %). The accumulated incidence of periodontal treatments was higher in female patients (n = 24,277; 28.7 %), than male patients (n = 17,825; 25.4 %) in the first quintile, similar for both sexes in the fourth quintile (38,661; 31.2 % and 37,042; 31.3 %), and higher in male patients (n = 49,286; 36.1 %), when compared to female patients (n = 47,107; 35.4 %), in the fifth quintile (Fig. 2b).

The incidence of periodontal treatments showed a tendency to increase in the NHIS group. In 2002, 7.5 % (37,368) of employees and 6.9 % (34,412) of self-employed individuals underwent periodontal treatments. In 2013, 18.1 % (124,315) of employees and 18.0 % (53,782) of self-employed individuals underwent treatment. However, from 2008 to 2011, the incidence of periodontal treatments increased sevenfold in the MAP group (n = 244; 1.9 % vs. n = 4,751; 13.9 %). In 2013 the period incidence in the MAP group was 17.3 % (n = 5,212), which was similar to that in the NHIS group (Fig. 3a). The accumulated incidence in the MAP group was 15.5 %, which was significantly lower than that in the NHIS group (32.8 % of employees and 30.8 % of self-employed). There was no difference between male and female patients in any of the groups (Fig. 3b).

The overall incidence of periodontal treatments increased from 2002 to 2013, to 19.7 % (7,688) in the minor disability group (Fig. 4a). The accumulated incidence of periodontal treatments differed with health status, and was 19.7 % in the major disability group, 31.4 % in the healthy group, and 34.2 % in the minor disability group. There were no significant differences between men and women in any of these groups (Fig. 4b).

The incidence of periodontal treatments increased from 2002 to 2013, for patients in both urban and rural areas. In 2013, the incidence was 18.0 % (170,124) for urban patients, and 17.2 % (13,188) for rural patients (Fig. 5a). The accumulated incidence of periodontal

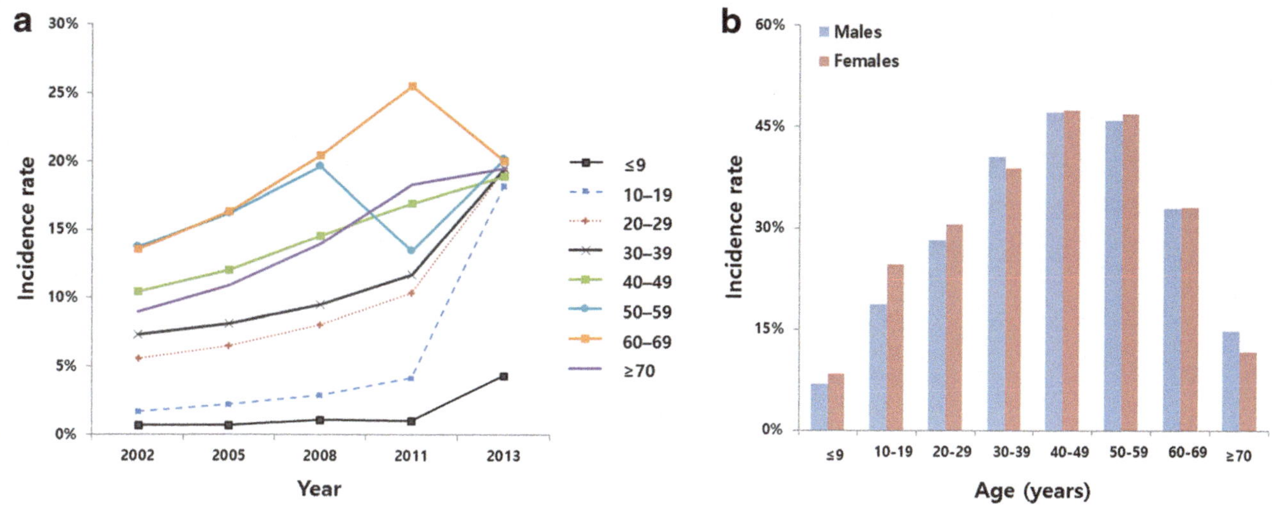

Fig. 1 Age-specific 1-year incidence rates of periodontal treatment (**a**); and sex-specific accumulated incidence rates of periodontal treatments (**b**) during 2002–2013 in South Korea

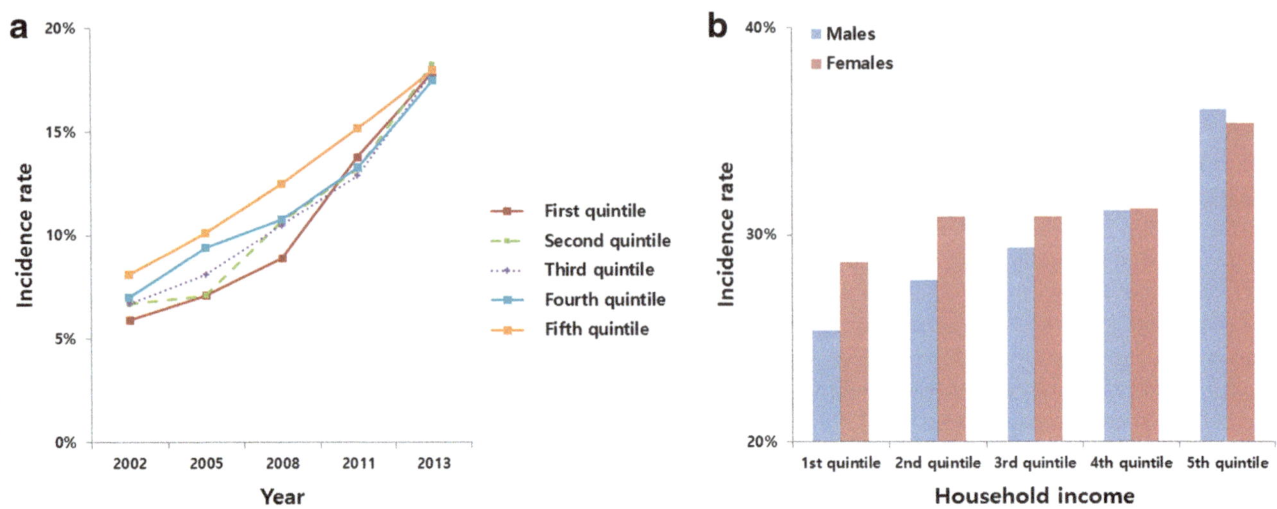

Fig. 2 Household income-specific 1-year incidence rates of periodontal treatment (**a**); and sex-specific accumulated incidence rates of periodontal treatment (**b**) during 2002–2013 in South Korea

treatments was 31.9 % in urban areas and 19.7 % in rural areas. There was no significant difference between the sexes (Fig. 5b).

Association of socio-demographic factors with periodontal treatments

The socio-demographic factors associated with periodontal treatments are shown in Table 2. Univariate analysis indicated that all socio-demographic factors investigated were significantly associated with periodontal treatments ($P < 0.001$); however, with multi-variant analysis, the only factor that was not statistically significant was sex ($P = 0.513$). Among all age groups, when using those ≤9 years of age as the reference, the OR for the incidence of periodontal treatments was highest among patients 40–49 years of age (OR = 9.58, 95 % CI = 9.36–9.81, $P < 0.001$). For household income, using the first quintile as the reference, the OR was 1.37 (95 % CI = 1.35–1.39, $P < 0.001$) for the fifth quintile. The incidence of periodontal treatments increased with household income. For insurance status, using the MAP group as the reference, the OR was 1.93 (95 % CI = 1.86–2.00, $P < 0.001$) for those in the NHIS (employees) group. For health status, using those in the healthy group as the reference, the major disability group had an OR of 0.61 (95 % CI = 0.58–0.64, $P < 0.001$) and the minor disability group had an OR of 0.94 (95 % CI = 0.91–0.97, $P < 0.001$). When using the urban-area group as the reference for living area, the

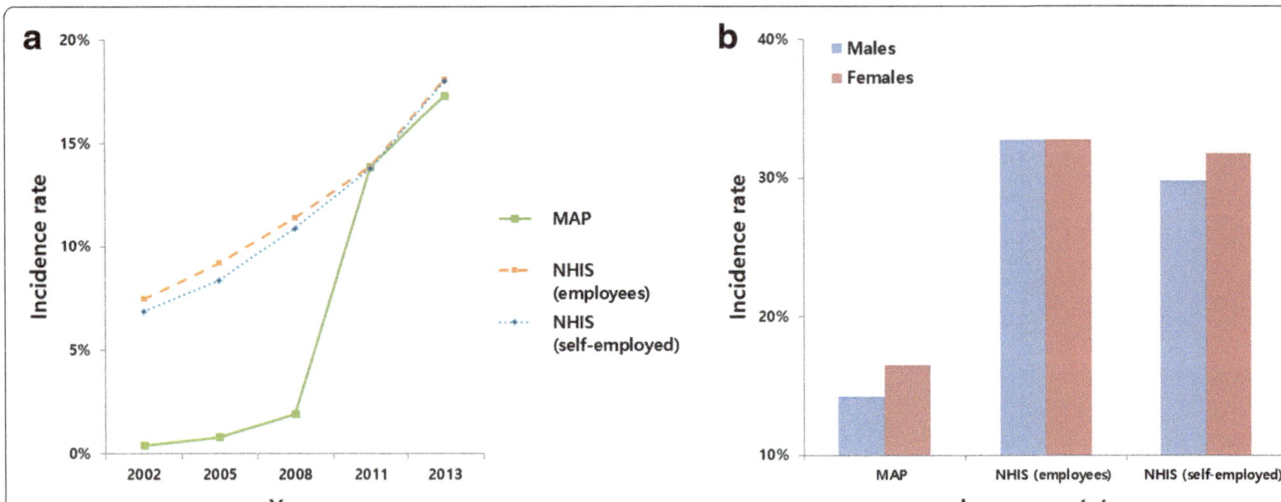

Fig. 3 Insurance status-specific 1-year incidence rates of periodontal treatment (**a**); and sex-specific accumulated incidence rates of periodontal treatment (**b**) during 2002–2013 in South Korea. NHIS, National Health Insurance Service; MAP, Medical Aid Program

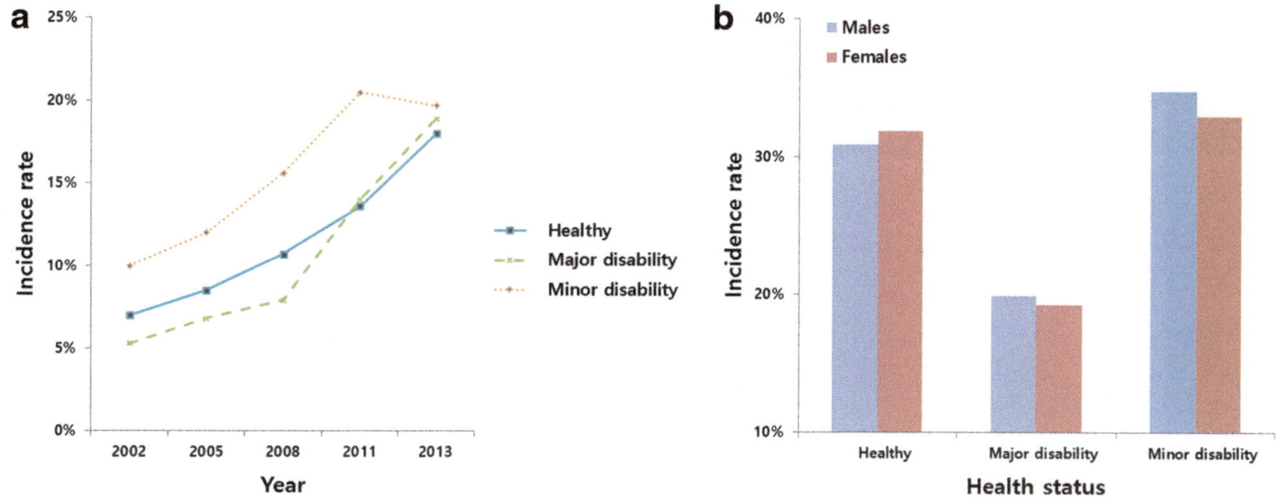

Fig. 4 Health status-specific 1-year incidence rates of periodontal treatment (**a**); and sex-specific accumulated incidence rates of periodontal treatment (**b**) during 2002–2013 in South Korea

rural-area group had an OR of 0.85 (95 % CI = 0.83–0.86, $P < 0.001$).

Discussion

Based on data in the KNHICD, our study shows that the incidence of periodontal treatments increased significantly from 2002 to 2013. The increase was seen in both male and female patients, and was due to both socio-demographic factors and the changes in national dental policies. Although there have been reports of sex differences in the incidence of periodontal treatments, this study found similar prevalence rates for both sexes, and that the prevalence for both sexes increased steadily. The incidence of periodontal treatments, according to age, have been influenced by changes in the national dental policies [16, 18]. From 2002 to 2011, the prevalence among individuals less than 20 years of age was similar to previously reported rates (5–8 %) [20, 21]. However, in 2013, the incidence of periodontal treatments among those 10 to 19 years of age increased by 18.2 %. This increase is likely attributable to expansion of insurance coverage for sealant treatment for those younger than 18 years of age, and to the improved accessibility to dental services, which resulted in an increase in the number of adolescents being diagnosed with periodontal disease.

The difference between the high-incidence age group and the low-incidence age group, excluding those less

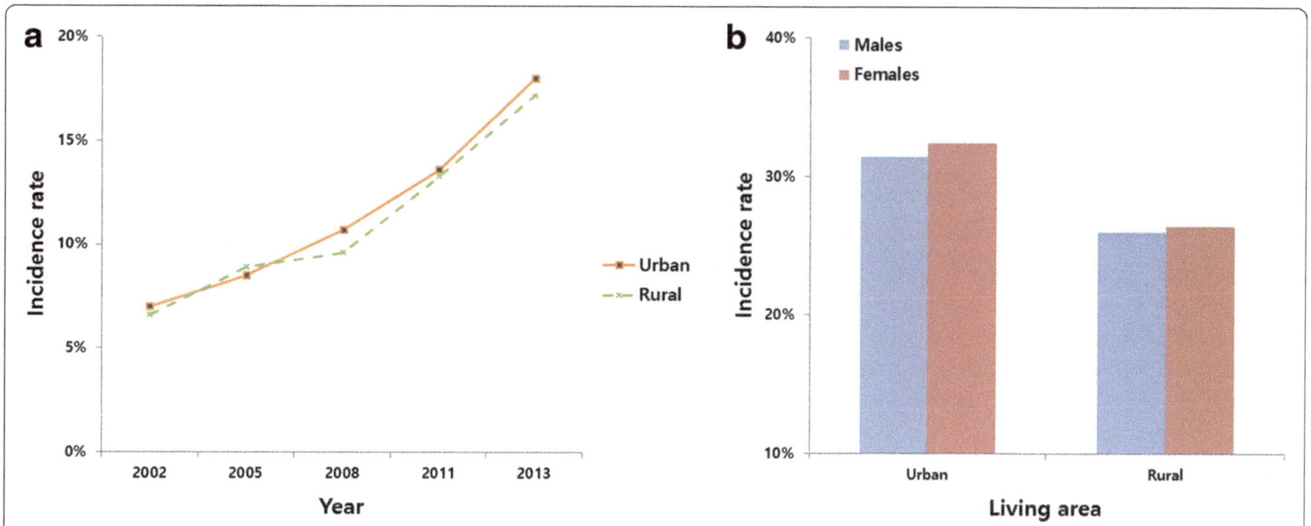

Fig. 5 Living area-specific 1-year prevalence rates of incidence rates of periodontal treatment (**a**); and sex-specific accumulated incidence rates of periodontal treatment (**b**) during 2002–2013 in South Korea

Table 2 Association of sociodemographic factors with periodontal treatments in univariate and multivariate analyses

	Univariate analysis				Multivariate analysis			
	OR		95 % CI	*P*	OR[a]		95 % CI	*P*
Sex								
Male	1.00	ref			1.00	ref		
Female	1.05		1.04–1.05	<0.001	1.00		1.00–1.01	0.513
Age group (years)								
≤ 9	1.00	ref			1.00	ref		
10–19	3.35		3.27–3.43	<0.001	3.50		3.41–3.58	<0.001
20–29	5.10		4.98–5.21	<0.001	5.19		5.07–5.32	<0.001
30–39	8.10		7.92–8.28	<0.001	7.72		7.55–7.90	<0.001
40–49	11.02		10.77–11.26	<0.001	9.58		9.36–9.81	<0.001
50–59	10.61		10.36–10.86	<0.001	8.39		8.18–8.60	<0.001
60–69	6.05		5.90–6.20	<0.001	4.67		4.54–4.80	<0.001
≥ 70	1.17		1.72–1.84	<0.001	1.64		1.58–1.70	<0.001
Household income								
First quintile	1.00	ref			1.00	ref		
Second quintile	1.11		1.09–1.13	<0.001	1.02		1.00–1.04	0.029
Third quintile	1.15		1.14–1.17	<0.001	1.10		1.08–1.12	<0.001
Fourth quintile	1.22		1.20–1.23	<0.001	1.18		1.16–1.20	<0.001
Fifth quintile	1.49		1.47–1.51	<0.001	1.37		1.35–1.39	<0.001
Insurance status								
MAP	1.00	ref			1.00	ref		
NHIS, employees	2.66		2.58–2.74	<0.001	1.93		1.86–2.00	<0.001
NHIS, self-employed	2.42		2.34–2.50	<0.001	1.65		1.59–1.71	<0.001
Health status								
Healthy	1.00	ref			1.00	ref		
Major disability	0.54		0.51–0.56	<0.001	0.61		0.58–0.64	<0.001
Minor disability	1.14		1.10–1.17	<0.001	0.94		0.91–0.97	<0.001
Living area								
Urban	1.00	ref			1.00	ref		
Rural	0.77		0.76–0.78	<0.001	0.85		0.83–0.86	<0.001

OR Odds ratio, *NHIS* National health insurance service, *MAP* Medical aid program
[a]OR, calculated by multivariate

than 9 years of age, can be explained by limited accessibility to dental services [7, 22]. In 2013, with the expansion of dental insurance coverage to include dentures and implants the incidence of periodontal treatments was expected to increase for individuals over 70 years of age. The incidence of periodontal treatments was lower in individuals with severe disabilities, and those living in rural areas. Although previous studies report the incidence of periodontitis was higher in the elderly and low-income individuals, the present study did not confirm these results. Decreased accessibility to dental services, due to individual socio-demographic characteristics, and lifestyle risk factors, may explain the different results [22]. Factors such as SES, health behaviors, and general health problems are associated with tooth loss. The main socio-demographic factors associated with tooth loss are, older age, low income, and low education level. Other oral-health-related factors, such as smoking, inadequate brushing habits, noncompliance with dental treatment, and poor dental knowledge, are also associated with tooth loss. General health factors related to tooth loss include coronary heart disease, diabetes, high blood sugar level, and limited physical activity [7, 8].

South Korea is an ethnically and culturally a homogeneous nation. In 2014, the population included only 3 % foreigners, mostly Mongoloid Chinese [23]. Therefore, unlike multiethnic countries, there are few racial barriers present in South Korea; hence, economic barriers are considered to be the most important factors restricting access to dental health-care services [24]. To overcome the SES disparities, various public health and insurance policies have been implemented. However, our study found that the disadvantaged groups still experience difficulties in accessing dental treatment. The incidence of periodontal treatments was 25.4 % among male patients in the first quintile of household income, and 36.1 % among those in the fifth quartile; the corresponding rates for female patients were 28.7 % and 35.4 %. This difference is attributed to an excessive number of voluntary non-reimbursable dental treatments, even when patients are covered by health insurance.

Prior to 2008, the incidence of periodontal treatments was significantly lower in the MAP group when compared to the NHIS group (comprising employees and self-employed). The incidence of periodontal treatments has increased in the MAP group since 2008, and it was similar (14.1 %) to that in the NHIS group. This increase is likely associated with 2008 changes in public health and insurance policies, which included the secondary poor population into the NHIS group. Policy changes were aimed at moderating the rapid increases in public expenditure on the MAP; however, these changes had no effect on the incidence of periodontal treatment in the MAP group.

Periodontal disease is characterized by chronic, irreversible, and progressive periodontal tissue destruction. Early detection of PD tends to be difficult, due to the absence of symptoms and lack of pain in early disease [25]. In addition, although still controversial, several studies have found a relationship between PD and comorbidities, such as cardiovascular disease, diabetes, premature birth, erectile dysfunction, and Alzheimer's disease [26, 27]. The incidence of periodontal treatments in the present study increased from 2002 to 2013. This increase is likely due to improvements in accessibility to dental health-care service, rather than an increase in the number of periodontally compromised patients.

The paradigm for dental insurance policies has changed in recent years, to focus on prevention and early diagnosis. Specifically, since 2013, there has been an expansion of dental insurance coverage to include periodontal scaling, dentures, and dental implants and it is expected that the incidence of periodontal treatments will continue to increase. Our study did not evaluate dental records or include detailed diagnostic codes, which limited the ability to diagnose the severity of PD. In addition, although there are still many uninsured voluntary non-reimbursable treatments for dental care, these data are not included in the KNHICD. These issues represent a limitation of the analysis performed in the present study. Nevertheless, in order to evaluate changes in the incidence of periodontal treatments, we used a precisely extracted cohort from the KNHICD, which includes data from all citizens of South Korea, as well as information from medical institutions. The results of this study suggest that national dental policies and socio-demographic factors are closely related to changes in the incidence of periodontal treatments, suggesting that this study will be useful in establishing dental policies that decrease the incidence of PD, and enhance the oral health of the entire population of South Korea.

Conclusions

Based on data in the KNHICD from 2002 to 2013, this study shows that the incidence of periodontal treatments has increased steadily, in both male and female patients, in South Korea. This study shows that the national dental policies and socio-demographic factors are clearly related to the incidence of periodontal treatments. Specifically, expansion of insurance coverage for dental treatments appears to be related to the increased incidence of periodontal treatment.

Abbreviations

DB: Database; ICD: International classification of disease; KCD: Korean classification of disease; KNHICD: Korean national health insurance cohort database; MAP: Medical aid program; NHANES: National health and nutrition examination survey; NHIS: National health insurance service; OECD: Organization for economic cooperation and development; PD: Periodontal disease; SES: Socioeconomic status

Acknowledgements

This study used a national sample cohort data of the National Health Insurance Service (NHIS-2016-3-005).

Funding

This research was supported by Wonkwang University in 2016.

Authors' contributions

JHL prepared the initial drafts of the manuscript. All authors contributed to the study design and oversight. JHL, JSL, JKC, HIK, YTK, and SHC conducted the data collection. JHL and JKC conducted the analyses. YTK and SHC are supervisor of the study and assisted in drafting of the manuscript. All authors contributed to the manuscript refinement and are responsible for its content. All authors read and approved the final manuscript.

Authors' information

JHL, Department of Periodontology, Daejeon Dental Hospital, Wonkwang University College of Dentistry, JSL and SHC, Department of Periodontology, Research Institute for Periodontal Regeneration, Yonsei University College of Dentistry, JKC, Department of Health Insurance Research, Ilsan Hospital, National Health Insurance Service, HIK and YTK, Department of Periodontology, Ilsan Hospital, National Health Insurance Service.

Competing interests

The authors declare that they have no competing interests.

Consent for publication

Not applicable.

Ethics approval and consent to participate
All cohort data was anonymous and the project was approved by the NHIS Ilsan Hospital, Goyang, Korea. An ethical approval was also obtained by the NHIS Ilsan Hospital (approval #2016-03-019).

Author details
[1]Department of Periodontology, Daejeon Dental Hospital, Wonkwang University College of Dentistry, Daejeon 35233, South Korea. [2]Department of Periodontology, Research Institute for Periodontal Regeneration, Yonsei University College of Dentistry, 50 Yonsei-ro, Seodaemun-gu, Seoul 03722, South Korea. [3]Department of Health Insurance Research, Ilsan Hospital, National Health Insurance Service, Goyang 10444, South Korea. [4]Department of Periodontology, Ilsan Hospital, National Health Insurance Service, 100 Ilsan-ro Ilsan-donggu, Goyang 10444, South Korea.

References
1. Petersen PE. The World Oral Health Report 2003: Continuous improvement of oral. Community Dent Oral Epidemiol. 2003;31(1):3–23.
2. Vettore MV, Faerstein E, Baker SR. Social position, social ties and adult's oral health: 13 year cohort study. J Dent. 2016;44:50–6.
3. Kim DW, Park JC, Rim TT, Jung UW, Kim CS, Donos N, et al. Socioeconomic disparities of periodontitis in Koreans based on the KNHANES IV. Oral Dis. 2014;20:551–9.
4. Akhter R, Hassan NMM, Aida J, Zaman KU, Morita M. Risk indicators for tooth loss due to caries and periodontal disease in recipients of free dental treatment in an adult population in Bangladesh. Oral Health Prev Dent. 2008;6:199–207.
5. Tonetti MS, Chapple ILC, Jepsen S, Sanz M. Primary and secondary prevention of periodontal and peri-implant diseases Introduction to, and objectives of the 11th European Workshop on Periodontology consensus conference. J Clin Periodontol. 2015;42 Suppl 16:1–4.
6. Outpatient disease statistics [Internet]. Health Insurance Review & Assessment Service. Available at http://opendata.hira.or.kr/op/opc/olapHifrqSickInfo.do. Accessed 17 Oct 2016.
7. Celeste RK. Contextual effect of socioeconomic status influences chronic periodontitis. J Evid Based Dent Pract. 2007;7:29–30.
8. Celeste RK, Nadanovsky P, De Leon AP, Fritzell J. The individual and contextual pathways between oral health and income inequality in Brazilian adolescents and adults. Soc Sci Med. 2009;69:1468–75.
9. Gil-Montoya JA, De Mello ALF, Barrios R, Gonzalez-Moles MA, Bravo M. Oral health in the elderly patient and its impact on general well-being: a nonsystematic review. Clin Interv Aging. 2015;10:461–7.
10. Moore PA, Weyant RJ, Mongelluzzo MB, Myers DE, Rossie K, Guggenheimer J, et al. Type 1 diabetes mellitus and oral health: assessment of periodontal disease. J Periodontol. 1999;70:409–17.
11. Steele J, Shen J, Tsakos G, Fuller E, Morris S, Watt R, et al. The interplay between socioeconomic inequalities and clinical oral health. J Dent Res. 2015;94:19–26.
12. Tseveenjav B, Suominen AL, Vehkalahti MM. Oral health-related behaviours among dentate adults in Finland: findings from the Finnish Health 2000 Survey. Eur J Oral Sci. 2012;120:54–60.
13. Morales A, Carvajal P, Romanelli H, Gomez M, Loha C, Esper ME, et al. Prevalence and predictors for clinical attachment loss in adolescents in Latin America: Cross-sectional study. J Clin Periodontol. 2015;42:900–7.
14. Kossioni AE. Current status and trends in oral health in community dwelling older adults: a global perspective. Oral Health Prev Dent. 2013;11:331–40.
15. Korean statistical information service [Internet]. Statistics Korea. accessed on 17 October 2016; Available at Outpatient disease statistics [Internet]. Health Insurance Review & Assessment Service. Available at http://kosis.kr/statisticsList/statisticsList_01List.jsp?vwcd=MT_ZTITLE&parmTabId=M_01_01. Accessed 17 Oct 2016.
16. Eke PI, Dye BA, Wei L, Slade GD, Thornton-Evans GO, Borgnakke WS, et al. Update on prevalence of periodontitis in adults in the United States: NHANES 2009 to 2012. J Periodontol. 2015;86:611–22.
17. Laaksonen M, Prattala R, Lahelma E. Sociodemographic determinants of multiple unhealthy behaviours. Scand J Public Health. 2003;31:37–43.
18. Lee MY, Chang SJ, Kim CB, Chung WG, Choi EM, Kim NH. Community periodontal treatment needs in South Korea. Int J Dent Hyg. 2015;13:254–60.
19. Armitage GC. Development of a classification system for periodontal diseases and conditions. Ann Periodontol. 1999;4:1–6.
20. Jenkins WM, Papapanou PN. Epidemiology of periodontal disease in children and adolescents. Periodontol. 2001;26:16–32.
21. Albandar JM, Tinoco EM. Global epidemiology of periodontal diseases in children and young persons. Periodontol. 2002;29:153–76.
22. Jung SH, Ryu JI, Jung DB. Association of total tooth loss with socio-behavioural health indicators in Korean elderly. J Oral Rehabil. 2011;38:517–24.
23. Kim SH, Han MS, Kim W, Kim W. Y chromosome homogeneity in the Korean population. Int J Legal Med. 2010;124:653–7.
24. Long SK, Karpman M, Kenney GM, Wissoker D, Anderson N, Zuckerman S. Taking Stock: Health Insurance Coverage under the ACA as of December 2014. Urban Institute. 2015.
25. Pihlstrom BL, Michalowicz BS, Johnson NW. Periodontal diseases. Lancet. 2005;366:1809–20.
26. Kebschull M, Demmer RT, Papapanou PN. "Gum bug, leave my heart alone!"–epidemiologic and mechanistic evidence linking periodontal infections and atherosclerosis. J Dent Res. 2010;89:879–902.
27. Lee JH, Lee JS, Park JY, Choi JK, Kim DW, Kim YT, et al. Association of lifestyle-related comorbidities with periodontitis: a nationwide cohort study in Korea. Medicine (Baltimore). 2015;94:e1567.

9

A pilot randomised controlled trial evaluating mini and conventional implant retained dentures on the function and quality of life of patients with an edentulous mandible

Sarra Jawad[1*], Craig Barclay[1], William Whittaker[2], Martin Tickle[3] and Tanya Walsh[3]

Abstract

Background: Total tooth loss (edentulism) can be a debilitating condition, impacting on ability to chew, speak and interact with others. The most common treatment is with complete removable dentures, which may be successful, but in the lower jaw, bone resorption that worsens over time makes denture-wearing difficult. Two dental implants in the mandible to retain the lower denture has been advocated as the gold standard of treatment, but has not been universally provided due largely to financial constraints and also patient fear. Mini implants (MI) are cheaper and less invasive than conventional implants (CI), but may not have equivalent longevity. Therefore, it is unknown whether they represent a cost-effective treatment modality over time. The aim of this pilot randomised controlled trial was to assess the feasibility of carrying out a trial on this cohort of patients, and to inform the study design of a large multicentre trial.

Methods: Forty-six patients were randomly allocated to receive either two mini implants or two conventional implants in the mandible to retain their lower dentures. Quality of life (QoL) questionnaires, pain and anxiety scores, and an objective "gummy jelly" chewing test were carried out at multiple timepoints, along with detailed health economics information. Implants were placed one-stage, and an early loading protocol was utilised. Patients were reviewed 8 weeks post-placement, and finally at 6 months. Implant failure, recruitment and retention rates were recorded and analysed.

Results: The pilot study demonstrated that it is possible to recruit, randomise and retain edentulous (mainly elderly) patients for an implant trial. We recruited to target and retention rates were acceptable. The large number of questionnaires was onerous for participants to complete, but the distribution of scores and feedback from participants helped inform the choice of primary and secondary outcomes in a full trial. The chewing test was time-consuming and inconsistent. Implant failure rate was low (1/46). The data on indirect costs gathered at every visit was viewed as repetitive and unnecessary, as there was little or no change between visits.

Conclusions: The pilot study has shown that acceptable recruitment and retention rates are achievable in this population of patients for this intervention. The results provide valuable information for selection of outcome variables and sample size calculations for future trials.
(Continued on next page)

* Correspondence: sarra.jawad@manchester.ac.uk
[1]Department of Restorative Dentistry, University Dental Hospital of Manchester, Higher Cambridge Street, Manchester M15 6FH, UK
Full list of author information is available at the end of the article

(Continued from previous page)

Trial registration: (ISRCTN): 87342238 Trial registration date: 05/07/2013.

Keywords: Dental implant, Edentulous, Complete overdenture, Randomised controlled trial, Mini implant, Quality of life, Masticatory efficiency

Background

The World Health Organisation (WHO) considers edentulism (total tooth loss) a physical disability [1, 2]. The majority of edentulous patients are able to chew their food with complete dentures but over time, the lower jaw becomes resorbed and there is less bone to retain the lower denture. This makes it more difficult to retain the denture which causes problems for the denture-wearer, such as difficulties in eating and speaking, which may lead to a change in lifestyle, as those affected become embarrassed to socialise and eat with friends [3]. Furthermore, their inability to chew results in poorer food choices [4, 5] with many opting for highly calorific softer foods that are easier to eat. This undoubtedly affects their nutrition and thus general health. All of these factors have been shown to impact greatly on a patient's quality of life [6].

The dental literature is awash with papers showing significant improvements in quality of life in edentulous patients who have two dental implants placed in their lower jaw to secure their lower dentures [6–15]. Indeed there are national and international consensus statements that this treatment modality should be the first line of treatment for patients with an edentulous mandible [16, 17]. However, this treatment is costly for both individual patients and health services around the world to provide. Furthermore, surgery to place implants is invasive [18], and this can pose a barrier to treatment even when provided free of charge [19, 20]. Edentulous patients are often older people (over 65 years) and may have significant bone resorption in their lower jaw and complex medical histories, which may affect their suitability for implant treatment.

Mini dental implants have been in use for the last 12 years [21–36] and offer a number of advantages over conventional implants: they have a smaller diameter (<2.4 mm) and are often made of a titanium alloy (Ti 6Al-4 V ELI) as opposed to commercially pure titanium (type 4) used in conventional dental implants. They are often placed using a minimally invasive technique, resulting in less post-operative pain [37]; and are therefore approximately a quarter of the cost of current conventional alternatives [21, 22]. These advantages need to be considered against a potentially higher failure rate [38] when compared to conventional implants, which have an impressively high survival rate over 10 years [15], and possibly a need for more intensive on-going maintenance [39].

There is a lack of high quality evidence of the effects of mini implants compared to conventional implants in retaining mandibular complete dentures [39, 40]. The primary aim of this study was to assess the feasibility of conducting a large surgical randomized controlled trial of mini versus conventional implants in a population of patients who can benefit from an implant- retained lower denture. The identified key areas of uncertainty to be explored in this trial focused upon the processes of recruitment and retention of participants, choice of clinical, quality of life and cost outcome measures and their method of capture. The objectives were specifically to determine:

- The proportion of referred patients that were eligible to participate, consented to the trial and provided data at all time-points;
- Whether masticatory functional ability could be measured using a validated 'gummy jelly' chewing test;
- The completeness and variability of using different instruments to collect data on pain, QoL, implant failure; and
- How to collect and measure costs

Methods

Design and eligibility criteria

The pilot trial was a two-arm parallel group randomised controlled pilot trial. Full ethical approval was obtained from the National Health Service Health Research Authority, National Research Ethics Service, Research Ethics Committee (ref: REC 13/NW/0384), and the study clinicians collected informed consent. All edentulous patients experiencing difficulties with their lower dentures, referred to the University Dental Hospital of Manchester or from internal referrals from hospital consultants, were initially screened for eligibility from the referral letters. Potentially eligible participants were booked onto consultation clinics for full medical history and clinical examination. Patients with an edentulous mandible, with residual mandibular ridge Cawood and Howell Class V or VI [41] with continued difficulties eating, even after the provision of new dentures, were eligible to participate. Patients with a history of bisphosphonate therapy or implant treatment, requiring sedation or general anaesthetic for implant placement, smokers, or patients unable to maintain adequate levels of oral hygiene were excluded.

Randomisation

The Clinical Trials Unit centrally randomised patients to one of two treatment groups with a 1:1 allocation ratio using random permuted blocks. A study clinician enrolled participants onto the trial and assigned participants to interventions according to the randomisation. The clinician performing the implant placement and health economist could not be blinded to treatment allocation; the research nurse (who collected masticatory efficiency and patient rated outcome data) and the trial statistician were blinded.

Treatment procedures

All patients were given an oral loading dose of 2 mg Amoxicillin (or 600 mg Clindamycin if allergic to penicillin) as per best current evidence [42]. All patients were asked to rinse for 60 s with Chlorhexidine (0.2%) mouthwash (with both dentures removed) and given local anaesthetic using 2% lignocaine + 1:80,000 adrenaline infiltrated into the anterior mandible.

Mini-implant (MI)

Two mini implants (3 M® 2.1 mm diameter, 10 mm length one-piece implant with a square collar and ball abutment) were placed transmucosally (flapless) in the interforamina region of the edentulous mandible.

Conventional implant (CI)

Two conventional (ASTRA TECH® Osseospeed 3 mm diameter, 11 mm length) implants were placed in the interforamina region of the edentulous mandible. These were placed after raising soft tissue flaps and drilling directly into bone. Ball abutments were placed on the conventional implants in a one-stage surgery approach to mimic the mini-implant attachment system.

Following surgery, all patients were given oral and written post-operative instructions and advised not to wear their lower dentures for 1 week. All patients were given 24 × 500 mg Paracetamol tablets to take as required. At 1 week postoperatively participants' lower dentures were hollowed out chair-side so they could fit over the exposed ball abutments. Therefore, lower dentures could be worn but the implants were not directly loaded. At the 2-month review appointment an impression was taken of the implant ball abutments using a polyether impression material (Impregum™ Penta™ 3 M ESPE) in the patient's lower complete denture. The denture was retrofitted with stud attachments on the same day by dental laboratory technicians using heat-cured acrylic.

Outcomes

Multiple outcome measures were assessed in accordance with the objectives of the study and as per the schedule below (Table 1). The primary outcomes of this study were feasibility outcomes. The feasibility of a main trial using the same study design and protocol was assessed according to the objectives of the pilot trial: recruitment and retention of trial participants; use of outcome measures and collection of cost data.

- The feasibility of recruitment was measured in terms of eligibility (the proportion of eligible patients from the number of screened patients), recruitment (the proportion of recruited patients from the number of eligible patients), and whether the required sample size could be met within the designated 12-month recruitment period. The success of patient retention was measured in terms of compliance with randomisation (the proportion of participants receiving their allocated treatment) completeness of follow-up (the proportion of patients providing 6 month follow up data). The denominator was the number of patients randomised.
- The feasibility of using masticatory efficiency as an effectiveness outcome was assessed as the number of 'gummy jelly' samples that were provided, and were able to be analysed.
- The appropriateness of the different outcome measures was assessed quantitatively in terms of proportion of completed questionnaires, and qualitatively in variation, absence of floor or ceiling effects and variability of responses over time.
- The feasibility and appropriateness of collecting cost information was assessed based on the proportions of completed patient questionnaires (patient costs) and completed health care costs, and the recording of unanticipated resource use.

Formal hypothesis testing for effectiveness was not be undertaken as the aim of a pilot trial is not to assess effectiveness and as such the study is underpowered for this purpose.

Sample size

As this was a pilot trial a formal sample size calculation was not appropriate. We estimated that of those patients screened and meeting the inclusion criteria, 50% would agree to participate. A total of 44 patients (22 in each arm) would have a 95% confidence interval ranging from 35% to 65% of patients who will agree to participate. A recruitment target was set at 44 patients or 1 year of recruitment, whichever endpoint was reached soonest.

Statistical analysis

It was not our intention to compare treatment groups and we did not test hypotheses. Cumulative and monthly (to assess season variation) recruitment figures were

Table 1 Outcome measures and timing of measurement

	Baseline	At operation	24 h	1 week	2 months	6 months
Anxiety: Modified Dental Anxiety Scale [64]	X					
Quality of Life: Oral Health Impact-Profile-EDENT [53, 65] Euroqol-5D(EQ-5D) [44, 66] SF-12 [67]	X				X	X
Satisfaction with dentures: The University of Newcastle 'Assessment of Prosthesis' questionnaire	X				X	X
Masticatory function: 'gummy jelly' chewing test	X				X	X
Pain: Visual Analogue Scale (VAS) or Verbal Rating Scale (VRS) (0–10)		X	X	X		
Use of analgesics (professionally and self prescribed) and antibiotics	X		X	X	X	X
Direct costs-staffing[a]		X				
Direct costs-equipment[a]		X				
Direct costs-consumables[a]		X				
Indirect costs[a]		X		X		
Healthcare utilisation[a]		X	X	X	X	X
Assessment of adverse events[a]		X	X	X	X	X
Assessment for possible implant failure				X	X	X

[a]data also to be collected at unscheduled visits

calculated, as were loss to follow up at 2 and 6 months post-surgery. Descriptive analyses were undertaken for a 12 month period (covering the period 6 months prior to the study start and the 6 months follow up) to identify the total number of referrals, the number and proportion of participants who attended for assessment, and the number and proportion of patients who required implants after fitting a new set of conventional complete dentures. Simple descriptive statistics involving calculation of ranges, frequency distributions and measures of central tendency and dispersion were used to assess the completeness and variability of clinical, quality of life and cost outcome measures collected at each time point.

The health economics analysis presents the resources recorded and their respective unit costs. Costs were calculated from the National Health Service (NHS) and social care provider perspective, secondary analysis includes costs from the patient perspective, and this approach approximates a societal perspective. The time trade-off (TTO) measurement for weighting the EQ-5D was used, as this is the recommended utility weight advocated by the National Institute for Health and Care Excellence NICE [43]. The TTO weights are obtained from Dolan (1997) [44]. The SF-12 was mapped onto the SF-6D (since the SF-6D has Health-Related QoL weights). SF-6D weights were obtained from Brazier and Roberts (2004) [45].

Results

The recruitment and retention of participants from screening through to 6-month follow-up is shown in Fig. 1. Of note is that only 81/181 of those referred were eligible for the study, and of the 73 patients for whom new complete dentures were made, 12 were relatively satisfied with their new lower denture and declined further treatment. Furthermore, only four patients who were dissatisfied with their new denture did not want to be randomised, having a preference for mini-implants (three patients) or conventional implants (one patient). Of the 46 patients randomized 43 (93.5%) completed the trial.

Although the initial plan was to recruit a maximum of 44 participants or as many participants as possible in the planned 1-year recruitment period, in total 46 patients were recruited and randomised (further ethical approval was provided to recruit the additional participants). The median number of patients recruited per month was three and the monthly and cumulative recruitment figures are summarised in Fig. 2. The maximum number of patients recruited in a single month was six patients

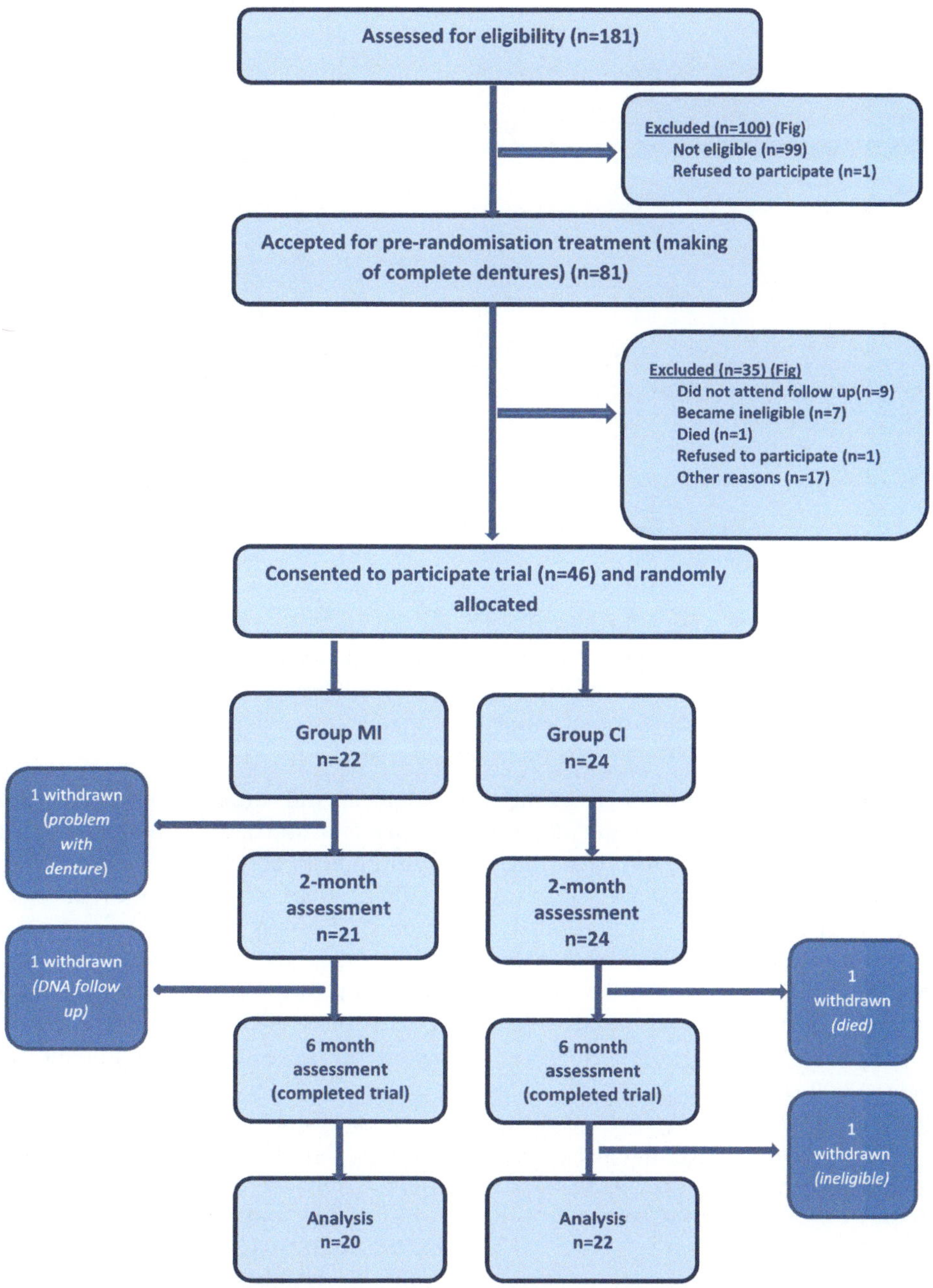

Fig. 1 Flow diagram showing recruitment and retention

(June 2014); the minimum number of patients recruited was one (February 2014 and September 2014).

During the trial there was one protocol violation. During analysis it transpired that one patient was taking bisphosphonates a concomitant medication that that was not fully disclosed at recruitment. This patient was not included in the analyses. Table 2 shows the baseline characteristics of the trial participants.

Table 3 presents the clinical and patient rates of oral health quality of life outcomes. No participants refused to take the 'gummy jelly' test and we were able to measure the glucose released from all samples. The pattern of results for the 'gummy jelly' test did not reflect those of the OHIP-20 or subjective assessment of chewing ability (see Fig. 5.) However, due to differences in batch composition the glucose released at 6 months was not comparable to baseline or 2 month measures.

Pain VAS scores recorded immediately post-op and after 1 week post-op are presented in Fig. 3. The range of scores was wider in the conventional implant group compared to the mini implant group; this difference in distribution was most notable 1 week post-operatively.

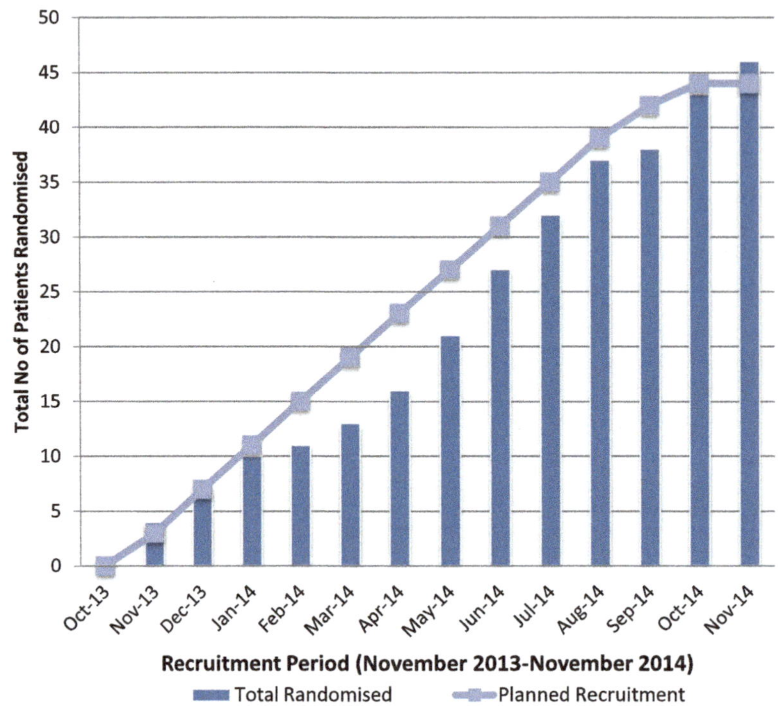

Fig. 2 Bar chart showing actual recruitment versus projected recruitment (line graph)

Clinician and patient reported analgesic consumption, at face value, was also higher in the CI group compared to the MI group during the surgical procedure and at 1 week post-surgery.

The results of the OHIP-20 scores are presented in Fig. 4. There was downward trend in OHIP QoL scores in both groups at 6-month follow up compared to baseline suggesting an improvement in oral health related quality of life.

The denture satisfaction questionnaire records different aspects of patient satisfaction with their prosthesis using a 100 mm VAS. The scales are anchored by the extremes of potential responses (e.g., not at all satisfied to extremely satisfied). Higher values indicate a positive response and improvement. The distributions of responses for each domain of the prosthesis assessment questionnaire are shown in Fig. 5.

Table 2 Summary statistics at baseline for patients analysed[a]

	Mini implants ($n = 22$)	Conventional implants ($n = 23$)	Total ($n = 45$)
Age	68.5 (9.5) 68.5, 63 to 74 52 to 88	68.1 (8.5) 71, 61 to 74 48 to 79	68.3 (8.9) 70, 62 to 74 48 to 88
Gender	10 male (45.5%)	9 male (39.1%)	19 male (42.2%)
Years edentulous	26.0 (20.8) 32, 3 to 45 1 to 58	20.2 (17.7) 14, 5 to 38 1 to 57	23.1 (19.3) 15, 5 to 40 1 to 58
Anxiety (Modified Dental Anxiety Scale)	10.8 (3.8) 11, 8 to 14 5 to 17	11.6 (6.6) 9, 6 to 15 5 to 25	11.2 (5.4) 10, 7 to 14 5 to 25

[a]Values are mean and standard deviation along with median, interquartile range, minimum and maximum for age, number of years edentulous and anxiety

There were no adverse events reported in the MI group. CI group had 4 adverse events (8.9%). One was due to pain, and three due to infection. All were treated medically with painkillers and antibiotics as appropriate. One patient died during the follow-up period, from a condition unrelated to treatment. No other Serious Adverse Events were recorded.

There was a total of 74 unscheduled visits in 45 patients (mean 1.7, range 0 to 6): In the MI group there were 23 implant-related visits, due primarily to problems with O-ring attachments, and 18 prosthesis-related visits; in the CI group there were 13 implant-related visits, 17 prosthesis related visits and 3 visits for other reasons.

The costs of the MI and C- groups are presented in Table 4. Mean NHS costs observed over the trial for MIs were lower than that for CIs (column 1 of Table 4, £296 vs. £688). The MI group had lower observed mean staff costs (£37 vs. £88), equipment and consumable costs (£181 vs. £532), and medication costs (£0.23 vs. £4.24). The MI group had higher observed mean unscheduled visits costs (£78 vs. £63) (a detailed analysis of all costs recorded and methods used to generate costs are contained in the Additional file 1).

There was a higher mean patient cost observed for the MI group (£193 vs. £156) (column 2 of Table 4). Missing

Table 3 Summary statistics for clinical and QoL outcomes

Outcome	Mini implants Baseline (n = 22)	Mini implants Operation (n = 22)	Mini implants 24 h (n = 22)	Mini implants 1 week (n = 22)	Mini implants 2 months (n = 20)	Mini implants 6 months (n = 19)	Conventional implants Baseline (n = 23)	Conventional implants Operation (n = 23)	Conventional implants 24 h (n = 23)	Conventional implants 1 week (n = 23)	Conventional implants 2 months (n = 23)	Conventional implants 6 months (n = 22)
Glucose Mean (sd)	145.18 (54.00)				193.95 (86.84)	198.84 (111.76)	185.35 (81.02)				189.21 (87.11)	187.86 (74.21)
Median (IQR)	132 (109 to 184)				172 (152 to 204)	170 (99 to 241)	164 (126 to 230)				161 (138 to 208)	180.5 (135 to 246)
Pain[a] Mean (sd)		6.5 (5.5)	3.05 (2.6)	16.8 (19.38)				11.58 (14.6)	4.3 (3.2)	38 (32.2)		
Median (IQR)		4 (3 to 10)	3 (0 to 5)	6.5 (2 to 27)				5 (3 to 15)	3 (1 to 7)	37 (7 to 69)		
Analgesic consumption		15/22 (68.18%)		8/22 (36.36%)				20/23 (86.96%)		16/23 (69.57%)		
OHIP-20[b] Mean (sd)	76.5 (20.1)				66.5 (28.3)	40.9 (18.1)	83.3 (23.1)				79.6 (24.9)	56.2 (29.6)
Median (IQR)	78.5 (60 to 92)				65 (43 to 80)	36 (25 to 58)	81 (64 to 100)				82 (58 to 105)	43 (29 to 81)
Affects general health[c]	14/22 (63.6%)				5/20 (25%)	5/19 (26.3%)	12/23 (52.2%)				7/23 (30.4%)	4/22 (18.2%)
Implant Failure					1	0					0	0

[a]Pain assessed at the end of surgery (100 mm VAS), 24 h post surgery (0 to 10 VRS) and 1 week (100 mm VAS)
[b]OHIP-20 has 20 items that are rated on six-point Likert type scales (range 1 = never to 6 = always). The total score of the scale ranges from 20 to 120 points, with lower scores indicating better oral health-related quality of life (OHRQoL). Total scores were calculated without item weighting
[c]One of the questions in the satisfaction questionnaire was whether the participants felt that their oral condition impacted on their general health

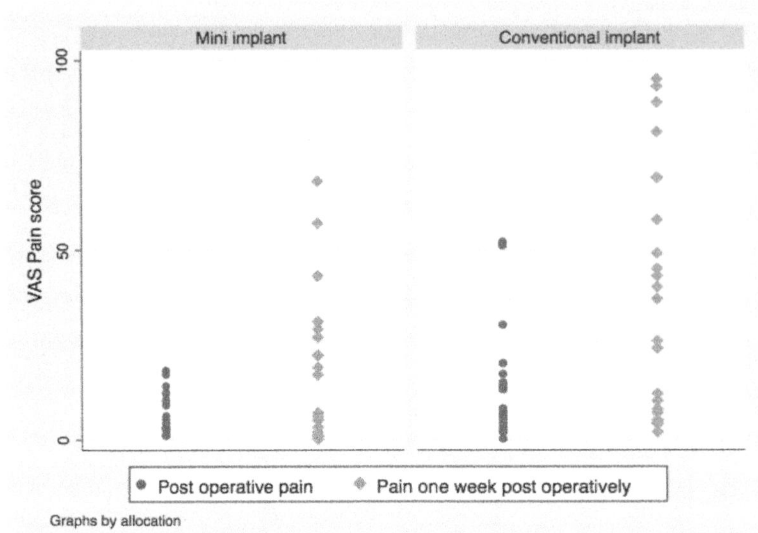

Fig. 3 Distributions of responses to pain outcome

data was evident in most patient costs; most patients reported the same costs at each visit and were perplexed that the same questions were asked at each visit. The compounding nature of missing data (since there are three instances of follow ups and numerous unscheduled visits) resulted in a final complete cost sample of 15 patients. Of these, the mean observed costs of MI were lower than that for CI (£481 vs. £814).

Table 5 presents the results of EQ-5D and SF-6D questionnaires at baseline and at 2 and 6 months assessment. A higher score represents higher health-related QoL (HRQoL). Data was complete in the sense that no missing data was apparent aside from those patients who did not complete the trial. At face value mean baseline EQ-5D and SF-6D scores were lower for the CI group compared to the MI group. Mean EQ-5D and SF-6D scores for both groups showed little variation at 6 months follow-up compared to baseline. Comparisons of changes in EQ-5D and SF-6D scores from baseline to 6 months assessment for those completing the trial suggest reductions in EQ-5D score for both implant groups. For SF-6D scores there appears to be higher mean SF-6D scores at 6 months compared to baseline for the CI group and a reduction in mean scores for the MI group.

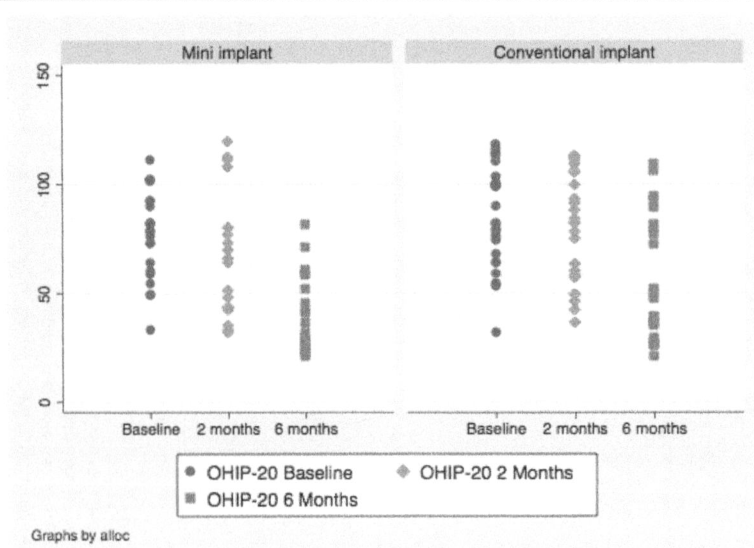

Fig. 4 Distributions of responses to OHIP-20 outcome

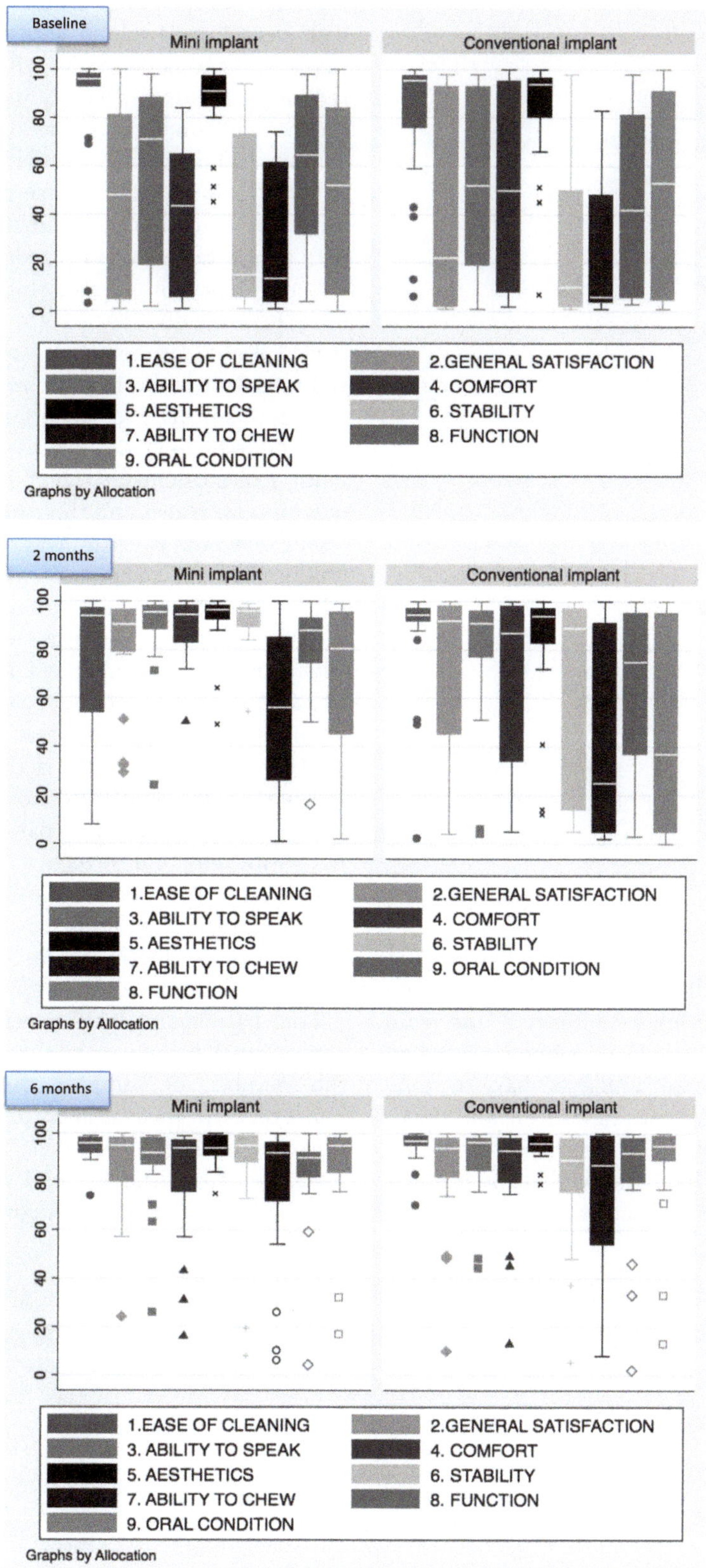

Fig. 5 Distributions for each domain of the prosthesis assessment questionnaire (Baseline, 2 months, 6 months)

Table 4 Cost information

	NHS cost	Patient cost	NHS and patient cost
Mini implants			
Mean	296.09	193.22	480.60
Sd	126.93	119.91	249.89
Count	22	7	7
Median	237.33	178.58	389.19
IQR	218.19 to 370.16	112.70 to 248.09	330.81 to 635.33
Range	194.41 to 736.72	62.73 to 430.23	277.90 to 984.82
Conventional implants			
Mean	688.30	155.57	813.99
Sd	124.17	70.68	93.62
Count	23	8	8
Median	655.31	157.89	823.17
IQR	628.13 to 687.45	106.73 to 198.26	750.10 to 860.51
Range	585.75 to 1189.69	54.07 to 264.72	676.53 to 967.84
Overall			
Mean	496.56	173.14	658.41
Sd	233.90	95.07	246.54
Count	45	15	15
Median	607.63	170.26	696.81
IQR	239.68 to 656.03	112.70 to 222.36	389.19 to 847.45
Range	194.41 to 1189.69	54.07 to 430.23	277.90 to 984.82

Discussion

Overview of the findings

This paper reports the findings of a National Institute for Health Research (NIHR)-funded pilot trial, the main purpose of which was to inform the design and conduct of future trials. Conventional implants have a long history and their clinical outcomes have been well documented [46–50]. Over the last 30 years, successive Adult Dental Health Surveys [51] have shown that the number of edentulous patients has fallen dramatically. The inability to retain a mandibular denture is debilitating, with dental need falling across the whole population a case could be made in the UK for NHS resources to be redirected to address the significant needs of this patient group. Mini implants could offer the NHS an effective and affordable means of providing care for this group of patients as a first line course of treatment. But to make a convincing case a high-quality, large, multi-centre trial with adequate follow up is required.

The primary aim of this study was to assess the feasibility of a conducting a large surgical randomised controlled trial as proposed in a population of patients who can benefit from an implant retained lower denture. The identified key areas of uncertainty to be explored in this trial focused upon the processes of recruitment and retention of participants, choice of clinical, QoL and cost outcome measures and their method of capture.

Our concerns over the willingness of this cohort to be randomized to different surgical options proved to be unfounded. We reached our required sample size within the pre-specified recruitment period, and very few eligible patients declined to take part in the trial because of a strong patient preference or unwillingness to be randomised. These results suggest that recruitment of participants through a major, secondary referral centre is feasible. Moreover, attrition over the 6 months duration was minimal (43 out of 46 patients (93.5%) completed the trial) with only four adverse events reported, all minor in nature and related to the surgery. However, follow up in this pilot study was limited to 6-months; in trials with a predominantly elderly sample some attrition from mortality unrelated to the intervention can be expected.

Trial participants were accepting of the test of masticatory function ('gummy jelly' test [52]) as evidenced by the number of samples provided, but the lack of consistency in measurement over time suggests that this measure is underdeveloped. Further development and evidence of repeatability and reliability is needed before the test could be used with confidence in a clinical trial.

Table 5 Health-Related Quality of Life HRQoL measures

	Mini implants				Conventional implants			
Outcome	Baseline ($n = 22$)	2 months ($n = 20$)	6 months ($n = 19$)	Baseline (complete cases, $n = 19$)	Baseline ($n = 23$)	2 months ($n = 23$)	6 months ($n = 22$)	Baseline (complete cases, $n = 22$)
EQ-5D Mean (sd)	0.7224 (0.3276)	0.7289 (0.3598)	0.7127 (0.2968)	0.7146 (0.3524)	0.6401 (0.3639)	0.5840 (0.4489)	0.6241 (0.3715)	0.6458 (0.3715)
Median (IQR)	0.7960 (0.7250 to 1.0000)	0.8050 (0.6380 to 1.000)	0.7270 (0.6200 to 1.0000)	0.7960 (0.7250 to 1.0000)	0.6560 (0.5160 to 1.0000)	0.7960 (0.0880 to 1.0000)	0.8220 (0.1890 to 1.0000)	0.6905 (0.5160 to 1.0000)
SF-6D Mean (sd)	0.7153 (0.2060)	0.6844 (0.2465)	0.6943 (0.2404)	0.7220 (0.2149)	0.6714 (0.2158)	0.6720 (0.2130)	0.7263 (0.2117)	0.6767 (0.2193)
Median (IQR)	0.7670 (0.6150 to 0.9220)	0.7580 (0.4055 to 0.8715)	0.8000 (0.4070 to 0.8800)	0.8000 (0.6150 to 0.9220)	0.7190 (0.4530 to 0.8630)	0.6900 (0.4670 to 0.8630)	0.8000 (0.4670 to 0.9220)	0.7645 (0.4530 to 0.8630)

Values are mean, standard deviation, count, median, interquartile range

All participants provided responses to pain outcome at all time-points. The data suggests we could expect to find a large difference in short-term post-operative pain scores between the groups in a definitive trial. Descriptively, the pain scores of participants in the CI group were substantially higher than participants in the MI group at 24 h and 7 days post-surgery. It would seem that 7 days post-surgery would be the optimal time for measurement and little is to be gained from measuring at both 24 h and 7 days.

Our Public Patient Involvement (PPI) group strongly recommended QoL as a primary outcome measure for any future trials in this area. Adherence to the NICE guidance for health technology appraisal requires health effects to be expressed in Quality Adjusted Life Years [43]. A key finding from our research is that the components of the generic EQ-5D and SF-6D HRQoL measures seem to show poor responsiveness to oral health-related changes in quality of life and many participants queried the relevance of the questions in these measures to an oral health intervention. A full trial may wish to utilise only one of the HRQoL measures, our data suggests SF-6D may provide some variability in the different implant groups but the EQ-5D is the preferred measure of HRQoL to aid in consistency when comparing the health effects across appraisals and so should be the measure of choice to use in future trials [43].

Data indicated that the OHIP-20 measure [3, 53, 54] and the individual items of the Assessment of Prosthesis scale [7] were sensitive to changes before and after placement of implants. The Assessment of Prosthesis scale performed as expected, with improvements between pre and post implant placement in both groups, but no apparent distinction between the two groups regarding ease of general satisfaction, cleaning, aesthetic and oral conditions. Satisfaction level was high in both groups after fitting the implants. Ability to speak, the level of comfort, stability of the dentures, perception of the chewing ability and function showed similar improvement in both groups pre and post implant placement. From a trials design perspective the lack of a single summary statistic to summarise each individual's response means that this instrument in its entirety cannot be used to calculate a trial sample size but the individual items of this measure particularly, subjective assessment of chewing ability, can provide valuable information as a secondary outcome measure in the absence of well-validated objective measures.

Responses to the OHIP questionnaire illustrated the expected improvement in oral health-related QoL and the pattern of responses in each group was very similar. This could indicate either that the effects of the interventions are indeed very similar, or that the instrument is insufficiently sensitive to detect any differences between the groups. Our view is that survival should be the primary outcome measure of a future multi-centre trial. This is the primary outcome measure of the majority of implants trials reported in Cochrane systematic reviews [42, 55–59] and will be the key determinant of clinical and economic outcomes. The literature suggests that mini implants have a lower survival rate than conventional implants [29, 34, 38, 40, 60, 61] but from the data we present seem less expensive to place and also to replace if they fail. Studies [34, 60, 61] also suggest that if an implant is going to fail it is likely to happen in the first 2–3 years, suggesting that follow up period for future trials could be confined to 3 years, which would help contain costs. Although in this pilot trial follow-up was limited to 6 months, implant failure was rare, with only one failure of a single implant in the mini implant group and no failures in the conventional implant group. A subsequent audit of longevity of mini implants placed, involving all cases completed in University Dental Hospital of Manchester Restorative Department over a 92-month period, indicates that most failures occur in the first 2–3 years following placement. A low event rate would mean that a substantial number of participants would be required to achieve adequate power for a Randomised Controlled Trial (RCT) if implant failure is the primary outcome.

The pilot trial provided important information with regard to the health economics of implant-retained dentures. Any difference in costs appears to be driven by the differences in implant (materials) costs and staff costs (reflected in staff time). Large differences in staff costs, equipment and consumable costs were evident between the groups but little difference in medication costs. The number of unscheduled visits amount to 41 for the mini implant group and 33 for the conventional implant group. Our PPI group recommended a shorter, single measure of indirect (patient-borne) costs should be used in a full trial. Unscheduled visit costs to the NHS and medication costs did not substantially differ between groups and neither did patient costs (travel, time off work etc.). This strongly suggests that in future studies measurement of costs should be mainly restricted to direct costs of treatment, whether that is borne by the state, insurance companies or individual patients. One issue that our PPI group raised, which is important for future trials to consider, is the costs of ongoing maintenance of implants in primary care. Patients reported difficulty in finding providers of ongoing care and also the high costs of maintenance both of which need to be measured and factored into health economic analyses of future trials.

Strengths and limitations

This trial had narrow inclusion criteria; only patients with the most atrophic mandibles were invited to participate (Cawood and Howell Class V or VI [41]). However, in the screening process summarised in the CONSORT flow diagram (Fig. 1.) of the 99 patients who were ineligible for inclusion 48 were excluded because their mandibular ridge was Class IV or better, but these patients still had problems retaining their lower denture. Also there is evidence [62] to demonstrate that placement of implants slows down bone resorption and so reduces the clinical problems faced by surgeons and prosthodontists. These findings strongly suggests that many more patients could benefit from implants than patients with Class V or VI ridges and points to the need for widening inclusion criteria in future large, multi-centre pragmatic trials. Broadening inclusion criteria exclusion criteria could result in a higher recruitment rate and increase applicability of findings.

Other than implant failure and chewing ability, we limited our measurements to patient reported outcomes. The rationale behind this choice was that we wanted to ensure that in addition to clinically important outcomes, we captured outcomes that were important to patients. There was uncertainty as to what patient reported outcomes would be acceptable and useable with elderly people in a secondary care setting. Conversely, there is a consensus on clinically important outcomes such as failure of the denture superstructure retained by the implants (total replacement or refurbishment needed), quality and quantity of peri-implant bone. Such measurements are routinely taken in secondary care (where the full trial would be undertaken) and so uncertainty surrounding the use of these outcome measures within an RCT is minimal.

Although the standard practice is the placement of four or more mini implants in the interforaminal region [26, 28–30, 32, 36], this study trialled the use of two, which has been shown in clinical case studies and in previous studies [25, 31] to provide equivalent retention to the recommended four. A recent RCT compared 4 mini implants with 2 mini implants with 2 conventional [63]. Further trials are required to assess the costs effectiveness of 2 versus 4 implant retained lower dentures. Although it could be argued that if mini implants fail they can be readily and cheaply replaced, however this assumption needs to be robustly evaluated in future trials.

This was a pilot trial; its purpose was to ascertain whether a full trial would be feasible and justified and to collect information to inform the design and conduct of subsequent trials. Our trial has shown that a full evaluation of 'which is more cost-effective, mini implants or conventional implants to retain a lower denture?' using the proposed design and methods we employed is feasible. The data suggest that mini implants are cheaper, have less post-operative pain and less complications than conventional implants whilst producing similar QoL improvements. However, the follow up period was too short to assess implant survival and long term cost effectiveness. The study was also restricted to one site and to have greater external validity, multi-centre trials are required in different populations with different care providers.

Conclusions

Recruitment and retention of sufficient, eligible patients to a trial within a realistic timescale is possible. There are limitations in using generic and 'disease-specific' QoL measures to evaluate effectiveness in this context. Implant survival is important for patients and has a major impact on clinical effectiveness and costs and should therefore be considered as a primary outcome measure. Outcomes should be assessed at 7 days post operatively (pain) and 6 monthly intervals (implant survival) following implant placement.

Abbreviations

CI: Conventional Implants; EQ-5D: Euroqol-5D questionnaire; HRQoL: Health-Related Quality of Life; IQR: Interquartile range; MI: Mini implants; NHS: National Health Service; NICE: National Institute for Health and Care Excellence; NIHR: National Institute for Health Research; OHIP: Oral Health Impact Profile; OHRQoL: Oral health-Related Quality of Life; PPI: Public Patient Involvement; QoL: Quality of Life; RCT: Randomised Controlled Trial; RfPB: Research for Patient Benefit; SD: Standard deviation; SF: Short Form; TTO: Time Trade-Off; VAS: Visual Analogue Scale; VRS: Verbal Rating Scale; WHO: World Health Organisation

Acknowledgements

We would like to acknowledge Dr Mark Harrison, Health Economist, for his contribution to the rationale for health economics analysis and for devising the health economics questionnaires. We would also like to acknowledge Ronnie Polak as our PPI lead. We would also like to thank members of our PPI group made up of previous implant patients who provided advice and opinions on the proposed research. We would also like to acknowledge Takahiro Ono who kindly provided the gummy jelly for the masticatory test.

Funding

The study was funded by the (NIHR) Research for Patient Benefit (RfPB) stream (£250,000) Competition 18 in May 2012 (ref: PBPG021227050). The funding body peer reviewed the study prior to its commence and made comments that contributed to its design. It had no role, however in data collection, analysis or interpretation nor in the writing of this manuscript.

Availability of data and materials

The datasets used and/or analysed during the current study available from the corresponding author on reasonable request.

Authors' contributions

All authors contributed substantially to the design and execution of the pilot study. The manuscript was prepared, revised, edited and approved by SJ, TW, MT, WW and CB. All authors are accountable for the information contained herein. All authors read and approved the final manuscript.

Competing interests
The authors all declare no competing interests in relation to this research.

Consent for publication
Not applicable.

Ethics approval and consent to participate
Full ethical approval was obtained from the National Health Service Health Research Authority, National Research Ethics Service, Research Ethics Committee (ref: REC 13/NW/0384), and the study clinicians collected informed consent from all participants in writing.

Author details
[1]Department of Restorative Dentistry, University Dental Hospital of Manchester, Higher Cambridge Street, Manchester M15 6FH, UK. [2]Division of Population Health, Health Services Research and Primary Care, School of Health Sciences, University of Manchester, Manchester, UK. [3]Division of Dentistry, Faculty of Biology, Medicine and Health, University of Manchester, Manchester, UK.

References

1. Organization WH. International classification of functioning, disability and health: ICF: World Health Organization. 2001.
2. Petersen PE, Bourgeois D, Ogawa H, Estupinan-Day S, Ndiaye C. The global burden of oral diseases and risks to oral health. Bull World Health Org Suppl. 2005;83(9):661–9.
3. Heydecke G, Locker D, Awad MA, Lund JP, Feine JS. Oral and general health-related quality of life with conventional and implant dentures. Community Dent Oral Epidemiol. 2003;31(3):161–8. Epub 2003/05/20. eng.
4. De Marchi RJ, Hugo FN, Padilha DM, Hilgert JB, Machado DB, Durgante PC, et al. Edentulism, use of dentures and consumption of fruit and vegetables in south Brazilian community-dwelling elderly. J Oral Rehabil. 2011;38(7): 533–40. Epub 2011/01/05. eng.
5. Gunne H-SJ, Wall A-K. The effect of new complete dentures on mastication and dietary intake. Acta Odontol. 1985;43(5):257–68.
6. Emami E, Heydecke G, Rompre PH, de Grandmont P, Feine JS. Impact of implant support for mandibular dentures on satisfaction, oral and general health-related quality of life: a meta-analysis of randomized-controlled trials. Clin Oral Implants Res. 2009;20(6):533–44. Epub 2009/06/12. eng.
7. Allen PF, Thomason JM, Jepson NJ, Nohl F, Smith DG, Ellis J. A randomized controlled trial of implant-retained mandibular overdentures. J Dent Res. 2006;85(6):547–51. Epub 2006/05/26. eng.
8. Awad MA, Lund JP, Dufresne E, Feine JS. Comparing the efficacy of mandibular implant-retained overdentures and conventional dentures among middle-aged edentulous patients: satisfaction and functional assessment. Int J Prosthodont. 2003;16(2):117–22. Epub 2003/05/10. eng.
9. Kapur KK, Garrett NR, Hamada MO, Roumanas ED, Freymiller E, Han T, et al. Randomized clinical trial comparing the efficacy of mandibular implant-supported overdentures and conventional dentures in diabetic patients. Part III: comparisons of patient satisfaction. J Prosthet Dent. 1999;82(4):416–27. Epub 1999/10/08. eng.
10. Fueki K, Kimoto K, Ogawa T, Garrett NR. Effect of implant-supported or retained dentures on masticatory performance: a systematic review. J Prosthet Dent. 2007;98(6):470–7. Epub 2007/12/07. eng.
11. Rashid F, Awad MA, Thomason JM, Piovano A, Spielberg GP, Scilingo E, et al. The effectiveness of 2-implant overdentures - a pragmatic international multicentre study. J Oral Rehabil. 2011;38(3):176–84. Epub 2010/08/14. eng.
12. Boerrigter EM, Geertman ME, Van Oort RP, Bouma J, Raghoebar GM, van Waas MA, et al. Patient satisfaction with implant-retained mandibular overdentures. A comparison with new complete dentures not retained by implants-a multicentre randomized clinical trial. Br J Oral Maxillofac Surg. 1995;33(5):282–8. Epub 1995/10/01. eng.
13. Meijer HJ, Raghoebar GM, Van't Hof MA, Visser A, Geertman ME, Van Oort RP. A controlled clinical trial of implant-retained mandibular overdentures; five-years' results of clinical aspects and aftercare of IMZ implants and Branemark implants. Clin Oral Implants Res. 2000;11(5):441–7. Epub 2001/02/13. eng.
14. Meijer HJ, Geertman ME, Raghoebar GM, Kwakman JM. Implant-retained mandibular overdentures: 6-year results of a multicenter clinical trial on 3 different implant systems. J Oral Maxillofac Surg. 2001;59(11):1260–8. discussion 9–70. Epub 2001/11/01. eng.
15. Meijer HJ, Raghoebar GM, Batenburg RH, Visser A, Vissink A. Mandibular overdentures supported by two or four endosseous implants: a 10-year clinical trial. Clin Oral Implants Res. 2009;20(7):722–8. Epub 2009/06/06. eng.
16. Thomason JM, Feine J, Exley C, Moynihan P, Muller F, Naert I, et al. Mandibular two implant-supported overdentures as the first choice standard of care for edentulous patients-the York Consensus Statement. Br Dent J. 2009;207(4):185–6. Epub 2009/08/22. eng.
17. Feine JS, Carlsson GE, Awad MA, Chehade A, Duncan WJ, Gizani S, et al. The McGill consensus statement on overdentures. Mandibular two-implant overdentures as first choice standard of care for edentulous patients. Gerodontology. 2002;19(1):3–4. Epub 2002/08/08. eng.
18. Fortin T, Bosson JL, Isidori M, Blanchet E. Effect of flapless surgery on pain experienced in implant placement using an image-guided system. Int J Oral Maxillofac Implants. 2005;21(2):298–304.
19. Walton JN, MacEntee MI. Choosing or refusing oral implants: a prospective study of edentulous volunteers for a clinical trial. Int J Prosthodont. 2005; 18(6):483–8. Epub 2005/12/13. eng.
20. Pommer B, Mailath-Pokorny G, Haas R, Busenlechner D, Fürhauser R, Watzek G. Patients' preferences towards minimally invasive treatment alternatives for implant rehabilitation of edentulous jaws. Eur J Oral Implantol. 2014;7:91–109.
21. Christensen GJ. The 'mini'-implant has arrived. J Am Dent Assoc. 2006; 137(3):387–90. Epub 2006/03/31. eng.
22. Sendax V. Mini implant strategy offers a broad range of uses. Dent today. 1995;14(1):227–32.
23. Vigolo P, Givani A. Clinical evaluation of single-tooth mini-implant restorations: a five-year retrospective study. J Prosthet Dent. 2000;84(1):50–4.
24. Vigolo P, Givani A, Majzoub Z, Cordioli G. Clinical evaluation of small-diameter implants in single-tooth and multiple-implant restorations: a 7-year retrospective study. Int J Oral Maxillofac Implants. 2003;19(5):703–9.
25. Morneburg TR, Proschel P. Success rates of microimplants in edentulous patients with residual ridge resorption. Int J Oral Maxillofac Implants. 2008;23(2):270.
26. Griffitts TM, Collins CP, Collins PC. Mini dental implants: an adjunct for retention, stability, and comfort for the edentulous patient. Oral Surg Oral Med Oral Pathol Oral Radiol Endod. 2005;100(5):e81–4.
27. Ahn M-R, An K-M, Choi J-H, Sohn D-S. Immediate loading with mini dental implants in the fully edentulous mandible. Implant Dent. 2004;13(4):367–72.
28. Lerner H. Minimal invasive implantology with small diameter implants. Implant Pract. 2009;2(1):30–5.
29. Scepanovic M, Calvo-Guirado JL, Markovic A, Delgardo-Ruiz R, Todorovic A, Milicic B, et al. A 1-year prospective cohort study on mandibular overdentures retained by mini dental implants. Eur J Oral Implantol. 2011;5(4):367–79.
30. Mundt T, Schwahn C, Stark T, Biffar R. Clinical response of edentulous people treated with mini dental implants in nine dental practices. Gerodontology. 2013;32(3):179–87.
31. Jofre J, Hamada T, Nishimura M, Klattenhoff C. The effect of maximum bite force on marginal bone loss of mini-implants supporting a mandibular overdenture: a randomized controlled trial. Clin Oral Implants Res. 2010; 21(2):243–9. Epub 2010/01/15. eng.
32. Preoteasa E, Meleşcanu-Imre M, Preoteasa CT, Marin M, Lerner H. Aspects of oral morphology as decision factors in mini-implant supported overdenture. Rom J Morphol Embryol. 2010;51(2):309–14.
33. Preoteasa E, Marin M, Imre M, Lerner H, Preoteasa CT. Patients' satisfaction with conventional dentures and mini implant anchored overdentures. Rev Med Chir Soc Med Nat Iasi. 2012;116(1):310–6. Epub 2012/10/20. eng.
34. Preoteasa E, Imre M, Preoteasa CT. A 3-Year Follow-up Study of Overdentures Retained by Mini-Dental Implants. Int J Oral Maxillofac Implants. 2013;29(5):1170–6.
35. Melescanu Imre M, Preoteasa E, Tancu A, Preoteasa CT. Imaging technique for the complete edentulous patient treated conventionally or with mini implant overdenture. J Med Life. 2013;6(1):86–92. Pubmed Central PMCID: 3624656, Epub 2013/04/20. eng.
36. Tomasi C, Idmyr BO, Wennstrom JL. Patient satisfaction with mini-implant stabilised full dentures. A 1-year prospective study. J Oral Rehabil. 2013; 40(7):526–34. Epub 2013/04/05. eng.
37. Ribeiro A, Della Vecchia M, Cunha T, Sorgini D, Reis A, Muglia V, et al. Short-term post-operative pain and discomfort following insertion of mini-implants for retaining mandibular overdentures: a randomized controlled trial. J Oral Rehabil. 2015;42(8):605–14.

38. Bidra AS, Almas K. Mini implants for definitive prosthodontic treatment: a systematic review. J Prosthet Dent. 2013;109(3):156–64. Epub 2013/03/26. eng.
39. Elsyad MA. Patient satisfaction and prosthetic aspects with mini-implants retained mandibular overdentures. A 5-year prospective study. Clin Oral Implant Res. 2015;27(7):926–33.
40. Bulard RA, Vance JB. Multi-clinic evaluation using mini-dental implants for long-term denture stabilization: a preliminary biometric evaluation. Compend Contin Educ Dent. 2005;26(12):892–7. Epub 2006/01/05. eng.
41. Cawood JI, Howell RA. A classification of the edentulous jaws. Int J Oral Maxillofac Surg. 1988;17(4):232–6. Epub 1988/08/01. eng.
42. Esposito M, Grusovin MG, Worthington HV. Interventions for replacing missing teeth: antibiotics at dental implant placement to prevent complications. Cochrane Database Syst Rev. 2013;7:CD004152. Epub 2013/08/02. eng.
43. NICE. Process and methods guide: Guide to the methods of technology appraisal. 2013. https://www.nice.org.uk/process/pmg9/chapter/foreword. Accessed 19 Jan 2017.
44. Dolan P. Modeling valuations for EuroQol health states. Med Care. 1997;35(11):1095–108.
45. Brazier JE, Roberts J. The estimation of a preference-based measure of health from the SF-12. Med Care. 2004;42(9):851–9.
46. Meijer HJ, Raghoebar GM, Batenburg RH, Vissink A. Mandibular overdentures supported by two Branemark, IMZ or ITI implants: a ten-year prospective randomized study. J Clin Periodontol. 2009;36(9):799–806. Epub 2009/07/01. eng.
47. Branemark PI, Adell R, Albrektsson T, Lekholm U, Lundkvist S, Rockler B. Osseointegrated titanium fixtures in the treatment of edentulousness. Biomaterials. 1983;4(1):25–8. Epub 1983/01/01. eng.
48. Branemark PI, Hansson BO, Adell R, Breine U, Lindstrom J, Hallen O, et al. Osseointegrated implants in the treatment of the edentulous jaw. Experience from a 10-year period. Scand J Plast Reconstr Surg Suppl. 1977;16:1–132. Epub 1977/01/01. eng.
49. Curtis DA, Sharma AB, Finzen FC. The use of dental implants to improve quality of life for edentulous patients. J Calif Dent Assoc. 2008;36(4):275–80. Epub 2008/05/17. eng.
50. Adell R, Lekholm U, Rockler B, Brånemark P-I. A 15-year study of osseointegrated implants in the treatment of the edentulous jaw. Int J Oral Surg. 1981;10(6):387–416.
51. Office for National Statistics. Social Survey Division and Information Centre for Health and Social Care ADHS. 2009 [computer file]. 2nd Edition. Colchester, Essex: UK Data Archive [distributor], August 2012. SN: 6884, http://dx.doi.org/10.5255/UKDA-SN-6884-2.
52. Ikebe K, Morii K, Matsuda K-i, Hazeyama T, Nokubi T. Reproducibility and accuracy in measuring masticatory performance using test gummy jelly. Prosthodont Res Pract. 2005;4(1):9–15.
53. Allen PF, McMillan AS, Locker D. An assessment of sensitivity to change of the Oral Health Impact Profile in a clinical trial. Community Dent Oral Epidemiol. 2001;29(3):175–82. Epub 2001/06/21. eng.
54. Allen F, Locker D. A modified short version of the oral health impact profile for assessing health-related quality of life in edentulous adults. Int J Prosthodont. 2002;15(5):446–50.
55. Esposito M, Ardebili Y, Worthington HV. Interventions for replacing missing teeth: different types of dental implants. Cochrane Database Syst Rev. 2014;7:CD003815. Epub 2014/07/23. eng.
56. Esposito M, Grusovin MG, Chew YS, Coulthard P, Worthington HV. Interventions for replacing missing teeth: 1- versus 2-stage implant placement. Cochrane Database Syst Rev. 2009;3:CD006698. Epub 2009/07/10. eng.
57. Esposito M, Grusovin MG, Maghaireh H, Worthington HV. Interventions for replacing missing teeth: different times for loading dental implants. Cochrane Database Syst Rev. 2013;3:CD003878. Epub 2013/04/02. eng.
58. Esposito M, Grusovin MG, Polyzos IP, Felice P, Worthington HV. Timing of implant placement after tooth extraction: immediate, immediate-delayed or delayed implants? A Cochrane systematic review. Eur J Oral Implantol. 2010;3(3):189–205. Epub 2010/09/18. eng.
59. Esposito M, Maghaireh H, Grusovin MG, Ziounas I, Worthington HV. Soft tissue management for dental implants: what are the most effective techniques? A Cochrane systematic review. Eur J Oral Implantol. 2012;5(3):221–38. Epub 2012/09/25. eng.
60. Shatkin T, Petrotto C. Mini dental implants: a retrospective analysis of 5640 implants placed over a 12-year period. Compend Contin Educ Dent. 2011;33:2–9.
61. Shatkin TE, Shatkin S, Oppenheimer BD, Oppenheimer AJ. Mini dental implants for long-term fixed and removable prosthetics: a retrospective analysis of 2514 implants placed over a five-year period. Compend Contin Educ Dent. 2007;28(2):92–9. quiz 100–1.
62. Jemt T, Lekholm U. Implant treatment in edentulous maxillae: a 5-year follow-up report on patients with different degrees of jaw resorption. Int J Oral Maxillofac Implants. 1995;10(3):303–11.
63. de Souza R, Ribeiro A, Della Vecchia M, Costa L, Cunha T, Reis A, et al. Mini vs. Standard Implants for Mandibular Overdentures A Randomized Trial. J Dent Res. 2015;94(10):1376–84.
64. Humphris G, Morrison T, Lindsay S. The Modified Dental Anxiety Scale: UK norms and evidence for validity. Community Dent Health. 1995;12(3):143–50.
65. Allen F, Locker D. A modified short version of the oral health impact profile for assessing health-related quality of life in edentulous adults. Int J Prosthodont. 2001;15(5):446–50.
66. Group TE. EuroQol-a new facility for the measurement of health-related quality of life. Health Policy. 1990;16(3):199–208.
67. Ware Jr J, Kosinski M, Turner-Bowker D, Gandek B. How to score version 2 of the SF-12 Health Survey (with a supplement documenting version 1). Lincoln: QualityMetric. Inc; 2002.

10

Patient-Reported oral health outcome measurement for children and adolescents

Honghu Liu[1*], Ron D. Hays[2], Marvin Marcus[1], Ian Coulter[1], Carl Maida[1], Francisco Ramos-Gomez[3], Jie Shen[1], Yan Wang[4], Vladimir Spolsky[1], Steve Lee[5], Li Cai[6] and James Crall[1]

Abstract

Background: Oral health is an important component of daily functioning and well-being. A comprehensive patient-reported oral health measure is needed to gauge the impact of oral health status on children and adolescents. This study aims to develop oral health item banks and associated short-form surveys for children and adolescents 2–17 year olds.

Methods: Using children and adolescents, ages 2–17 years, selected from diverse dental sites in Greater Los Angeles Area, we propose to develop state-of-the-science methods to create oral health item banks to effectively measure oral health outcomes for children and adolescents. Methods include a literature review of existing measures, focus groups, cognitive interviews, drafting and field testing of survey items, and evaluation of the psychometric properties of the measures.

Results: Based on the systematic literature search and focus groups, we identified core (physical health, mental health, and social function domains) and peripheral (e.g., need and access) oral health domains. We then drafted survey items and revised them based on 66 cognitive interviews (27 children/adolescents and 39 parents) with 39 families. The revised items will be administered in a field test of 500 children and adolescents ages 2–17, and their parents.

Conclusions: The qualitative methods used in the initial phases of the project (focus group and cognitive interviews) are the initial steps in the development of oral health item banks and associated short-form surveys for children and adolescents. The oral health items can potentially be used to create effective computerized adaptive test and/or create ad hoc short forms targeting specific areas of oral health to survey large populations of children with much less cost compared with traditional clinical oral health examination.

Keywords: Oral health, Children, Adolescent, Longitudinal survey, Patient-reported outcomes

Background

Oral health is an important component of daily functioning and well-being. Healthy People 2020 [1] notes the importance of prevention and control of oral and craniofacial diseases, conditions, and injuries, and of enhancing access to preventive services and dental care. The 2000 Surgeon General's Report on Oral Health in America [2] showed that early childhood caries is one of the most serious and costly health conditions among young children. The need for oral health care is the most prevalent unmet healthcare need among children and adolescents [3]. Pediatric oral disorders have a negative effect on children's health-related quality of life [4]. The adolescent years could be a difficult emotional period when dental and medical needs may be neglected [5]. Understanding and assessing children and adolescents is complex as they are not a stable target, rather in the stage of emerging-developmental skills and functions.

Patient-reported outcomes (PROs) are important for assessing oral health status and evaluating the impact of dental care. Prior researches have shown that children 8 years and older are mature enough to be able to accurately self-report health issues [6–8], and respond appropriately to questions regarding their functioning and

* Correspondence: hhliu@dentistry.ucla.edu
[1]Division of Public Health & Community Dentistry, School of Dentistry, University of California, Los Angeles (UCLA), Los Angeles, CA, USA
Full list of author information is available at the end of the article

well-being [9]. More recently, Tsakos et al. (2012)'s study has shown that children as young as 5 years old can provide accurate reports of the impact of oral disorders on their quality of life [10].

Obtaining PROs directly from children, adolescents, and their parents is possible; however, effective assessment requires consideration of developmental issues such as the rapid change in children's cognitive capacities. Self-reports are the primary method of assessment, supplemented by parent or guardian proxy report when a child is unable to accurately self-report (e.g., too young) [11]. The Patient-Reported Outcome Measurement Information System (PROMIS®) was initiated in 2004 to develop and evaluate health-related quality of life measures. The PROMIS Network's overall goal is to develop a publicly available set of standardized instruments for measuring major self-reported health domains that are affected by many chronic illnesses [12].

Several questionnaires for measures of oral health-related quality of life have been produced for use with children or using parents as proxies. These generic questionnaires are designed to cover a variety of oral conditions such as dental caries, malocclusion and craniofacial anomalies. The most frequently used measures for self-completion by children are the Child Perceptions Questionnaire (CPQ) [13–15], Child Oral Impacts on Daily Performances Index (C-OIDP) [16], Child Oral Health Impact Profile (COHIP) [17], and PedsQL Oral Health Scale.

This paper describes the approaches, methods and process of our study for the creation, administration and evaluation of oral health items for children and adolescents 2–17, selected from diverse dental sites in Greater Los Angeles Area. The PROMIS methodologies and framework were adopted in this study, as detailed below.

Methods

Measurement framework

Our proposed framework for conceptualizing and addressing oral health domains is summarized in Fig. 1. Children and adolescent characteristics have an impact on oral health determinants, which in turn have an impact on oral health outcomes. Social environmental factors also have an impact on both oral health determinants and oral health outcomes. This model builds upon our previous work on the multi-level influences of oral health [18]. It integrates the life-course concept into the dynamics of oral health by including genetic, biological, behavioral, social, and economic contexts that change as a person develops through childhood, adolescence, young adulthood and later adult life [19].

The study has four carefully designed and well-connected operational phases: (1) a systematic review of the literature to identify instruments and survey items associated with oral health; (2) focus groups, cognitive interviews, item selection, and drafting of oral health items; and (3) field testing of subject surveys and dental examinations; and (4) psychometric analyses of oral health items. We have already completed Phase 1 and Phase 2 of the study and are now in the middle of Phase 3.

PHASE 1: Evaluate the relevance of PROMIS and conduct systematic literature review

We conducted systematic literature searches on existing oral health items previously used to measure oral health, particularly those for children and adolescent ages 2–17, as well as their parents, to capture the latest research, through exhaustive searches of PubMed, Google scholar, the Patient-Reported Outcome and Quality of Life Instruments Database, and the Dental, Oral, and Craniofacial Data Resource Center (DRC). The systematic review and search identified all surveys, instruments and items that have been used to date to measure oral health applicable to children and adolescents, ages 2–17. The DRC serves as a resource on dental, oral, and craniofacial data. We searched through DRC by criteria, which include survey title, acronym, sample design type, sample size, general variables, oral health variables, population, survey type, sponsor, and geographic region. Multiple items can be selected under each criterion. Records can be selected that match all or any of the criteria. Search results included survey overview, sample size, geographic region, population, year, interval, survey type, sample design, method/technique, reliability/validity, general variables, and oral health variables. Key instruments were identified to be considered "legacy" instruments. A modified Delphi approach was used to reach agreement on the domain, subdomains and elements for oral health within the PROMIS domain hierarchy framework. We adopted the PROMIS method of binning (identifying those items thought to represent distinct domains related to oral health) and winnowing (using a consensus process to exclude items that do not meet the domain definitions or are redundant, etc.), and ensure that the items are concise, simple, have the same item stem, and are targeted to appropriate reading level for the children and adolescents.

PHASE 2: Focus groups, cognitive interviews, and final item selection

Phase 2 involved convening focus groups with racially/ethnically and geographically diverse groups of children, parents, and oral health professionals, and was conducted to help conceptualize oral health PROs. The cut-off criteria used to separate age groups are based on

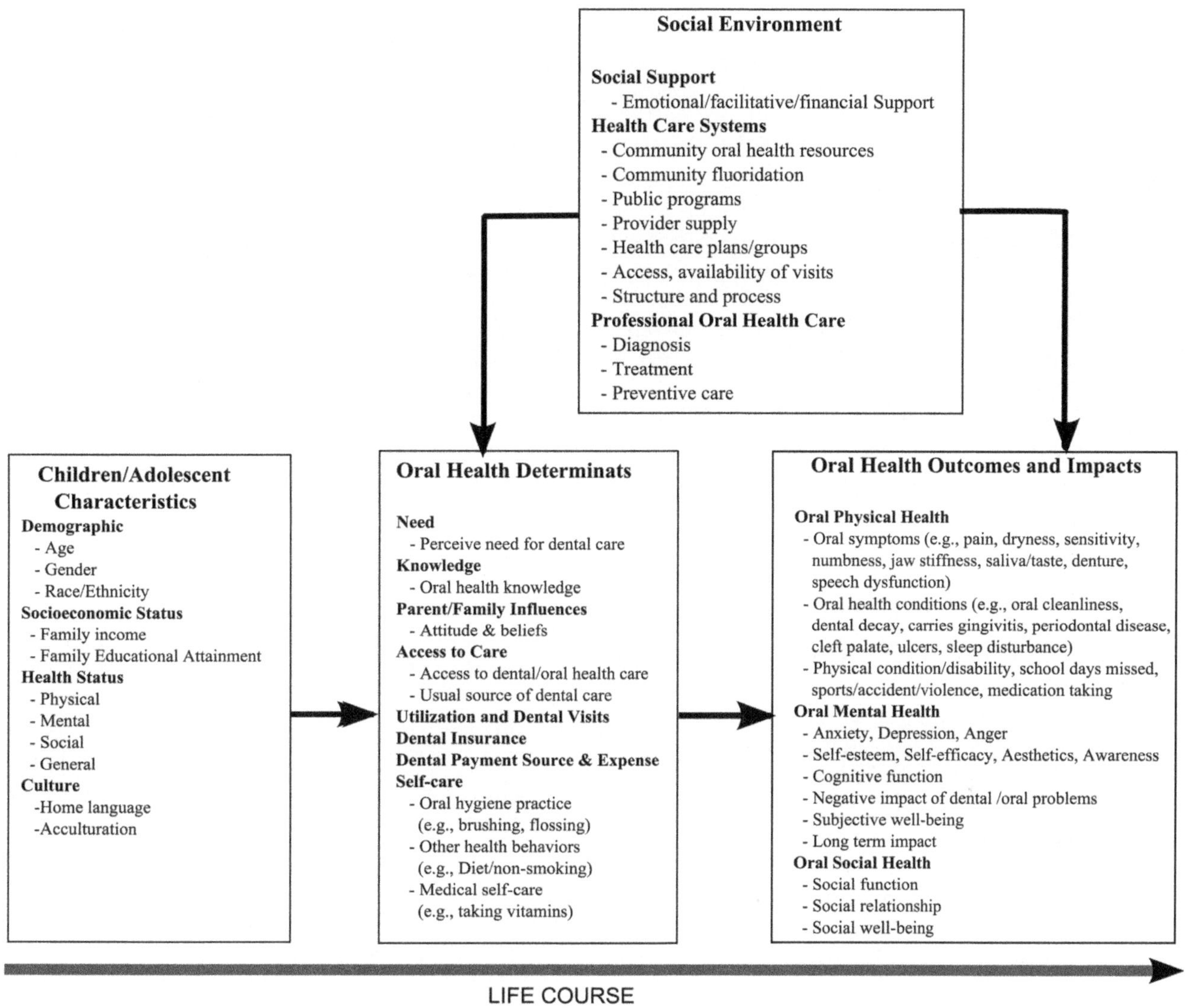

Fig. 1 Children/adolescent oral health measurement framework

children and adolescents' physical, mental and dental development that are pertinent to that specific age group. The basic age breakdown was related to dentition. In the 2–7 age group, children mainly had primary teeth; in the 8–12 age group, there is mixed dentition, including permanent and primary teeth; the 13–17 age group all have permanent teeth. Adolescents were also more likely to have full orthodontic treatment. We conducted focus group interviews with parents of children ages 2–7, 8–13, and 14–17, and with children/adolescents ages 8–13 and 14–17. These focus groups elicited perceptions of oral health in children and adolescents. Each focus group was digitally recorded and transcribed verbatim. The research team conducted thematic and narrative analysis to identify the terms used by the participants.

Following the focus groups, we drafted survey items and administered them in a series of face-to-face cognitive interviews with children and adolescents, parents and professionals. Cognitive interviewing provides a means to evaluate participants' responses to the items and test their understanding of the meaning of the items. For each candidate item, we probed the subject regarding the item content and response options [20]. We explored how respondents recall information, what time frame they use, and what time frame is beyond their recall. Cognitive interviews were conducted using intermittent and retrospective probes following completion of all items. Based on findings from cognitive interviews, items were then refined for the field test.

PHASE 3: Field test

The field test collects data to evaluate the oral health items identified through phases 1 and 2. We survey children's oral health perceptions and conduct dental clinical examination. Children ages 2–7 receive dental clinical examinations only, and their parents completed the survey as their child's proxy. Children 8–13 and 14–17 received both survey and dental clinical examinations, and their parents also completed surveys. We use a software program called Questionnaire Development System™ (QDS™), developed by Nova Research Company, to build and implement Audio Computer-Assisted Self-Interview Software (ACASI) interviews for child and patient surveys. Each of the surveys contains core items (e.g., demographics and pain) that are applicable to all three age groups and the targeted items that are pertinent only to that specific age group. With the ACASI surveys, each participant hears the same text-to-speech computer-generated voice reading the same instructions and questionnaire items.

Given the large age span of children from 2 to 17, in view of the varying nature of dentation and the level of maturity, we use different versions of the ACASI surveys: one for parents of children ages 2–7, one for children ages 8–17, and one for their parents. Each of the surveys contains core items (e.g., demographics and pain) that are applicable to all three age groups and age-group targeted items.

To evaluate responsiveness to change over time and estimate minimally important differences, a group of 150 randomly selected children and adolescents along with their parents will also complete a follow-up ACASI survey at 6 months from the initial survey to collect information about changes in oral health. They will also be given a follow-up clinical exam at the 6-month period. These children and adolescents will likely have changes, such as loss of primary teeth and body growth, which may affect their aesthetic concept and perception.

Clinical examination

A dental clinical examination is conducted on all participating children. The oral examination of the 2-7-year group is performed before or after the interview of their parent or caregiver. The clinical examination of the 2–7 year children consists of an examination of the oral mucosa, examination of the teeth for the presence of obvious decay and decalcification (white spots), the presence of plaque on the centrals and molars, when present, and bleeding on probing an inflammation of the gingiva. Oral clinical examinations for children ages 8–17 are performed before or after they have completed the survey. Starting with an examination of the oral mucosa, dental caries are assessed and followed by examination for the presence of plaque, gingivitis and calculus. In addition, the occlusion is assessed as well as orthodontic factors that characterize the position of the teeth, spacing within the arch and facial profile. Condition on tooth crowding, spaces and jaw relationships, such as overbite and overjet, are also noted. Photographs of the profile of front teeth are taken to assess aesthetics and tooth color.

The assessment of the oral mucosa is based on the format developed by the World Health Organization, which consists of a systematic assessment of the lips, labial mucosa and sulcus, commissures, buccal mucosa and sulcus, gingival and alveolar ridges, floor of the mouth, and hard and soft palate. The caries examination consists of a full mouth examination of all primary and permanent teeth. All of the coronal portions are assessed using the DFT/DMFT index, for the primary and permanent dentition, respectively. The measures included in the exam are also consistent with the Children's Oral Health Status Index [21, 22].

Sample size

Sample size will be 500 children/adolescents for the field test. The sample will be selected from diverse dental clinics and private practices throughout the Greater Los Angeles Area. With a sample size of 500, the standard error around a correlation is approximately 0.045. A sample size of 500 or more was recommended by Reeve and Fayers (2005) [23] for estimating the item response theory graded response model (2 parameter model).

Field test recruitment

Four hundred children and adolescents, and their parents will be recruited from community clinics and private practices throughout the Greater Los Angeles Area. These clinics and practices encompass community general clinics, safety-net clinics, group practices, solo general practices, and solo specialty practices with general dentists, pediatric dentists and specialists. These recruitment sites cover different geographic areas and communities, ranging from low-income underserved immigrant neighborhoods to high–income professional communities, with diverse race and ethnic compositions. Institutional review board approval for this study was obtained from the UCLA Office of the Human Research Protection Program.

Phase 4: Psychometric and statistical analysis

Using data collected from field test, psychometric and statistical analyses will be performed to evaluate oral health items and scales. We will evaluate the reliability and validity of the oral health scales by using item-level factor analytic methods to assess the dimensionality of the oral health scales, and estimate item response theory (IRT) parameters (e.g., threshold, discrimination). Psychometric evaluations will be completed sequentially using the following steps described in Reeve et al.'s paper [24].

Revision and finalization of item banks

Based on the findings from psychometric and statistical analyses, we will make revisions and adjustments to the selected oral health items to finalize the item banks. For example, we may modify the levels of response for some items or drop the items that do not show good psychometric properties (e.g., very low reliability).

Results

After comprehensive and systematic literature search on existing oral health items, surveys and instrument relative to children and adolescents, ages 2–17 and their parents, initial core domains for the oral health item banks to be developed are listed in Table 1, which include physical health domains, mental health domains, and social function domains. These initial domains were revised in light of data derived from focus group analysis, cognitive interview, team investigators, experts and analysis.

Table 2 lists domains that are related to oral health. Items related to access, behavior, etc., are critical to oral health, but do not yet fit into the current PROMIS framework.

Table 3 lists the PROMIS self-reported health domains. These results provided valuable information about core domains for the oral health item banks to be developed and generated content for new items and evaluated with cognitive interviews and in a field test.

Through focus groups, we identified three unique themes that the youth associated with their oral health status: (1) understanding the value of maintaining good oral health over the life course, with respect to longevity and quality of life in the adult years; (2) positive association between maintaining good oral health and interpersonal relationships at school, and dating, for older youth; and (3) knowledge of the benefits of orthodontic treatment to appearance and positive self-image, while holding a strong view as to the discomfort associated with braces [25].

We then drafted survey items and revised them based on 66 cognitive interviews (27 children/adolescents and 39 parents) with 39 families. We identified a number of issues from the cognitive interviews that informed subsequent item development. The first issue was guardian involvement in the interview and their reliability as proxies. The second issue was confusing wording of some of the new items created as a result of focus group discussions. The third issue was temporality. Certain items required parents to recall a time when they were concerned about a recent oral health problem or indicate any instances of dental anxiety or phobic reactions. We have completed additional cognitive interviews to test comprehensibility of 23 child/adolescent items and 35 parent items, notably those items that we changed through analysis and expert review of the results of original cognitive interviews, and also to test a few revised legacy items derived from the California Health Interview Survey (CHIS) [26, 27].

Table 1 Oral health domains

Domains	Measures
Physical Health	Physical Function
	Pain
	Physical Condition
	Sleep Disturbance/Pain
	Other Symptoms
	School Days Missed
	Sports/Accident/Violence
	Medication Taking
	Physical disability
	Function Limitation
	Oral health symptoms
	Halitosis
	Sensory Problem
	Lips/tongue
	Gums/tissues
	Saliva/Taste
	Natural teeth
	Denture
	Oral cleanliness
	Speech function
Mental Health	Anxiety
	Depression
	Anger
	Cognitive Function
	Negative Impact of Dental/Oral Problems
	Awareness
	Self-Esteem
	Self-Efficacy
	Aesthetics
	Sleep disturbance
	Subjective well-being Provided
Social Function	Social Function
	Social Relationship
	Social Well-being

Table 2 Oral health related domains

Domains	Measures
Need	Perceived need for dental care
Knowledge	Oral health Knowledge
	Awareness
Health Behavior	Oral hygiene practice
	Smoking
	Alcohol
	Substance abuse
Access	Access to dental/oral health care
	Usual Source of Dental Care
Utilization	Utilization of dental/oral health care
Diet	Diet
Community Level Measures	Community Oral Health Prevention and Intervention
Preventive Dental services	Immunizations, water fluoridation
	Oral health access
	Dental Visits
	Availability of Dentists
Health care delivery	Access, availability of visits
	Process – method by which oral health care is provided
	Outcome – the consequence of the healthcare Provided
	Structure– the environment in which healthcare is provided
Dental Visits	Last dental visits, first dental visits, frequency, type of provider seen.
Dental Insurances	Type of insurance
Dental Expense and Payment Source	Source of payment

Discussion

Children and adolescents are in the stage of emerging developmental skills and functions. Younger children are already capable of expressing a range of emotions (e.g., anxiety, happiness). However, due to limited level of maturity and responsibilities, children ages 8–17 are not able to answer all questions related to their oral health such as insurance co-pay or other financial questions, for which parents or guardians are the appropriate respondents. Therefore, it is necessary to assess self-reported oral health outcomes for children and adolescents with children surveys supplemented by parent interviews. Furthermore, given the young age of children, oral health outcomes will have profound long-term impacts on their future function and well-being for many years to come, and we need to use life course lens to view the process and impact. Focus groups can serve as an innovative approach to understanding children's experiences from a developmental perspective through children and parents' involvement.

The National Institute of Health is encouraging use of PROMIS measures in clinical practice and research through the Patient-Centered Assessment Resource: http://healthcaredelivery.cancer.gov/resource/. PROMIS has created an extensive library of item banks, but is still completely lacking oral health item banks. This project capitalized on innovations in modern measurement theory, qualitative methods for instrument development and computerized adaptive testing. In our field testing, we used ACASI approach that has very desirable measurement properties. A research staff is present to instruct the respondent in the use of the laptop computer that administers the questions. The questions are presented both visually on computer screen and audible through earphones so that even respondents with low levels of literacy can take part. ACASI combines the power, flexibility, and standardization of automation with the privacy of self-administration. The audio component of ACASI is particularly effective for participants with low literacy skills. Among the diverse participants and different clinical settings, the majority felt comfortable using the computer, liked the privacy, and faced few difficulties with its use. When they faced difficulties, research staff is present to help solve the technical issues. Weaknesses using ACASI are possible data loss if staff is not properly trained, or the children cannot focus on answering the questions, or the children are cognitively impaired to use the computers. We strived to train research staff and a knowledgeable data manager will be present onsite to troubleshoot so that these issues can be minimized.

Some important future steps are as follows. First, psychometric analyses on the field test data will be performed to construct oral health-targeted items and scales for children and adolescents, ages 2–17. We will use full-information item factor analysis methods [28, 29] to evaluate dimensionality [30–32], calibrate the selected items using the graded response model (GRM) [33], and assess differential item functioning (DIF) using the updated version of Lord's Wald test [34]. Second, we will estimate the minimally important differences (MID) for the new oral health measures using an anchor-based approach [35]. A subset of 150 patients with longitudinal data will be asked to assess changes in their oral health at second data point compared to baseline (e.g., retrospective global oral health rating: *a lot better, a little better, the same, a little worse*, or *a lot worse*). People who report either getting a "little better" or a "little worse" on oral health will constitute the minimal change subgroup. The change in oral health rating for this group will be used to estimate the MID. The change

Table 3 Self-reported health domains in PROMIS

Component	Subcomponent	Domain	Sub-domain
Physical Health	symptoms	Pain	Behavior*
			Interference
			Quality*
			Intensity*
			Impact
		Fatigue	Experience
			Impact
		Asthma Impact	
		Gastro-intestinal Symptoms*	
	Function	Physical Function	Upper Extremity
			Lower Extremity
			Central
			Activities*
			Mobility
		Sexual Function and Satisfaction	Global Satisfaction with Sex Life
			Interest in Sexual Activity
			Lubrication
			Vaginal Discomfort
			Erectile Function
			Orgasm
			Therapeutic Aids
			Sexual Activities
			Anal Discomfort
			Interfering Factors
		Sleep Function	Sleep Disturbance
			Sleep-related Impairment
			Wake Disturbance
		Wake Function	
		Physical Activity	
		Motor	Balance
			Dexterity
			Endurance
			Locomotion
			Strength
		Sensation	Audition
			Olfaction
			Pain
			Taste
			Vestibular
			Vision
	Affect		Anxiety
Mental Health		Negative (Emotional Distress)	Depression
			Anger
			Experience of Stress*
			Psychosocial Illness Impact - Negative
			Meaning & Spirituality
			Stress Response
			Self-concept
			Social Isolation
			Emotional and Behavioral Dyscontrol
			Stigma
			Fear
			Sadness
		Positive	Subjective Well-being*
			Psychosocial Illness Impact - Positive
			Meaning & Spirituality
			Coping
			Self-concept
			Social Connection
			Mastery & control (Self-efficacy)
			Subjective Well-being (positive affect) *
	Behavior	Substance Use/Alcohol	Alcohol Use
			Positive Consequences
			Positive Expectancies
			Negative Consequences
			Negative Expectancies
		Smoking	Nicotine Dependence
			Perceived Benefits: Affective/Hedonic
			Perceived Benefits: Coping
			Perceived Benefits: Social
			Perceived Benefits: Psychosocial

Table 3 Self-reported health domains in PROMIS *(Continued)*

			Perceived Benefits: Health
	Cognition	Applied Cognition - General Concerns	
		Applied Cognition - Abilities	
		Applied Cognition – Attention/ Executive Function	
		Self - efficacy	General
			Self-Efficacy with management of Chronic Disease*
		Episodic memory	
		Language	
		Processing speed	
		Working memory	
Social Health	Relationships	Social Isolation	
		Quality of Social Support	Companionship
			Emotional Support
			Informational Support
			Instrumental Support
			Social Isolation
		Peer Relationships	
			Interaction with peers
		Family Belongingness*	
		Communication	
	Function	Ability to Participate in Social Roles and Activities	Social Roles
			Discretionary Social Activities
		Satisfaction with Participation in Social Roles and Activities	Social Roles
			Discretionary Social Activities

* Under-development as indicated by http://www.assessmentcenter.net/documents/instrumentlibrary.pdf

in oral health self-reports will also be examined using clinical anchors of change (e.g. the difference in number of dental caries between baseline and follow-up by dental exams). Third, linking metrics and cross-walk tables will be created to estimate legacy scores from oral health domains and vice versa, and provide confidence interval around these estimates. Appropriate equity criteria such as the equipercentile equating procedure will be implemented to determine the linking method. Using the information in the item bank library, users will be able to create computerized adaptive tests or short forms tailored to their populations of interest or aspects of oral health (e.g., dental caries issue) of interest. Scores on these tailored measures can then be compared because the items have been mapped onto a common metric.

This study has several limitations. First, our study sample may not be representative of the U.S. general population in that it is comprised of children who are already under dental care and agreed to participate in this project. Second, there are many decisions involved in the evaluation and refinement of item banks. These decisions require extensive skill and experience and are inherently subjective, but the experience of our team will provide a system of checks and balances. Additionally, we will minimize the likelihood of bad decisions by performing a comprehensive set of psychometric and statistical analyses and balance empirical results with clinical input. We are aware of issues that arise when health-related constructs are fit to IRT models (e.g., extreme threshold parameters, very large discrimination parameters, and highly skewed information curves), and will test alternative models in order to find the best fit.

Conclusions

This project utilizes qualitative and state-of-the-science quantitative methods to develop oral health PROs for children and adolescents. The qualitative methods used in the initial phases of the project (focus group and cognitive interviews) are the initial steps in the development of oral health item banks and associated short-form surveys for children and adolescents. The oral health items can potentially be used to create effective computerized adaptive test and/or create ad hoc short forms targeting specific areas of oral health to survey large populations of children with much less cost compared with traditional clinical oral health examination. These surveys can be used by dentists, oral health researchers and professionals, and public policy makers for oral health screening, program assessment, oral health evaluation with large populations as well as oral health management and policy planning.

Abbreviations

ACASI: Audio computer-assisted self-interview software; COHIP: Child oral health impact profile; C-OIDP: Child oral impacts on daily performances index; CPQ: Child perceptions questionnaire; DIF: Differential item functioning; GRM: Graded response model; IRT: Item response theory; MID: Minimally important differences; PedsQL™: Pediatric Quality of Life Inventory™; PRO: Patient-reported outcomes; PROMIS: Patient-reported outcomes measurement information system

Acknowledgements

We thank the families for their participation in the study and contributing to the enhancement of oral health item back development. We also thank the field staff of the data collection and coordination sites. This research was supported by a NIDCR/NIH grant to the University of California, Los Angeles (UCLA) (U01DE022648).

Authors' contributions
HHL and JS drafted the manuscript. RDH MM IC CM FRG JS YW VS LC JC made substantial contributions to conception and design of the study and acquisition and analysis and interpretation of the data, were involved in revising the manuscript. SL made contributions to acquisition and analysis and interpretation of the data. All authors gave final approval for publication.

Competing interests
The authors declare that they have no competing interests.

Consent for publication
Not applicable.

Ethics approval and consent to participate
To participate in the study, each family member will provide active consent, as approved by the University of California Los Angeles Institutional Review Board (approval # 13–001330). All children gave consent to participate in the study. Moreover, each of their parents or guardians signed an informed consent form.

Author details
[1]Division of Public Health & Community Dentistry, School of Dentistry, University of California, Los Angeles (UCLA), Los Angeles, CA, USA. [2]UCLA Department of Medicine, David Geffen School of Medicine, Los Angeles, CA, USA. [3]UCLA Section of Pediatric Dentistry, Los Angeles, CA, USA. [4]UCLA Department of Biostatistics, Los Angeles, CA, USA. [5]UCLA Section of Restorative Dentistry, Los Angeles, CA, USA. [6]UCLA Department of Education, School of Education and Information Studies, Los Angeles, CA, USA.

References

1. Dye BA, Thornton-Evans G. Trends in oral health by poverty status as measured by Healthy People 2010 objectives. Public Health Rep. 2010;125: 817–30.
2. Oral health in America: a report of the Surgeon General. J Calif Dent Assoc. 2000;28:685–95.
3. Romer M, Dougherty N, Amores-Lafleur E. Predoctoral education in special care dentistry: paving the way to better access? ASDC J Dent Child. 2007;66:132–5.
4. Barbosa TS, Gavião MBD. Oral health-related quality of life in children: Part I. How well do children know themselves? A systematic review. Int J Dent Hyg. 2008;6:93–9.
5. Waldman HB, Perlman SP. Dental needs assessment and access to care for adolescents. Dent Clin North Am. 2006;50:1–16.
6. Walsh TR, Irwin DE, Meier A, Varni JW, DeWalt DA. The use of focus groups in the development of the PROMIS pediatrics item bank. Qual Life Res. 2008;17:725–35.
7. Varni JW, Seid M, Rode CA. The PedsQL (TM): Measurement model for the pediatric quality of life inventory. Med Care. 1999;37:126.
8. Matza LS, Patrick DL, Riley AW, Alexander JJ, Rajmil L, Pleil AM, et al. Pediatric patient-reported outcome instruments for research to support medical product labeling: report of the ISPOR PRO good research practices for the assessment of children and adolescents task force. Value Health. 2013;16:461–79.
9. Irwin DE, Varni JW, Yeatts K, DeWalt DA. Cognitive interviewing methodology in the development of a pediatric item bank: a patient reported outcomes measurement information system (PROMIS) study. Health Qual Life Outcomes. 2009;7:1–10.
10. Tsakos G, Blair YI, Yusuf H, Wright W, Watt RG, Macpherson LMD. Developing a new self-reported scale of oral health outcomes for 5-year-old children (SOHO-5). Health Qual Life Outcomes. 2012;10:62.
11. Irwin DE, Gross HE, Stucky BD, Thissen D, DeWitt EM, Lai JS, et al. Development of six PROMIS pediatrics proxy-report item banks. Health Qual Life Outcomes. 2012;10:22.
12. Cella D, Yount S, Rothrock N, Gershon R, Cook K, Reeve B, et al. The Patient-Reported Outcomes Measurement Information System (PROMIS): progress of an NIH Roadmap cooperative group during its first two years. Med Care. 2007;45:S3.
13. Jokovic A, Locker D, Tompson B, Guyatt G. Questionnaire for measuring oral health-related quality of life in eight- to ten-year-old children. Pediatr Dent. 2004;26:512–8.
14. Jokovic A, Locker D, Stephens M, Kenny D, Tompson B, Guyatt G. Validity and reliability of a questionnaire for measuring child oral-health-related quality of life. J Dent Res. 2002;81:459–63.
15. Jokovic A, Locker D, Guyatt G. Short forms of the Child Perceptions Questionnaire for 11-14-year-old children (CPQ11-14): development and initial evaluation. Health Qual Life Outcomes. 2006;4:4.
16. Gherunpong S, Tsakos G, Sheiham A. Developing and evaluating an oral health-related quality of life index for children; the CHILD-OIDP. Community Dent Health. 2004;21:161–9.
17. Broder HL, McGrath C, Cisneros GJ. Questionnaire development: face validity and item impact testing of the Child Oral Health Impact Profile. Community Dent Oral Epidemiol. 2007;35 Suppl 1:8–19.
18. Fisher-Owens SA, Gansky SA, Platt LJ, Weintraub JA, Soobader M-J, Bramlett MD, et al. Influences on children's oral health: a conceptual model. Pediatrics. 2007;120:e510–520.
19. Osler M. The life course perspective: a challenge for public health research and prevention. Eur J Public Health. 2006;16:230.
20. Christodoulou C, Junghaenel DU, DeWalt DA, Rothrock N, Stone AA. Cognitive interviewing in the evaluation of fatigue items: results from the patient-reported outcomes measurement information system (PROMIS). Qual Life Res. 2008;17:1239–46.
21. Koch AL, Gershen JA, Marcus M. A children's oral health status index based on dentists' judgment. J Am Dent Assoc. 1985;110:36–42.
22. Gershen JA, Marcus M, Koch A. Using dentists' judgments to identify the components of children's oral health. ASDC J Dent Child. 1980;47:419–24.
23. Reeve BB, Fayers P. Applying item response theory modeling for evaluating questionnaire item and scale properties. Assess. Qual. Life Clin. Trials Methods Pract. 2005;2:55–73.
24. Reeve BB, Hays RD, Bjorner JB, Cook KF, Crane PK, Teresi JA, et al. Psychometric evaluation and calibration of health-related quality of life item banks: plans for the Patient-Reported Outcomes Measurement Information System (PROMIS). Med Care. 2007;45:S22.
25. Maida CA, Marcus M, Hays RD, Coulter ID, Ramos-Gomez F, Lee SY, et al. Child and adolescent perceptions of oral health over the life course. Qual Life Res. 2015;24:2739–51.
26. CHIS 2011–2012 Child Questionnaire Version 12. 5 [Internet].Available from: http://healthpolicy.ucla.edu/chis/design/Documents/CHIS2011childquestionnaire.pdf. Accessed 2 Sept 2016.
27. CHIS 2011–2012 Adolescent Questionnaire Version 15. 3 [Internet]. Available from: http://healthpolicy.ucla.edu/chis/design/Documents/CHIS2011teenquestionnaire.pdf. Accessed 2 Sept 2016.
28. Cai L, Du Toit SHC, Thissen D. IRTPRO: Flexible, multidimensional, multiple categorical IRT modeling [Computer software]. Chicago: Scientific Software International; 2011.
29. Cai L, Thissen D, du Toit SHC. IRTPRO for Windows [Computer software]. Lincolnwood: Scientific Software International; 2011.
30. Cai L. A two-tier full-information item factor analysis model with applications. Psychometrika. 2010;75:581–612.
31. Cai L. Metropolis-Hastings Robbins-Monro algorithm for confirmatory item factor analysis. J Educ Behav Stat. 2010;35:307–35.
32. Cai L. High-dimensional exploratory item factor analysis by a Metropolis–Hastings Robbins–Monro algorithm. Psychometrika. 2010;75:33–57.
33. Samejima F. Estimation of latent ability using a response pattern of graded scores. Psychometrika. 1969;34:1–97.
34. Langer MM. A reexamination of Lord's Wald test for differential item functioning using item response theory and modern error estimation. Chapel Hill: The University of North Carolina; 2009.
35. Hays RD, Farivar SS, Liu H. Approaches and recommendations for estimating minimally important differences for health-related quality of life measures. COPD J Chronic Obstr Pulm Dis. 2005;2:63–7.

11

The relationship between children's oral health-related behaviors and their caregiver's social support

Rong Min Qiu[1,2], Ye Tao[1], Yan Zhou[1], Qing Hui Zhi[1] and Huan Cai Lin[1*]

Abstract

Background: Social support might play a role in helping people adopt healthy behaviors and improve their health. Stronger social support from mothers has been found to be positively related to higher tooth brushing frequency in 1- to 3-year-old children. However, little is known regarding the relationship between the caregiver's social support and the oral health-related behaviors of 5-year-old children in China. This study aimed to investigate this relationship.

Methods: A cross-sectional study was conducted among 1332 5-year-old children and their caregivers in Guangzhou, southern China. Data were collected using questionnaires that were completed by the caregivers and the children's caries status were examined. The caregivers' social support was measured using the Social Support Rating Scale. The measurements of the children's oral health-related behaviors included the frequencies of sugary snack intake and tooth brushing, utilization of dental services, and patterns of dental visits. Univariate and multiple logistic regression analyses were used to analyze the relationships between the variables.

Results: No association was found between the caregiver's social support and the child's oral health-related behaviors in a multiple logistic regression analysis. However, other factors, particularly the oral health-related behaviors of the caregiver, were found to be significantly linked to the child's oral health-related behaviors.

Conclusions: The oral health-related behaviors of 5-year-old children in Guangzhou are unrelated to the caregiver's social support but are related to other specific factors, particularly the caregiver's oral health-related behaviors.

Keywords: Child, Caregiver, Social support, Oral health-related behavior, Psychosocial factor

Abbreviations: dmft, decayed, missing and filled teeth; SSRS, Social support rating scale

Background

Despite great improvements in the oral health of people in many countries over the past few decades, dental caries in preschool children are a public health problem of great concern [1]. The occurrence of dental caries is strongly related to oral health behaviors, such as sugar consumption, tooth brushing habits and dental care [1, 2]. Understanding the factors that affect oral health behaviors is crucial for the development of programs to prevent dental caries.

Researchers studying dental health have documented the need to understand the role of oral health knowledge and attitudes in the oral health behaviors of individuals [3, 4]. However, a shift of focus toward the psychosocial determinants of oral health behaviors has become evident [5, 6]. Social support is a psychosocial factor that might help individuals cope with psychological distress, adopt healthy behaviors and improve their health [7, 8].

Social support is defined as "assistance and protection given to others, especially to individuals" [9]. It can essentially be divided into two categories [10]. The first is objective, visible or actual support, which reflects the material support that individuals might directly receive,

* Correspondence: lin_hc@163.net
[1]Department of Preventive Dentistry, Guanghua School of Stomatology, Guangdong Provincial Key Laboratory of Stomatology, Sun Yat-sen University, 56 Ling Yuan Road West, 510055 Guangzhou, Guangdong Province, China
Full list of author information is available at the end of the article

and the social network or the community that individuals belong to. The second is subjective and emotional support, which reflects the emotional experience and degree of satisfaction experienced when individuals feel respected, supported and understood. When individuals receive more social support, they may be better able to cope with psychological distress in their life, which could help them maintain better health. It has been reported that those who receive less social support or use their available social support less effectively are more likely to adopt unhealthy oral health behaviors, such as smoking and alcohol consumption, which could increase their risk of developing periodontitis [11].

Social support of children is provided by their caregivers. Access to and availability of social support from their caregivers could affect the oral health of children. Children from families with better access to social support are more likely to utilize dental services, have better oral health habits, and exhibit better oral health [12–14]. A mother's social support is significantly associated with the tooth brushing habits of children aged 1-3 years but not with those of children aged 4-5 years [15]. The reason for this might be that children younger than 3 years have no ability to live independently and are totally dependent on their caregivers. Thus far, little is known regarding the relationship between the social support of caregivers and the oral health-related behaviors of their children in China.

Our study is a further step in the exploration of the relationship between the social support of caregivers and the oral health-related behaviors of 5-year-old children in China. We hypothesized that a caregiver with more social support would have a child with better oral health-related behaviors, such as a lower frequency of sugary snack intake, more frequent tooth brushing and utilization of dental care services, and regular dental check-ups, than a caregiver with less social support.

Methods

This cross-sectional study was carried out from August 2011 to December 2011 in Guangzhou, China.

Study population

The target population of this study was 5-year-old children and their main caregivers in Guangzhou, China. The main caregiver was defined as the individual who was primarily in charge of the child on a day-to-day basis. For the purposes of this study, the main caregiver could be the child's mother, father or grandparent.

Sampling method

The sampling method was described in our previous study [16]. The sample size was calculated based on the prevalence of dental caries among 5-year-old children in Guangzhou, as reported in the third Chinese national oral health survey [17]. A standard error of 1.5 % was set as the precision of the estimate. Finally, a minimum sample size of 1067 children was calculated as the number needed to satisfy the requirements. The selection of participants was based on a two-stage area probability sample of the 12 administrative districts in Guangzhou. In the first stage, six randomly selected districts were the primary sampling units. In the second stage, four kindergartens were randomly selected in each of the selected administrative districts, and all of the 5-year-old children in the selected kindergartens and their main caregivers were invited to take part in the study. All the caregivers were fully informed of the study purpose in writing, and participation in the study was voluntary.

Instruments and measures

Information relating to the following data was collected using a questionnaire administered to the caregivers: the child's oral health-related behaviors, the caregiver's social support, the caregiver's oral health knowledge, the caregiver's oral health attitudes, the caregiver's oral health-related behaviors, the demographic and socioeconomic background of the participants. The questionnaire was distributed by the kindergarten teachers to the caregivers, who completed the questionnaire at home and returned it to the kindergarten teachers.

Oral health-related behaviors of children and caregivers

The oral health-related behaviors of 5-year-old children and their caregivers that were assessed in this study included the frequency of sugary snack intake (<once/day vs. ≥once/day), tooth brushing frequency (≤once/day vs. ≥twice/day), having used dental services ever (yes vs. no), and the pattern of dental visits for those children who had visited a dentist (for the treatment of dental problems vs. mainly for check-ups). The design of the oral health-related behavior assessment was described in our previous study [16].

Social support

Social support was measured via the Social Support Rating Scale (SSRS) proposed by Xiao [18]. The SSRS contains 10 items and measures the following dimensions of social support: objective support (3 items), subjective support (4 items), and the availability of support (3 items). Objective support reflects the degree of actual support that an individual received in the past, subjective support reflects the perceived interpersonal network that an individual can count on, and the availability of support refers to the pattern of behavior that an individual utilizes when seeking social support. The scores of the 10 items were summed to obtain the overall SSRS score. Thus, the SSRS score could range from 12 to 66, with higher scores indicating stronger social support. Objective support scores ranged from 1 to 22, subjective support scores ranged from 8 to 32, and the support availability scores ranged from 3 to 12. Cultural adaptation of the SSRS has been undertaken in China. The SSRS has been applied in a wide range of Chinese people and has been shown to have good reliability and validity [19, 20]. In this sample, the *Cronbach*'s alpha coefficient of the SSRS was 0.76.

Oral health knowledge and oral health attitudes of the caregivers

The oral health knowledge of the caregivers was measured using four questions regarding the causes and prevention of dental caries and periodontal disease, which were used in a previous study of adults in Guangdong [21]. The two questions relating to the causes and prevention of dental caries were as follows: "Which of the following statements do you believe describe a cause of dental caries?" and "Which of the following statements do you believe describe a method to prevent dental caries?". The two questions relating to the causes and prevention of periodontal disease were as follows: "Which of the following statements do you believe describe a cause of periodontal disease?" and "Which of the following statements do you believe describe a method to prevent periodontal disease?". A score of 1 was given for each correct answer to a question, and a score of 0 was given for an incorrect answer or for an answer of "I don't know". For each question, there were only four correct answers, and the maximum score was 4. The scores from the four questions were summed to obtain the overall oral health knowledge score, which could range from 0 to 16, with higher scores indicating better oral health knowledge.

To explore the attitudes of caregivers toward oral health, eight questions on dental health beliefs and the importance of oral health, retaining natural teeth, and the use of dental service were used, which were used in a previous study [22]. There were three possible responses to each statement: "agree," "disagree" or "neither". For each question, caregivers showing a positive attitude received a score of 1. The total scores for dental attitude were calculated by summing the scores of the eight questions. The final scores ranged from 0 to 8, with higher scores indicating a more positive attitude toward oral health.

Demographic and socioeconomic background

The demographic data included the gender of the child, single-child status, marital status of the parents, caregiver type and socioeconomic background data, including the mother's education and occupation, father's education and occupation, family income, and the child's dental insurance.

Clinical examination

Assessments of the caries status of each child who returned a fully answered questionnaire were carried out by a trained examiner. Decayed, missing and filled teeth (dmft) were recorded according to the recommended criteria of the World Health Organization [23]. The dmft value was set as one of the factors related to the child's dental service use and his/her pattern of dental visits.

Statistical analysis

Data analysis was conducted with SPSS for Windows (version 16.0, Chicago, IL, USA). In the analysis, the child's oral health-related behaviors were set as the outcomes, and the caregiver's social support was set as the independent variable. The caregiver's oral health knowledge and attitudes, the caregiver's oral health-related behaviors, and the child's demographic background, socioeconomic background and dmft value were set as the controlling variables.

The total SSRS score was analyzed as a continuous variable. First, in the univariate analysis, two-sample *t*-tests were used to analyze the relationship between the SSRS scores and the outcome variables, and the relationships between the controlling variables and the outcome variables were assessed via chi-square tests or *t*-tests. The controlling variables in the univariate analysis with a p value not higher than 0.20 were included in the multiple logistic regression analysis. Second, the effects of the independent variable and the controlling variables on the outcome variables were tested via multiple logistic regression analysis. For all of the statistical tests, a p value of 0.05 was set as the level of significance.

Results

In total, 1440 questionnaires were distributed; of these, 1332 were fully completed and returned, 46 were not returned, and 62 were returned incomplete and with most items unanswered. Thus, the data from 1332 caregivers (1141 mothers, 85.7 %; 72 fathers, 5.4 %; and 119 grandparents, 8.9 %) were used for the analysis of the relationship between the caregiver's social support and the child's oral health-related behaviors. Among the children of the 1332 caregivers, 54.9 % (731) were boys and 45.1 % (601) were girls.

The frequency distributions of the categorical variables and the values of the continuous variables are shown in Tables 1 and 2.

The caregivers' total SSRS scores ranged from 19 to 62, with a mean of 43.2 and a standard deviation of 6.6. The means and standard deviations of the SSRS scores of the different types of caregivers were, respectively, 43.4 and 6.6 for the mothers, 41.8 and 6.7 for the fathers, and 42.6 and 6.6 for the grandparents. No statistically significant differences were found in the total SSRS scores among the various types of caregivers ($p = 0.083$).

Table 1 Frequency distribution of the categorical variables

Variables	Number	Percentage
Gender		
Boy	731	54.9
Girl	601	45.1
Single child		
Yes	936	70.3
No	396	29.7
Caregivers		
Mother	1141	85.7
Father	72	5.4
Grandparent	119	8.9
Marital status of parents		
Cohabiting	1309	98.3
Not cohabiting	23	1.7
Mother's education		
≤ high school graduated	727	54.6
≥ university graduated	605	45.4
Mother's occupation		
Unemployed	248	18.6
Employee/non-professional	794	59.6
Employer/professional	290	21.8
Father's education		
≤ high school graduated	677	50.8
≥ university graduated	655	49.2
Father's occupation		
Unemployed	52	3.9
Employee/non-professional	846	63.5
Employer/professional	434	32.6
Family monthly income (per-capital)		
< 2000 RMB	262	19.7
2000-4999 RMB	546	41
≥ 5000 RMB	524	39.3
Child's dental insurance		
No	1056	79.3
Yes	276	20.7
Child's frequency of sugary snack intake		
< once/day	671	50.4
≥ once/day	661	49.6
Child's toothbrushing frequency		
≤ once/day	896	67.3
≥ twice/day	436	32.7
Child's dental service utilization		
No	923	69.3
Yes	409	30.7
Child's pattern of dental attendance		
For treatment of dental problem	348	85.1
Mainly for check-up	61	14.9
Caregiver's frequency of sugary snack intake		
< once/day	833	62.5
≥ once/day	499	37.5
Caregiver's toothbrushing frequency		
≤ once/day	405	30.4
≥ twice/day	927	69.6
Caregiver's dental service utilization		
No	381	28.6
Yes	951	71.4
Caregiver's pattern of dental attendance		
For treatment of dental problem	833	87.6
Mainly for check-up	118	12.4

The results show that the caregiver's social support was significantly associated with the child's tooth brushing frequency, utilization of dental care, and pattern of dental visits but not with the frequency of sugary snack intake. Children whose caregivers had higher SSRS scores had a higher frequency of tooth brushing ($p = 0.007$) and utilization of dental care ($p = 0.006$) than did the children whose caregivers scored lower on the SSRS. Among the children having received dental care, the children whose caregivers scored higher on the SSRS were more likely to visit the dentist mainly for check-ups than for treatment of a dental problem ($p = 0.009$) (Table 3).

Because the caregiver's social support was associated with the child's tooth brushing frequency, utilization of dental care, and pattern of dental visits, a further analysis was performed.

Social support and children's tooth brushing frequency

As shown in Table 4, it was found that the controlling variables of a child's gender, single-child status, type of caregiver, mother's education and occupation, father's education, family monthly income, caregiver's tooth

Table. 2 Values of the continuous variables

Variables	Mean	SD
Caregiver's social support	43.2	6.6
Caregiver's oral health knowledge	9.1	3.9
Caregiver's oral health attitudes	6.2	1.4
Child's dmft value	3.8	4.5

Table 3 Univariate analysis between the child's oral health-related behaviors and the caregiver's total social support ($n = 1332$)

Outcome variables	Number	Percentage	Social support Mean (SD)	P-value
Child's frequency of sugary snack intake				
< once/day	671	50.4	43.4 (6.5)	0.434
≥ once/day	661	49.6	43.1 (6.7)	
Child's toothbrushing frequency				
≤once/day	896	67.3	42.9 (6.7)	**0.007**
≥twice/day	436	32.7	43.9 (6.4)	
Child's utilization of dental care of children				
No	923	69.3	42.9 (6.7)	**0.006**
Yes	409	30.7	44.0 (6.2)	
Child's pattern of dental attendance				
For treatment of dental problem	348	85.1	43.7 (6.3)	**0.009**
Mainly for check-up	61	14.9	45.9 (5.9)	

A p value of 0.05 was set as the level of significance. Bold data is a p value set as the level of significance

brushing frequency, and caregiver's oral health knowledge and attitudes were significantly associated with the child's tooth brushing frequency.

After adjusting for the above controlling variables in a multiple logistic regression analysis, the caregiver's SSRS score was not significantly associated with the child's tooth brushing frequency. The child's tooth brushing frequency was significantly related to the child's sex, mother's and father's education, and caregiver's tooth brushing frequency and oral health knowledge. Girls were more likely to brush their teeth twice or more a day (OR = 1.30, $p = 0.034$). Children with a mother or father with a higher level of education brushed their teeth more frequently (OR = 1.39, $p = 0.035$; OR = 1.39, $p = 0.031$, respectively). Children whose caregivers brushed their teeth more frequently were more likely to brush their teeth more frequently (OR = 3.57, $p < 0.001$) (Table 5).

Table 4 Univariate analysis between the control variables and the child's toothbrushing frequency ($n = 1332$)

Variables	Frequency of toothbrushing		
	≤once/day n (%)	≥twice/day n (%)	P-value
Gender			
Boy	513 (57.3)	218 (50.0)	
Girl	383 (42.7)	218 (50.0)	**0.013***
Single child			
Yes	600 (67.0)	336 (77.1)	
No	296 (33.0)	100 (22.9)	**<0.001***
Caregivers			
Mother	755 (84.3)	386 (88.5)	
Father	53 (5.9)	19 (4.4)	
Grandparent	88 (9.8)	31 (7.1)	0.113*
Marital status of parents			
Cohabiting	878 (98.0)	431 (98.9)	
Not cohabiting	5 (2.0)	18 (1.1)	0.257*
Mother's education			
≤ high school graduated	545 (60.8)	182 (41.7)	
≥ university graduated	351 (39.2)	254 (58.3)	**<0.001***
Mother's occupation			
Unemployed	180 (20.1)	68 (15.6)	
Employee/non-professional	543 (60.6)	251 (57.6)	
Employer/professional	173 (19.3)	117 (36.8)	**0.004***
Father's education			
≤ high school graduated	509 (56.8)	168 (38.5)	
≥ university graduated	387 (43.2)	268 (61.5)	**<0.001***
Father's occupation			
Unemployed	37 (4.1)	15 (3.4)	
Employee/non-professional	585 (65.3)	261 (59.9)	
Employer/professional	274 (30.6)	160 (36.7)	0.079*
Family monthly income (per-capital)			
< 2000 RMB	195 (21.8)	67 (15.4)	**0.002***
2000-4999 RMB	374 (41.7)	172 (39.4)	
≥ 5000 RMB	327 (36.5)	197 (45.2)	
Caregiver's toothbrushing frequency			
≤ once/day	346 (38.6)	59 (13.5)	
≥ twice/day	550 (61.4)	377 (86.5)	**<0.001***
	Mean(SD)	Mean(SD)	
Caregiver's oral health knowledge score	8.7 (4.0)	9.9 (3.5)	**<0.001****
Caregiver's oral health attitude score	6.2 (1.4)	6.4 (1.3)	**0.010****

(*by Chi-square test; **by t-test). A p value of 0.05 was set as the level of significance Bold data is a p value set as the level of significance

Social support and children's use of dental care

As shown in Table 6, the controlling variables of the father's occupation, caregiver's utilization of dental care and the child's dmft value were significantly associated with the child's utilization of dental care.

After adjusting for the above controlling variables in a multiple logistic regression analysis, the caregiver's SSRS score was not significantly associated with the child's utilization of dental care. The child's utilization of dental care was significantly associated with the father's occupation, caregiver's utilization of dental care and child's dmft value. Children with more caries, children whose father was an employer/professional, and children whose caregiver had used dental care were more likely to have visited a dentist (all $p < 0.05$) (Table 7).

Table 5 Multiple logistic regression analysis between the caregiver's social support and the child's toothbrushing frequency ($n = 1332$)

Variables	Frequency of toothbrushing (≤once/day vs. ≥ twice/day)*	
	Adjusted OR (95 % CI)	*P*-value
Caregiver's social support	-	-
Gender		
Boy	1	
Girl	1.30 (1.02 ~ 1.67)	**0.034**
Single child		
Yes	1	
No	0.77 (0.58 ~ 1.02)	0.072
Caregivers		
Mother		
Father	-	-
Grandparent	-	-
Mother's education		
≤ high school graduated	1	
≥ university graduated	1.39 (1.02 ~ 1.88)	**0.035**
Mother's occupation		
Unemployed		
Employee/non-professional	-	-
Employer/professional	-	-
Father's education		
≤ high school graduated	1	
≥ university graduated	1.39 (1.03 ~ 1.87)	**0.031**
Father's occupation		
Unemployed		
Employee/non-professional	-	-
Employer/professional	-	-
Family monthly income (per-capital)		
< 2000 RMB		
2000-4999 RMB	-	-
≥ 5000 RMB	-	-
Caregiver's toothbrushing frequency		
≤ once/day	1	
≥ twice/day	3.57 (2.61 ~ 4.87)	**<0.001**
Caregiver's oral health knowledge score	1.04 (1.01 ~ 1.07)	**0.03**
Caregiver's oral health attitude score	-	

*in the multiple logistic regression analysis, "≤once/day" was set as the reference category. A *p* value of 0.05 was set as the level of significance
Bold data is a *p* value set as the level of significance

Social support and children's patterns of dental visits

As shown in Table 8, the controlling variables of family monthly income, a caregiver's pattern of dental visits and oral health attitude, and a child's dmft value were significantly associated with the pattern of a child's dental visits.

After adjusting for the above controlling variables in a multiple logistic regression analysis, the caregiver's SSRS score was not significantly linked to the child's utilization of dental care. The pattern of a child's dental care utilization was significantly associated with the pattern of the caregiver's dental care utilization and the dmft value of the child. Caregivers who visited the dentist primarily for check-ups had children who visited the dentist primarily for check-ups (OR = 5.78, $p < 0.001$). A child who had more teeth caries was not likely to have visited the dentist primarily for check-ups but rather for the treatment of dental problems (OR = 0.93, $p = 0.035$) (Table 9).

Discussion

This cross-sectional study shows that the associations between a caregiver's social support and a child's oral health-related behaviors, including the frequency of sugary snack intake, tooth brushing frequency, use of dental services and pattern of dental visits, were not significant.

In this study, the tooth brushing frequency of 5-year-old children was not related to the social support of their caregivers. This result is similar to that of a previous study [15]. The brushing frequency of 4-5-year-old children was not associated with their mother's social support and was positively associated with higher family income and dental insurance coverage; higher family income and improved insurance coverage could help increase access to needed services and foster dental health-promoting habits [15]. In our study, a child's tooth brushing frequency was linked to other factors, including the child's sex, the mother and father's education, and the caregiver's tooth brushing frequency and oral health knowledge. These results indicate that caregivers who were more knowledgeable regarding oral hygiene needs and who brushed their own teeth more frequently had children who brushed more frequently. Girls were found to brush their teeth more frequently, and it is possible that the girls received more attention from the caregivers than the boys. This result indicates that boys should receive more attention from programs aimed at promoting oral health behaviors in Guangzhou, China.

Research has shown that mothers with greater social support received more information regarding dental care from family members or friends and focused more on improving access to dental care for their younger children [14]. However, in our study, no significant association between the caregiver's social support and the child's utilization of dental care was found; the same result was found for the pattern of a child's utilization of dental care. In our study, approximately 30.7 % of the children had received dental care; only 14.9 % of the children had visited the dentist primarily for check-ups. We found that the children with more caries were more likely to have had dental visits and to have visited the dentist predominantly

Table 6 Univariate analysis between the control variables and the child's utilization of dental care ($n = 1332$)

Variables	Utilization of dental care		
	No	Yes	*P*-value
	n (%)	n (%)	
Gender			
Boy	514 (55.7)	217 (53.1)	
Girl	409 (44.3)	192 (46.9)	0.373*
Single child			
Yes	638 (69.1)	298 (72.9)	
No	285 (30.9)	111 (27.1)	0.169*
Caregivers			
Mother	783 (84.8)	358 (87.5)	
Father	51 (5.5)	21 (5.2)	
Grandparent	89 (9.7)	30 (7.3)	0.366*
Marital status of parents			
Cohabiting	905 (98.0)	404 (98.8)	
Not cohabiting	18 (2.0)	5 (1.2)	0.347*
Mother's education			
≤ high school graduated	505 (54.7)	222 (54.3)	
≥ university graduated	418 (45.3)	187 (45.7)	0.883*
Mother's occupation			
Unemployed	180 (19.5)	68 (16.6)	
Employee/non-professional	533 (57.8)	261 (63.8)	
Employer/professional	210 (22.8)	80 (19.6)	0.114*
Father's education			
≤ high school graduated	470 (50.9)	207 (50.6)	
≥ university graduated	453 (49.1)	202 (49.4)	0.917*
Father's occupation			
Unemployed	45 (4.8)	7 (1.7)	
Employee/non-professional	584 (63.3)	262 (64.1)	
Employer/professional	294 (31.9)	140 (34.2)	**0.02***
Family monthly income (per-capital)			
< 2000 RMB	184 (19.9)	78 (19.1)	0.929*
2000-4999 RMB	378 (41.0)	168 (41.1)	
≥ 5000 RMB	361 (39.1)	163 (39.9)	
Child's dental insurance			
No	719 (77.9)	337 (82.4)	
Yes	204 (22.1)	72 (17.6)	0.062*
Caregiver's dental insurance			
No	676 (73.2)	303 (74.1)	
Yes	247 (26.8)	106 (25.9)	0.748*
Caregiver's utilization of dental care			
No	295 (32.0)	86 (21.0)	
Yes	628 (68.0)	323 (79.0)	**<0.001***
	Mean(SD)	Mean(SD)	

Table 6 Univariate analysis between the control variables and the child's utilization of dental care ($n = 1332$) *(Continued)*

Caregiver's oral health knowledge score	9.0 (3.8)	9.3 (4.0)	0.258**
Caregiver's oral health attitude score	6.2 (1.4)	6.3 (1.4)	0.628**
dmft	3.0 (4.0)	5.4 (5.2)	**<0.001****

(*by Chi-square test; **by t-test). A *p* value of 0.05 was set as the level of significance
Bold data is a *p* value set as the level of significance

for treatment of dental problems. These findings indicate that the occurrence of dental caries was the principal reason for children to visit a dentist. Additionally, our study revealed that a child's utilization of dental care and their pattern of dental care use were strongly linked to the caregiver's utilization of dental care and pattern of dental care use, respectively. Most of the caregivers had dental visits that were predominantly for dental problems, indicating that caregivers neglect the importance of regular dental check-ups in their own and their children's oral health. The severe shortage of pediatric dentists was a limitation leading to the lack of utilization of dental care for children and the lack of information and assistance provided to caregivers by dentists.

Table 7 Multiple logistic regression analysis between the caregiver's social support and children's the child's utilization of dental care ($n = 1332$)

Variables	Utilization of dental care (No vs. Yes)*	
	Adjusted OR (95 % CI)	*P*-value
Caregive's social support	1.02(0.99 ~ 1.04)	0.094
Single child		
Yes		
No	-	-
Mother's occupation		
Unemployed	1	0.082
Employee/non-professional	1.01 (0.79 ~ 1.54)	0.575
Employer/professional	0.74 (0.48 ~ 1.14)	0.171
Father's occupation		**0.025**
Unemployed		
Employee/non-professional	2.67 (1.14 ~ 6.23)	**0.023**
Employer/professional	3.35 (1.40 ~ 7.98)	**0.006**
Child's dental insurance		
No		
Yes	-	-
Caregiver's utilization of dental care		
No	1	
Yes	1.75 (1.31 ~ 2.33)	**<0.001**
dmft	1.12 (1.09 ~ 1.15)	**<0.001**

*in the multiple logistic regression analysis, "No" was set as the reference category. A *p* value of 0.05 was set as the level of significance
Bold data is a *p* value set as the level of significance

Table 8 Univariate analysis between the control variables and the child's pattern of dental attendance ($n = 409$)

Variables	Pattern of dental attendance		
	For treatment of dental problem	Mainly for check-up	*P*-value
	n (%)	n (%)	
Gender			
Boy	185 (55.2)	32 (52.5)	0.919*
Girl	163 (46.8)	29 (47.5)	
Single child			
Yes	251 (72.1)	47 (77.0)	0.425*
No	97 (27.9)	14 (23.0)	
Caregiver			
Mother	303 (87.1)	55 (90.2)	0.728*
Father	18 (5.2)	3 (4.9)	
Grandfather or grandmother	27 (7.7)	3 (4.9)	
Marital status of parents			
Cohabiting	193 (55.5)	659 (98.2)	0.862*
Not cohabiting	11 (1.7)	12 (1.8)	
Mother's education			
≤ high school graduated	193 (55.5)	29 (47.5)	0.252*
≥ college graduated	155 (44.5)	32 (52.5)	
Mother's occupation			
Unemployed	57 (16.4)	11 (18.0)	0.478*
Employee/non-professional	226 (64.9)	35 (57.4)	
Employer/professional	65 (18.7)	15 (24.6)	
Father's education			
≤ high school graduated	183 (52.6)	24 (39.3)	0.056*
≥ college graduated	165 (47.4)	37 (60.7)	
Father's occupation			
Unemployed	7 (2.0)	0 (0)	0.202*
Employee/non-professional	227 (65.2)	35 (57.4)	
Employer/professional	114 (32.8)	26 (42.6)	
Family monthly income (per-capital)			
< 2000 RMB	69 (19.8)	9 (14.8)	**0.048***
2000-4999 RMB	149 (42.8)	19 (31.1)	
≥ 5000 RMB	130 (37.4)	33 (54.1)	
Child's dental insurance			
No	293 (84.2)	44 (72.1)	**0.022***
Yes	55 (15.8)	17 (27.9)	
Caregiver's pattern of dental attendance			
For treatment of dental problem	245 (90.4)	31 (59.6)	**<0.001***
Mainly for check-up	26 (9.6)	21 (40.4)	
	Mean(SD)	Mean(SD)	
Caregiver's oral health knowledge score	9.2 (4.0)	100 (3.8)	0.117**
Caregiver's oral health attitude score	6.2 (1.4)	6.6 (1.3)	**0.027****
Child'sdmft value	5.7 (5.3)	3.6 (4.4)	**0.005****

(* by Chi-square test; ** by t-test). A *p* value of 0.05 was set as the level of significance
Bold data is a *p* value set as the level of significance

No research has been conducted to explore the relationship between a caregiver's social support and a child's frequency of sugary snack intake. In this study, the caregiver's social support was not significantly associated with a child's frequency of sugary snack intake. The frequency of sugary snack intake by children was predominantly related to the caregiver's frequency of sugary snack intake and other factors, which was also shown in our previous study [16, 22]. In addition, these findings revealed that a child's sugary snack intake habits are influenced by his/her caregiver's sugary snack intake habits.

In Guangzhou, China, a child's oral health-related behaviors were associated with his/her caregiver's oral health-related behaviors and not with his/her caregiver's social support. The reason that the social support of the caregiver was not related to the child's oral health-related

Table 9 Multiple logistic regression analysis between the caregiver's social support and children's and the child's pattern of dental attendance ($n = 409$)

Variables	Pattern of dental attendance	
	(For treatment of dental problem vs. Mainly for check-up)*	
	Adjusted OR (95 % CI)	*P*-value
Caregive's social support	-	-
Father's education		
≤ high school graduated		
≥ college graduated	-	-
Family monthly income (per-capital)		
< 2000 RMB		
2000-4999 RMB	-	-
≥ 5000 RMB	-	-
Children's dental insurance		
No		
Yes	-	-
Caregiver's pattern of dental attendance		
For treatment of dental problem		
Mainly for check-up	5.78 (2.89-11.6)	**<0.001**
Caregiver's oral health attitude score	-	-
Child's dmft value	0.93 (0.87-0.99)	**0.035**

*in the multiple logistic regression analysis, "for treatment of dental problem" was set as the reference category. A *p* value of 0.05 was set as the level of significance
Bold data is a *p* value set as the level of significance

behaviors is not clear. Other research has shown that the social support of individuals is associated with their oral health-related behaviors [7, 8]. In the present study, the caregiver's oral health-related behaviors were related to the child's oral health-related behaviors; the social support of a caregiver could indirectly influence a child's oral health-related behaviors through influences on the caregiver's own oral health-related behaviors. This is a hypothesis that needs further study.

Some further points should be noted with respect to this study. Adoption of consistent behavioral habits in childhood occurs at home, and caregivers could be the primary models for children's behavior. Caregivers with good personal oral hygiene skills are more likely to understand the importance of a child's oral health than caregivers with poor oral hygiene skills and would likely be more effective in controlling proper tooth brushing, sugary snack intake and other oral health behaviors of their children [24, 25]. We have demonstrated that caregivers who have better oral health habits are more likely to have children with better oral health habits. Young children depend on their caregivers to take care of their oral health needs, and caregivers play a key role in influencing the habits and health status of their children. Therefore, more attention should be paid to improving the oral health-related behaviors of caregivers for the promotion of children's oral health.

This study was the first to explore the relationship between the social support of caregivers and their children's oral health behaviors, and it has some limitations. First, the data in this study were cross-sectional, which precludes drawing inferences regarding the causal relationships between the social support of caregivers and the oral health behaviors of their children. Further work on this topic should adopt a longitudinal approach. Second, further research should be conducted to explore whether the social support of a caregiver might influence his/her oral health-related behaviors, thus indirectly influencing his/her child's oral health-related behaviors.

Conclusions

These findings indicate that the oral health-related behaviors of 5-year-old children in Guangzhou are unrelated to the social support of their caregivers and are instead related to other specific factors, particularly the caregiver's oral health-related behaviors. The potential for caregivers to play a significant role in the oral health of their children should be considered in the development of programs to promote oral health.

Acknowledgements

Support for this study was provided by the Department of Preventive Dentistry, Guanghua School of Stomatology, and Guangdong Provincial Key Laboratory of Stomatology, Sun Yat-sen University. We would like to acknowledge the Department of Education of Guangzhou; the administrators, teachers and public health officials affiliated with the kindergartens that participated in the study; and the children and their caregivers for their cooperation

Funding

No funding was obtained for this study.

Authors' contributions

RMQ: study design, data collection and manuscript writing. YT, YZ and QHZ: data collection and analysis. HCL: study design, fieldworker training and supervision, and critical revision of the manuscript for important intellectual content. All of the authors read and approved the final manuscript.

Competing interests

The authors declare that they have no competing interests.

Consent for publication

Not applicable.

Ethics approval and consent to participate

Before beginning the study, the protocol was approved by the Ethics Committee of Guanghua School of Stomatology, Sun Yat-sen University, and written informed consent for participation was obtained from the caregiver participants.

Author details

[1]Department of Preventive Dentistry, Guanghua School of Stomatology, Guangdong Provincial Key Laboratory of Stomatology, Sun Yat-sen University, 56 Ling Yuan Road West, 510055 Guangzhou, Guangdong Province, China. [2]Department of Pediatric Dentistry, College of Stomatology, Guangxi Medical University, Nanning, China.

References

1. Petersen PE. Global policy for improvement of oral health in the 21st century–implications to oral health research of World Health Assembly 2007, World Health Organization. Community Dent Oral Epidemiol. 2009;37(1):1–8.
2. Sgan-Cohen HD. Oral hygiene improvement: a pragmatic approach based upon risk and motivation levels. BMC Oral Health. 2008;8:31.
3. Al-Ansari J, Honkala E, Honkala S. Oral health knowledge and behavior among male health sciences college students in Kuwait. BMC Oral Health. 2003;3(1):2.
4. Poutanen R, Lahti S, Hausen H. Oral health-related knowledge, attitudes, and beliefs among 11 to 12-year-old Finnish schoolchildren with different oral health behaviors. Acta Odontol Scand. 2005;63(1):10–6.
5. Dorri M, Sheiham A, Hardy R, Watt R. The relationship between Sense of Coherence and toothbrushing behaviours in Iranian adolescents in Mashhad. J Clin Periodontol. 2010;37(1):46–52.
6. Silva AN, Mendonça MH, Vettore MV. A salutogenic approach to oral health promotion. Cad Saude Publica. 2008;24 Suppl 4:s521–530.
7. Merchant AT, Pitiphat W, Ahmed B, Kawachi I, Joshipura K. A prospective study of social support, anger expression and risk of periodontitis in men. J Am Dent Assoc. 2003;134(12):1591–6.
8. Vered Y, Soskolne V, Zini A, Livny A, Sgan-Cohen HD. Psychological distress and social support are determinants of changing oral health status among an immigrant population from Ethiopia. Community Dent Oral Epidemiol. 2011;39(2):145–53.
9. Shumaker SA, Bronwell A. Toward a theory of social support: closing conceptual gaps. Journal of Social Issues. 1984;40(4):11–33.
10. Kessler RC, Price RH, Wootman CB. Social factors in psychopathy: stress, social support and coping stress. Ann Rev Psychology. 1985;36:532–72.
11. Handley ED, Chassin L. Stress-induced drinking in parents of adolescents with externalizing symptomatology the moderating role of parent social support. Am J Addict. 2008;17(6):469–77.

12. Reisine S, Ajrouch KJ, Sohn W, Lim S, Ismail A. Characteristics of African-American male caregivers in a study of oral health in Detroit–a brief communication. J Public Health Dent. 2009;69(3):197–200.
13. Tellez M, Sohn W, Burt BA, Ismail AI. Assessment of the relationship between neighborhood characteristics and dental caries severity among low-income African-Americans: a multilevel approach. J Public Health Dent. 2006;66(1):30–6.
14. Nahouraii H, Wasserman M, Bender DE, Rozier RG. Social support and dental utilization among children of Latina immigrants. Health Care Poor Underserved. 2008;19(2):428–41.
15. Finlayson TL, Siefert K, Ismail AI, Sohn W. Maternal self-efficacy and 1-5-year-old children's brushing habits. Community Dent Oral Epidemiol. 2007;35(4):272–81.
16. Qiu RM, Wong MC, Lo ECM, Lin HC. Relationship between children's oral health-related behaviors and their caregiver's sense of coherence. BMC Public Health. 2013;13:239.
17. Qi XQ. Report of the third national oral health survey in China [In Chinese]. Beijing: People's Medical Publishing House; 2007. p. 20–4.
18. Xiao S. Social support rating scale. In: Wang X, editor. Mental Health Scale (Suppl). Beijing: Chinese Mental Health Publishing House; 1999. p. 127–33.
19. Xie RH, He G, Koszycki D, Walker M, Wen SW. Prenatal social support, postnatal social support, and postpartum depression. Ann Epidemiol. 2009;19(9):637–43.
20. Ke X, Liu CJ, Li NX. Social support and quality of life: a crosssectional study on survivors eight months after the 2008 Wenchuan earthquake. BMC Public Health. 2010;10:573.
21. Lin HC, Wong MCM, Wang ZJ, Lo EC. Oral health Knowledge, attitudes, and practices of Chinese adults. J Dent Res. 2001;80(5):1466–70.
22. Qiu RM, Lo ECM, Zhi QH, Zhou Y, Tao Y, Lin HC. Factors related to children's caries: a structural equation modeling approach. BMC Public Health. 2014;14:1071.
23. World Health Organization. Oral health surveys: basic methods. 4th ed. Geneva: World Health Organization; 1997.
24. Poutanen R, Lahti S, Tolvanen M, Hausen H. Parental influence on children's oral health-related behavior. Acta Odontol Scand. 2006;64(5):286–92.
25. Vanagas G, Milasauskiene Z, Grabauskas V, Mickeviciene A. Associations between parental skills and their attitudes toward importance to develop good oral hygiene skills in their children. Medicina (Kaunas). 2009;45(9):718–23.

12

Management of Dentin Hypersensitivity by National Dental Practice-Based Research Network practitioners: results from a questionnaire administered prior to initiation of a clinical study on this topic

Dorota T. Kopycka-Kedzierawski[1*], Cyril Meyerowitz[1], Mark S. Litaker[2], Sidney Chonowski[3], Marc W. Heft[4], Valeria V. Gordan[4], Robin L. Yardic[5], Theresa E. Madden[6], Stephanie C. Reyes[7], Gregg H. Gilbert[2] and National Dental PBRN Collaborative Group

Abstract

Background: Dentin hypersensitivity (DH) is a common problem encountered in clinical practice. The purpose of this study was to identify the management approaches for DH among United States dentists.

Methods: One hundred eighty five National Dental Practice-Based Research Network clinicians completed a questionnaire regarding their preferred methods to diagnose and manage DH in the practice setting, and their beliefs about DH predisposing factors.

Results: Almost all dentists (99%) reported using more than one method to diagnose DH. Most frequently, they reported using spontaneous patient reports coupled with excluding other causes of oral pain by direct clinical examination (48%); followed by applying an air blast (26%), applying cold water (12%), and obtaining patient reports after dentist's query (6%). In managing DH, the most frequent first choice was desensitizing, over-the-counter (OTC), potassium nitrate toothpaste (48%), followed by fluorides (38%), and glutaraldehyde/HEMA (3%). A total of 86% of respondents reported using a combination of products when treating DH, most frequently using fluoride varnish and desensitizing OTC potassium nitrate toothpaste (70%). The most frequent predisposing factor leading to DH, as reported by the practitioners, was recessed gingiva (66%), followed by abrasion, erosion, abfraction/attrition lesions (59%) and bruxism (32%).

Conclusions: The majority of network practitioners use multiple methods to diagnose and manage DH. Desensitizing OTC potassium nitrate toothpaste and fluoride formulations are the most widely used products to manage DH in dental practice setting.

Keywords: Dentin hypersensitivity, National Dental Practice-Based Research Network

* Correspondence: Dorota_KopyckaKedzierawski@urmc.rochester.edu
[1]Eastman Institute for Oral Health, University of Rochester, 625 Elmwood Ave, Rochester, NY 14620, USA
Full list of author information is available at the end of the article

Background

Dentin hypersensitivity (DH) has been defined as a "short, sharp pain arising from exposed dentin in response to stimuli, typically thermal, evaporative, tactile, osmotic or chemical, and that cannot be ascribed to any other form of dental defect or pathology" [1]. One of the most frequent patient complaints is related to cold stimuli, although pain may also occur when consuming acidic foods (mainly fruit), sweets and salty foods. Tactile stimulus provocation frequently occurs when patients brush their teeth or rub the sensitive area with a finger nail [2].

DH is a relatively common problem encountered in clinical practice. It may disturb patients during eating, drinking and brushing. The prevalence of DH has been reported to be in the range of 8 to 57% [1, 3–11]. The wide range could be related to different methods used to diagnose this condition and whether prevalence was assessed by clinical examination and/or questionnaires [12].

For example, among 780 patients from the Health Examination Center of National Taiwan University Hospital, the prevalence of DH was 32% [9]. The self-reported prevalence of DH among regular attenders in three general dental practices in the United Kingdom was 52%; DH was most prevalent among 30–40 year old patients and it was more common among female patients [10]. A cross-sectional study conducted by 19 dental practitioners in the United Kingdom examined 4841 patients in one calendar month and found that 4.1% of patients were diagnosed with DH based on the dentist examination. Upper premolars were the most commonly affected, and cold drinks initiated DH most often. More sensitive teeth were found in patients with periodontal disease who also smoked [13].

Based on a cross-sectional survey of 787 adult patients from 37 general dental practices within the Northwest PRECEDENT Practice Based-Research Network (PBRN), the prevalence of DH was 12.3% [11]. Patients with hypersensitivity had, on average, 3.5 hypersensitive teeth. The prevalence was highest among patients who were 18–44 years of age and lowest among patients who were 65 years of age or older. The prevalence was higher among women, patients with gingival recession and patients who used at home tooth whitening products [11].

No clear consensus among Northwest PRECEDENT dentists existed for successfully treating DH, but fluoride varnishes and gels apparently were most widely employed. Dentists also expressed high levels of interest in testing fluoride varnishes and gels, as well as glutaraldehyde/HEMA and restorative treatments, in future studies [14].

DH affects patients of any age with its peak occurrence in middle-aged adults. It may affect any tooth, but most often affects canines and first premolars, probably because they are prominent in the arch and they are exposed to higher pressure during tooth brushing. It may present clinically on any tooth surface, but most often occurs on the buccal cervical margins of teeth. Several theories of DH have been proposed. These include hydrodynamic, odontoblast transduced mechanism and direct innervation theories [7]. None of these mechanisms fully explain this phenomenon. Although dentin sensitivity appears to be prevalent, no universally used or highly reliable desensitizing agents or treatment modalities have been identified [15, 16].

Recently the Practitioners Engaged in Applied Research and Learning Network (PEARL Network) conducted a randomized clinical trial in the practice setting to assess the outcomes of noncarious cervical lesion treatment choices [17]. The overall objective was to determine the efficacy of three randomly assigned treatments for hypersensitive noncarious lesions: chemoactive dentifrice use, dentin bonding agent with sealing and flowable resin-based composite restoration. The secondary outcomes were tubule occlusion, retention of resin coating, retention of restoration and change in lesion size. Results suggest that placement of the sealant or resin restoration was effective in reducing hypersensitive noncarious cervical lesions over the 6-month study period.

According to a survey of dental practitioners conducted by the Canadian Advisory Board on Dentin Hypersensitivity, approximately 50% of the respondents reported lack of confidence in managing patients' pain due to DH [1]. The Canadian Advisory Board on Dentin Hypersensitivity suggested that providers initiate management of this condition by applying desensitizing treatment that is noninvasive; i.e., desensitizing toothpaste and/or topical agents. Some dental providers use a stepped approach to treatment with multiple visits; others apply and prescribe multiple treatments at one time. Invasive treatments of DH are also performed by placing a restoration on an otherwise healthy tooth [1].

Although DH has been studied previously in the practice-based research setting, there have been wide differences among clinicians as to the methods used to diagnose and manage DH; furthermore the prior data were constrained to one region of the US. Therefore, the purpose of this study was to identify in a broader national context the preferred methods to diagnose and manage DH in the practice setting and to assess practitioners' beliefs about DH predisposing factors. In addition, we assessed whether practitioner and practice characteristics were associated with practitioners' selected treatments and approaches to care.

Methods

As an initial phase of a prospective, multicenter cohort study of patients with DH, 185 National Dental Practice-Based Research Network (National Dental PBRN) clinicians answered an online questionnaire related to the diagnostic methods, treatment modalities and predisposing factors of DH. The questionnaire is publicly available and it is enclosed in a supplementary file with the manuscript [18]. The current paper reports the results of the online questionnaire that was administered prior to initiation of a cohort study on this topic. The network is a consortium of dental practices and organizations that participate in clinical research studies and comprises six regions across the US [18, 19].

Initially, the study investigators pilot tested the questionnaire with six practitioners to assess its length, acceptability, and internet browser compatibility. Based on practitioner feedback, the study investigators administered a revised questionnaire to 24 additional practitioners to quantify test-retest reliability for 94 items (text items were not evaluated). Agreement between responses was calculated for each of 24 practitioners. For each practitioner, if there was no response for an item at both test and retest, this item was not included in the evaluation. Percentage agreement was calculated as the number of items for which the test and retest responses were the same, divided by the number of items for which the practitioner provided responses, multiplied by 100. Descriptive statistics were calculated for the practitioner-level agreement values. The mean number of items for which responses were provided was 37.63, minimum 19, maximum 48. The mean number of items showing agreement was 24.33, minimum 13, maximum 33. The mean agreement across the 24 practitioners was 65.01%. The minimum and maximum agreement for individual practitioners was 45.65 and 100%. The questionnaire was not modified after testing. The test-retest questionnaires were completed in February 2015. Practitioners also complete an enrollment questionnaire that describes characteristics about themselves and their practice(s). Selected questions from the enrollment questionnaire were used to explore which characteristics were associated with practitioners' treatments and approaches to DH care. Practitioner variables included: age, gender, race/ethnicity and dental specialty. Practice variables included: practice size, location and practice type.

The study participants were invited to enroll in the study in March 2015. Any National Dental PBRN practitioner (i.e., general dentist and specialist) who was enrolled in the network at the full participation level was eligible to participate in the study. One hundred eighty five practitioners were study-ready by the end of July 2015, having completed all necessary human subjects and conflict of interest training as required by the National Dental PBRN procedures.

Statistical Analysis

Sample size considerations were based on precision of estimation of percentages, represented by the widths of 95% confidence intervals adjusted for the effect of clustered sampling due to enrolment of multiple patients per dental practice. Adjustment for clustering used variance inflation factors calculated for a range of likely values of intracluster correlation (ICC). Power to detect a difference between proportions of dentists using each of the treatment modalities was estimated based on cluster-adjusted chi-square tests to approximate the power of the proposed GEE analysis. Based on this analysis, the target sample size of the study was set at 180 practitioners.

Descriptive statistics including frequencies, means, medians, standard deviations and quartiles were calculated. The chi-square and Fisher's exact tests were used to compare distributions of categorical variables. Analysis of variance and the Kruskal-Wallis test were used for the analysis of continuous variables. The Tukey and Wilcoxon rank sums tests were used for post-hoc comparisons. The analysis was conducted using SAS® Release 9.4 statistical software. *P*-values less than 0.05 were considered statistically significant.

Results

Practitioners' characteristics, practice location and practice type

Among the 185 practitioners who completed the questionnaire, 34 represented the Western region, 29 represented the Midwest region, 30 represented the Southwest region, 30 represented the South Central region and 31 practitioners each represented the South Atlantic and Northeast regions of the National Dental PBRN. Table 1 summarizes practitioners' characteristics, practice location and type. One hundred nineteen practitioners were male (64%) and 66 (36%) were female. The majority (79%) identified themselves as White, 4% as African-American, 10% as Asian and 7% as other racial category. Practitioners' ages differed significantly by network region ($p = 0.02$). Practitioners in the Northeast and the South Central regions were the oldest (mean (SD) age of 56.1 (11.15) years) and practitioners from the South Atlantic region were the youngest (mean (SD) age of 48.7 (12.17) years; $p = 0.02$, ANOVA).

Diagnosis of Dentin Hypersensitivity

Table 2 summarizes the most frequent methods practitioners reported using when diagnosing DH. Spontaneous patient report confirmed by the dental examination, was chosen most frequently as the first choice (48%). This was followed by applying air blast (26%), scratching dentin with a dental explorer (12%), patient report after dentist's query (6%), using other methods, most likely applying endo-ice (4%), and applying cold water (2%).

Table 1 Characteristics of participating practitioners and their practice(s) ($N = 185$)

Practitioner and practice characteristics	
Gender	N (%)
Male	119 (64)
Female	66 (36)
Race	N (%)
White	146 (79)
African-American	8(4)
Asian	18 (10)
Other	12 (7)
Age	Years (SD)
Mean	52 (11.4)
Median	55
Range	27–58
Practice location	%
Inner City of Urban Area	9
Urban Area	27
Suburban	50
Rural	14
Practice type	%
Owner of a private practice	73
Associate/employee of a private practice	10
Health Partners Dental Group	4
Permanente Dental Associates	7
Other managed care/preferred provider	1
Public health practice	3
Dental School/academic institution	2
Specialty	N (%)
General Dentist	173 (94)
Specialist	12 (6)

Table 2 Most frequent choices used when diagnosing DH ($N = 182$)

Most frequent methods used when diagnosing DH	N (%)
Spontaneous patient report confirmed by the dental exam	88 (48)
Applying air blast	47 (26)
Scratching dentin with dental explorer	22 (12)
Obtaining patient report after dentist's query	11 (6
Other (most likely using endo ice)	8 (4)
Applying cold water	4 (2)
Requesting numeric rating of pain	2 (1)

Treatment Modalities

As shown in Table 3, the practitioners reported using multiple products when managing DH. Almost all practitioners (97%) reported routine use of fluoride formulations, followed by desensitizing over-the-counter (OTC) potassium nitrate toothpaste (94%). Glutaraldehyde/HEMA products were reported as being used routinely by 42% participating in the survey. Interestingly, bonding agents and restorative treatments were reported to be used routinely respectively by 52 and 64% of the practitioners when treating DH.

As shown in Table 4, practitioners reported that the most frequent, practitioner reported, first choice of products used when managing DH was: OTC potassium nitrate toothpaste (48%), followed by fluoride formulations (38%) and glutaraldehyde/HEMA products (3%). Four percent of the practitioners reported giving advice (i.e., related to diet and dental habits) to their patients as their first choice of treatment modality. A total of 86% of the respondents reported using a combination of products when treating DH, most frequently fluoride varnish and desensitizing OTC potassium nitrate toothpaste (70%).

Predisposing Factors

As summarized in Table 5, practitioners indicated their first choice of potential factors that may be related to dentin hypersensitivity. Recessed gingiva was chosen by 66% of the practitioners, followed by abrasion, erosion, abfraction and/or attrition lesions (59%). Thirty two percent indicated that bruxism contributes to DH and that it was their first choice of predisposing factors. Excessive tooth whitening and frequent consumption of citric juices and/or carbonated drinks were chosen by 17 and 15% of practitioners, respectively, as first choices for predisposing factors of DH.

Table 3 Treatment modalities routinely used when treating Dentin Hypersensitivity (Practitioners had options to check multiple answers)

Treatment modality	N (%)
Fluoride formulations (gels, varnishes, pasted and rinses)	180 (97)
Desensitizing over-the counter (OTC) potassium nitrate toothpastes	173 (94)
Glutaraldehyde/HEMA products	78 (42)
Bonding agents	97 (52)
Sealants	30 (16)
Restorative treatments	119 (64)
Lasers	6 (3)
Oxalates	21 (11)
Advice	41 (22)
Other	35 (19)

Table 4 Most frequent products used when managing DH (these were first choices of products indicated by the practitioners)

Most frequent products used when managing DH	N (%)
OTC potassium nitrate toothpaste	88 (48)
Fluoride formulations	70 (38)
Giving advice (related to diet and dental habits)	7 (4)
Other	7 (4)
Glutaraldehyde/HEMA	6 (3)
No treatment	2 (1)
Restorative treatments	1 (2)
Bonding agents	1 (.5)
Lasers	1 (.5)
Oxalates	1 (.5)

Diagnosis, management and predisposing factors, by network region and practitioners' characteristics

Practitioners' diagnostic and management methods did not differ significantly across the six network regions. There were no age differences in diagnostic methods, except for using "other methods" to diagnose DH ($p < 0.0001$, Fisher's exact test). Only 2% of practitioners in the younger age category (younger than 55 years) indicated using "other methods", compared to 20% in the older age category (55 years of age and older). Most of the responses in the "other" category suggested using soft bristle toothbrushes, recommending gingival grafting, occlusal adjustments, and fabricating occlusal guards.

There were no practitioner gender differences in diagnostic methods, except when using an explorer ($p = 0.015$, Fisher's exact test). More male dentists than female dentists use a dental explorer to diagnose DH (84 versus 68%).

There were no regional differences in dentists' beliefs regarding predisposing factors to DH, except for bruxism ($p = 0.047$, chi-square test). The highest percentage of practitioners from the South Atlantic region (87%) had chosen bruxism as one of the predisposing factors of DH; the lowest percentage was chosen by practitioners from the Western region (53%).

Table 5 Most frequent predisposing factors of DH as indicated by the practitioners (Practitioners indicated their first choice of predisposing factors)

Predisposing factor	N (%)
Recessed gingiva	122 (66)
Abrasion, erosion, abfraction and/or attrition lesions	109 (59)
Bruxism	59 (32)
Excessive tooth whitening	31 (17)
Frequent consumption of citrus juices and/or carbonated drinks	28 (15)

The practice locations did not differ significantly across the 6 regions, however the practice type did differ significantly by region ($p < 0.0001$, chi-square test). Almost 87% of practitioners from the Southwest and the South Central regions identified themselves as owners of a private practice, 83% practitioners from the South Atlantic region, 74% practitioners from the Northeast region, 59% practitioners from the Western region and 52% of practitioners from the Midwest region.

Discussion

These results suggest that when diagnosing DH practitioners most frequently rely on spontaneous patient report, confirmed by the dental examination, followed by applying an air blast and scratching dentin with a dental explorer. Our finding is consistent with the 2008–2009 study by Northwest PRECEDENT practitioners, which suggested that the most frequently reported diagnostic method was spontaneous patient report [14]. Patient reports, prompted by a query from the dentist, were also common, but used less frequently. Additionally, dentists employed a dental explorer or air blast to assess DH [14]. Our findings indicate that practitioners confirm their patients' reports with a dental examination to diagnose DH. The diagnosis of DH is thus made by excluding other oral conditions that may explain pain and discomfort in the oral cavity.

These findings also suggest that fluoride formulations and OTC potassium nitrate toothpastes were the most frequent products used to treat DH. Almost 97% of practitioners reported routinely using fluoride formulations and 94% reported routinely using OTC potassium nitrate toothpastes. Almost half (48%) used OTC potassium nitrate toothpaste and 38% used fluoride formulations as their first choice when treating DH. This finding is consistent with the PRECEDENT study, wherein dentists reported using fluoride formulations most commonly and it was the only treatment modality used by more than 50% of respondents. Almost half the PRECEDENT dentists (47%) reported using OTC potassium nitrate toothpastes when managing DH [14]. Our findings also suggest that 86% of respondents used a combination of products when treating DH, most frequently using fluoride varnish and desensitizing OTC potassium nitrate toothpaste (70%); suggesting that most practitioners combine in-office treatment with at-home treatment.

When reporting predisposing factors of DH, 66% of practitioners reported that recessed gingiva was their first choice, followed by abrasion, erosion, abfraction and/or attrition lesions (59%) and bruxism (32%). This finding is supported by the most accepted theory related to DH, the hydrodynamic theory, which proposes that stimuli (thermal, physical or osmotic changes) cause displacement of the fluid that exists within the dentinal tubules and this mechanical disturbance activates the nerve endings in the pulp [20]. This requires that the dentin must be exposed to the oral cavity. In addition to using fluoride varnish and desensitizing OTC potassium nitrate toothpaste, the majority of practitioners indicated restorative treatments when managing DH, most likely restoring abfraction lesions. Older practitioners were more likely than younger practitioners to report occlusal adjustments and fabricating occlusal guards as "other" treatment when managing DH.

Regarding practitioner and practice characteristics that are associated with managing DH, our results suggest that younger and older dentists use similar methods when diagnosing DH. More male practitioners than female practitioners reported using a dental explorer when diagnosing DH. Practitioners 55 years of age or older more often suggested gingival grafting, occlusal adjustments and fabrication of occlusal guards when indicating treatment options used for DH. One of the possible explanations that older practitioners suggested more options when managing DH could be that they had more experience in managing DH than younger practitioners. There are regional differences in beliefs regarding predisposing factors for DH. Most practitioners from the South Atlantic region (87%) indicated bruxism as one of the predisposing factors, while only 53% dentists from the Western region reported this.

Practitioners reported using similar methods when diagnosing and managing DH in their offices, regardless of their practice location, practice type, and network region. As mentioned above, there were a few differences in diagnostic methods and treatment options offered when comparing younger to older practitioners and male to female practitioners; however, the differences were not significantly different between the six network regions.

This study does have some limitations; and interpretation of its conclusions should take these into account. This study relied on questionnaire data rather than direct observation of clinical procedures. Although network practitioners have much in common with dentists at large, it is possible that their reports on diagnosis and treatment of DH and their beliefs about DH predisposing factors are not representative of dentists at large [21, 22]. Additionally, network members are not recruited randomly; their participation in the network (*e.g.*, an interest in participating in clinical research studies) may make them unrepresentative of dentists at large. While we cannot assert that network dentists are entirely representative of US dentists, we can state that they have much in common with dentists at large, while also offering substantial diversity in these characteristics. This assertion is warranted because: 1) substantial percentages of network dentists are represented in the various response categories of the characteristics in the Enrollment Questionnaire; 2) findings from several network studies document that network dentists report patterns of diagnosis and treatment that are similar to patterns determined from non-network dentists [23–25] and 3) the similarity of network dentists to non-network dentists using the best available national source, the 2010 ADA Survey of Dental Practice [26].

Conclusions

The majority of network practitioners use multiple methods to diagnose and manage DH. Desensitizing OTC potassium nitrate toothpaste and fluoride formulations are the most widely reported products used to manage DH in the practice setting. The majority reported that recessed gingiva, followed by the abrasion/erosion; abfraction/attrition lesions and bruxism most likely contribute to DH.

Abbreviations

MDH: Management of dentin hypersensitivity; National Dental
PBRN: National Dental Practice-Based Research Network

Acknowledgments

An Internet site devoted to details about the nation's network is located at http://nationaldentalpbrn.org. We are very grateful to the network's Regional Coordinators who worked with network practitioners to conduct the study:
Kimberly Johnson, RDH, MDH; Midwest Region
Stephanie Hodge, MA; Western Region
Rita Cacciato, RHD, MS; Northeast Region
Deborah McEdward, RDH, BS, CCRP; South Atlantic Region
Claudia Carcelén, MPH, Shermetria Massengale, MPH, CHES, Ellen Sowell, BA; South Central Region
Meredith Buchberg, MPH, Colleen Steward MPH; Southwest Region
Camille Baltuck, RDH; Western Region
Opinions and assertions contained herein are those of the authors and are not to be construed as necessarily representing the views of the respective organizations or the National Institutes of Health.
National Dental PBRN Collaborative Group:
The National Dental PBRN Collaborative Group comprises practitioner, faculty, and staff investigators who contributed to this network activity. A list of these persons is at http://www.nationaldentalpbrn.org/collaborative-group.php; University of Alabama at Birmingham, Birmingham, AL.

Funding

This work was supported by NIH/NIDCR grant U-19-DE-22516.

Authors' contributions

DKK-drafted the manuscript. DKK, CM, MWH, SC, GHG, VVG, SCR, RLY, TEM have made substantial contributions to conception and design, and/or acquisition of data, and interpretation of data. MSL- has made substantial contributions to data analysis and interpretation of data. All authors read and approved the final manuscript.

Competing interests

The authors declare that they have no competing interests.

Consent for publication

N/A.

Ethics approval and consent to participate

The study was approved by the University of Rochester Research Subject Review Board (approval number RSRB 00053321) and also by the IRBs of the remaining five study sites. The informed consent of all human subjects who participated in this investigation was obtained after the nature of the procedures had been explained fully. As per regional IRB requirements written informed consents were used in the Midwest, South Atlantic and Northeast regions of the network and verbal informed consents were used in South Central, Western and Southwestern regions of the network.

Author details

[1]Eastman Institute for Oral Health, University of Rochester, 625 Elmwood Ave, Rochester, NY 14620, USA. [2]University of Alabama at Birmingham, Birmingham, AL, USA. [3]Private practice of general dentistry, Morristown, NJ, USA. [4]University of Florida, Gainesville, FL, USA. [5]Health Partners, Minneapolis, MN, USA. [6]Private practice of periodontics, Olympia, WA, USA. [7]University of Texas Health Science Center at San Antonio, San Antonio, TX, USA.

References

1. Canadian Advisory Board on Dentin Hypersensitivity. Consensus-based recommendations for the diagnosis and management of dentin hypersensitivity. J Can Dent Assoc. 2003;69:221–6.
2. Porto IC, Andrade AK, Montes MA. Diagnosis and treatment of dentinal hypersensitivity. J Oral Sci. 2009;51:323–32.
3. Amarasena N, Spencer J, Ou Y, Brennan D. Dentine hypersensitivity - Australian dentists' perspective. Aust Dent J. 2010;55:181–7.
4. Amarasena N, Spencer J, Ou Y, Brennan D. Dentine hypersensitivity in a private practice subject population in Australia. J Oral Rehabil. 2011;38:52–60.
5. Chu CH, Lam A, Lo EC. Dentin hypersensitivity and its management. Gen Dent. 2011;59:115–22. quiz 123–4.
6. Cummins D. Advances in the clinical management of dentin hypersensitivity: A review of recent evidence for the efficacy of dentifrices in providing instant and lasting relief. J Clin Dent. 2011;22:100–7.
7. Parolia A, Kundabala M, Mohan M. Management of dentinal hypersensitivity: A review. J Calif Dent Assoc. 2011;39:167–79.
8. Poulsen S, Errboe M, Lescay Mevil Y, Glenny AM. Potassium containing toothpastes for dentine hypersensitivity. Cochrane Database Syst Rev. 2006; 3:CD001476.
9. Liu HC, Lan WH, Hsieh CC. Prevalence and distribution of cervical dentin hypersensitivity in a population in Taipei, Taiwan. J Endod. 1998;24:45–7.
10. Gillam DG, Seo HS, Bulman JS, Newman HN. Perceptions of dentine hypersensitivity in a general practice population. J Oral Rehabil. 1999;26: 710–4.
11. Cunha-Cruz J, Wataha JC, Heaton LJ, Rothen M, Sobieraj M, Scott J, Berg J. The prevalence of dentin hypersensitivity in general dental practices in the Northwest United States. J Am Dent Assoc. 2013;144:288–96.
12. Dababneh RH, Khouri AT, Addy M. Dentine hypersensitivity - an enigma? A review of terminology, mechanisms, aetiology and management. Br Dent J. 1999;187:606–11. discussion 603.
13. Rees JS, Addy M. A cross-sectional study of dentine hypersensitivity. J Clin Periodontol. 2002;29:997–1003.
14. Cunha-Cruz J, Wataha JC, Zhou L, Manning W, Trantow M, Bettendorf MM, Heaton LJ, Berg J. Treating dentin hypersensitivity: Therapeutic choices made by dentists of the northwest PRECEDENT network. J Am Dent Assoc. 2010;141:1097–105.
15. Holland GR, Narhi MN, Addy M, Gangarosa L, Orchardson R. Guidelines for the design and conduct of clinical trials on dentine hypersensitivity. J Clin Periodontol. 1997;24:808–13.
16. Orchardson R, Gillam DG. Managing dentin hypersensitivity. J Am Dent Assoc. 2006;137:990–8. quiz 1028–9.
17. Veitz-Keenan A, Barna JA, Strober B, Matthews AG, Collie D, Vena D, Curro FA, Thompson VP. Treatments for hypersensitive noncarious cervical lesions: a Practitioners Engaged in Applied Research and Learning (PEARL) Network randomized clinical effectiveness study. J Am Dent Assoc. 2013;144:495–506.
18. The National Dental Practice-Based Research Network, the nation's network. http://www.nationaldentalpbrn.org/. Accessed 30 June 2016.
19. Gilbert GH, Williams OD, Korelitz JJ, Fellows JL, Gordan VV, Makhija SK, Meyerowitz C, Oates TW, Rindal DB, Benjamin PL, Foy PL, National Dental PBRN Collaborative Group. Purpose, structure and function of the United States National Dental Practice-Based Research network. J Dent. 2013;41: 1051–9.
20. Brannstrom A, Astrom A. The hydrodynamics of dentin and its possible relationship to dentinal pain. Int Dent J. 1972;22:219–27.
21. Makhija SK, Gilbert GH, Rindal DB, Benjamin P, Richman JS, Pihlstrom DJ, Qvist V, DPBRN Collaborative Group. Practices participating in a dental PBRN have substantial and advantageous diversity even though as a group they have much in common with dentists at large. BMC Oral Health. 2009;9:26.
22. Makhija SK, Gilbert GH, Rindal DB, Benjamin PL, Richman JS, Pilhstrom DJ, DPBRN Collaborative Group. Dentists in practice-based research networks have much in common with dentists at large: evidence from the Dental Practice-Based Research Network. Gen Dent. 2009;57:270–5.
23. Gordan VV, Garvan CV, Heft MW, Fellows JL, Qvist V, Rindal DB, Gilbert GH, DPBRN Collaborative Group. Restorative treatment thresholds for interproximal primary caries based on radiographic images: findings from the Dental Practice-Based Research Network. Gen Dent. 2009;57:654–63. quiz 64–6, 595, 680.
24. Gordan VV, Garvan CW, Richman JS, Fellows JL, Rindal DB, Qvist V, Heft MW, Williams OD, Gilbert GH, DPBRN Collaborative Group. How dentists diagnose and treat defective restorations: evidence from the dental practice-based research network. Oper Dent. 2009;34:664–73.
25. Norton WE, Funkhouser E, Makhija SK, Gordan VV, Bader JD, Rindal DB, Philstrom DJ, Hilton TJ, Frantsve-Hawley J, Gilbert GH, NDPBRN Collaborative Group. Concordance between clinical practice and published evidence: findings from The National Dental Practice-Based Research Network. J Am Dent Assoc. 2014;145:22–31.
26. American Dental Association Survey Center. The 2010 Survey of Dental Practice. Chicago: American Dental Association; 2012.

13

A randomized, double-blind, placebo-controlled clinical trial of fluoride varnish in preventing dental caries of Sjögren's syndrome patients

Weini Xin[1], Katherine Chiu Man Leung[2*], Edward Chin Man Lo[3], Mo Yin Mok[4] and Moon Ho Leung[5]

Abstract

Background: Sjögren's syndrome (SS) patients are prone to caries development due to reduction of salivary flow. Topical fluoride is commonly prescribed for caries prevention.

Methods: In this 24-month randomized, double-blind, placebo-controlled clinical trial, SS patients were randomly assigned to receive either fluoride varnish or placebo gel quarterly. Development and arrest of caries at the coronal and root surfaces were recorded at 12-month and 24-month and compared to that of the baseline. Effect of fluoride varnish on oral Candida and lactobacilli colonization was explored by comparing baseline oral microbiological assessments to data obtained at 12-month and 24-month.

Results: Seventy-eight SS patients (mean age = 50 years, 2 men) completed this trial. At 24-month, the mean new coronal enamel caries were 1.6 surfaces in both groups, and new dentin caries were 1.4 and 2.7 surfaces in the fluoride and placebo group respectively ($p > 0.05$). Mean arrested caries were 0.6 and 0.7 surfaces for fluoride and placebo groups respectively and that of root caries were 0.3 and 0.1 surfaces ($p > 0.05$). The mean oral Candida count was reduced by 30% in the fluoride group but increased 61% in the placebo group while no change in oral lactobacilli counts in both groups at 24 months ($p > 0.05$). SS patients receiving fluoride varnish were significantly less likely to develop dentin caries ($p < 0.05$). In contrast, those with high baseline DMFS scores ($p = 0.05$), harbored mixed Candida species ($p < 0.05$), or unstimulated whole saliva at low pH ($p < 0.01$) were significantly more likely to develop dentin caries.

Conclusions: Results of this randomized clinical trial did not provide clear evidence to support or refute that quarterly applications of fluoride varnish can prevent development of dental caries in people with Sjögren's syndrome.

Trial registration: This study was retrospectively registered at the ISRCTN registry (ISRCTN85164658) on 9 Sept 2016 and was funded by the Research Grant Council of Hong Kong.

Keywords: Sjögren's syndrome, Fluoride varnish, Dental caries, Oral Candida, Oral lactobacilli

* Correspondence: kcmleung@hku.hk
[2]Prosthodontics, Faculty of Dentistry, The University of Hong Kong, Hong Kong SAR, China
Full list of author information is available at the end of the article

Background

Sjögren's syndrome (SS) is a slowly progressive autoimmune disorder of exocrine glands which is characterized by intense lymphocytic infiltration [1]. Salivary and lacrimal glands are the most commonly affected exocrine glands, resulting in reduced secretion of saliva (hyposalivation) and tears [2].

SS patients often complain of dry mouth (xerostomia). Reduction in salivary flow rate and high caries occurrence have also been reported in previous studies [3]. In addition, there is a high prevalence of SS sufferers presented with oral colonization of pathological microorganisms such as lactobacilli and Candida [4].

Prevention of dental caries in SS patients is important. Topical fluoride has been extensively used to prevent caries in children and elderly people, however, little evidence is available for its efficacy in SS patients at present. Most fluoride varnishes contain 22600 ppm fluoride. It has been reported to effectively prevent enamel caries and dentin caries, and to arrest initial caries lesions in children and adolescent [5, 6]. The Sjögren's Syndrome Foundation Clinical Practice Guidelines Committee strongly recommends the use of topical fluoride [7]. The American Dental Association (ADA) suggests that people at moderate risk should receive fluoride varnish or gel applications at 6-month intervals and higher-risk patients at three- to 6-month intervals [8].

The current study reports a randomized, double-blind, placebo-controlled clinical trial with the primary aim of investigating the efficacy of fluoride varnish in preventing dental caries in Chinese patients with SS. The effect of fluoride varnish on oral colonization of Candida and lactobacilli in Chinese patients with SS over a 24-month period will also be investigated.

Methods

Study design and participants

This was a parallel study. Randomized, double-blind, placebo-controlled clinical trial design which lasted for 24 months was employed. Dental records of 15 SS patients were randomly selected from those who had participated in previous consecutive studies revealed a mean caries increment of 3.5 surfaces (SD = 2.8) over 24 months [3]. Assuming the caries preventive fraction of fluoride varnish was 35% [9], the estimated 24-month mean caries increment of the fluoride group would be 2.3 surfaces (SD = 1.8). The estimated minimum sample size was 48 per group to achieve $\alpha = 0.05$ and $\beta = 80\%$. Allowing for a 10% annual dropout, 120 SS patients was planned.

SS patients were recruited from the Rheumatology Clinics of the Queen Mary Hospital (QMH) and Queen Elizabeth Hospital (QEH), Hong Kong. These two hospitals were selected because they were the two largest public hospitals in Hong Kong and are within 30 minutes travelling time to the Prince Philip Dental Hospital (PPDH). Patients from QMH and QEH are comparable in terms of ethnic origin, diet and culture. Diagnosis of SS was established using the American-European Consensus Group (AECG) criteria [10] at least 6 months before the commencement of this study. Potential recruits were excluded if they were under 18 years of age, had less than 8 natural teeth, had severe periodontal disease (e.g., periodontal pockets were deeper than 6 mm at two or more sextants), had received therapeutic irradiation to the head and neck region, had concurrent systemic illness (except connective tissue disorder associated with sSS), were taking medication that altered salivary flow, or had participated in a clinical trial within 6 months before commencement of this trial. Socio-demographic information regarding education level, employment status, and oral hygiene measures were obtained. To ensure comparability of the characteristics of the subjects in the intervention and control groups, a stratified block randomization method with a block size of four was applied so that a similar number of pSS and sSS subjects were allocated to each group [11]. Concealment of participant allocation was kept by a clinical staff who was not involved in the trial. Topical applications of fluoride varnish or placebo gel were carried out by one hospital dentist who was not involved in research team. Blinding of the participants and the examiner was maintained until all clinical data were collected at 24-month.

All recruited subjects were invited to attend a pre-baseline full-mouth oral and dental examination at the PPDH. Bitewing radiographs were taken to aid diagnosis of caries. Standard oral hygiene instruction on toothbrushing and flossing was given and participants were advised to brush twice a day and floss every day. Dental treatments including scaling, tooth extraction, root canal treatment, periodontal therapy and dental prosthesis were provided if indicated. Restorations were provided except for initial caries lesion and arrested non-cavitated caries lesions. The use of fluoride-releasing restorative materials was avoided. All treatments were completed at least 14 days before commencement of the baseline data collection.

Clinical procedure

All clinical procedures were carried out between 9:00 am and 12:00 noon in a surgery room at the PPDH. Participants were advised to refrain from food or beverage intake (except water) one hour before the attending dental examination. They were asked to rinse their mouth with 10 ml of sterile phosphate-buffered saline (PBS; 0.01 M; pH = 7.2) for 30s prior to collection in a sterile container. Dentures, if present, were retained during rinsing. The oral rinse sample was then sent for microbiological analysis. After resting for 5 min and voiding the mouth, a sterile, pre-weighed plastic vial was provided for collection of unstimulated whole saliva (UWS). Over a period of 5 min, all saliva was drained into the vial by drooling or gentle spitting. For stimulated whole saliva (SWS) collection, subjects were instructed to chew on a piece of sterilized silicone rubber tubing (2 mm × 8 mmØ) and to spit all the saliva into another sterile, pre-weighed plastic vial for 5 min. The weights of vials were recorded and UWS and SWS flow rates were determined and expressed as g/min. Immediately after saliva collection, pH values and buffer capacity of UWS and SWS were determined at chair side using a pH meter (Sentron 501 Pocket FET pH meter, Sentron, WA, USA) and a commercial strip (CRT® buffer, Vivadent, Liechtenstein) respectively. Supra-gingival dental plaque was collected from all accessible coronal tooth surfaces of the whole mouth using a sterile sickle scaler and then dispersed into a pre-weighed vial containing 500 μl PBS.

The examiner was trained and calibrated before the start of the baseline examination and recalibrated at 6-month, 12-month, 18-month and 24-month. The examiner received training through the "ICDAS E-Learning Course" in the ICDAS official website. After calibration, data collection was performed by the calibrated examiner. To assess intra-examiner reliability, duplicate examinations were carried out on one in ten subjects.

The Silness-Löe plaque index [12] was modified where score 0 denoted no plaque accumulation, and score 1 dental plaque accumulation when a WHO probe (Guilin Woodpecker Medical Instrument Co., Ltd) was run along the gingival margins of the index teeth. Plaque index was expressed as the percentage of examined sites with plaque accumulation.

After air-drying and plaque removal, all exposed coronal and root surfaces were evaluated using a WHO probe according to the modified International Caries Detection and Assessment System (ICDAS) [13]. Molars and premolars were considered to have five coronal surfaces and canines and incisors were considered to have four. Codes were given as follows: sound (code 0), visual change on enamel (code 1), distinct visual change on enamel (code 2), caries extended to dentin (code 3), filled without decay (code 4), filled with decay (code 5), arrested caries (code 6), missing (code 7), crowned (code 8). Decayed, missing, or filled surface (DMFS) score at baseline was computed by summing the number of caries, missing and filled surfaces related to caries. The exposed root surfaces were coded as sound (code 0), no cavitation with discolored area (code 1), cavitation with discolored area (code 2), or arrested caries (code 6). Dental examination was carried out at 12-month and 24-month.

Microbiological assessment

Lactobacilli were explored in the SWS and dental plaque samples. The SWS and dental plaque samples were vortexed for 30s at maximum setting (Autovortex Mixer SA2, Stuart Scientific, London, UK) and then serially diluted (10^{-2} and 10^{-3}) with 0.01 M sterile PBS (pH = 7.2). A 50-μl aliquot of the 1:100 and the 1:1000 dilutions were duplicately spiral-plated (Spiral Systems Autoplate 4000 Spiral plater, Spiral Biotech, Norwood, Mass) on Rogosa agar (Difco, Detroit, MI, USA). The Rogosa agar plates were incubated for 3 days in an anaerobic chamber (37 °C, 5% CO_2 and 95% N_2). Following incubation, a stereomicroscope (Olympus TL, Tokyo, Japan) was used to verify the presence of colonies. The colonies were subcultured using blood agar plates (Oxoid, Basingstoke, Hampshire, UK), which contained 5% defibrinated blood, 0.0005% (5 mg/L) haemin and menadione, to obtain pure isolates for identification. Identification for lactobacilli was confirmed by colony morphology, gram-stain reaction, Candida was explored in the oral rinse and dental plaque samples.

Candida were explored in the oral rinse and dental plaque samples. The samples were vortexed for 30s at maximum setting and 1:10 diluted with 0.01 M sterile PBS (pH = 7.2). To estimate the level of Candida in each sample, a 50-μl aliquot of the undiluted (oral rinse samples) and dilution samples (oral rinse and dental plaque samples) were duplicately spiral-plated by using the spiral plater onto the Sabouraud dextrose agar (SDA; Oxoid, Unipath Ltd, Basingstoke, Hampshire, UK) and CHROMagar (Becton Dickinson Europe, Le Pont de Claix, France). All plates were incubated for 2 days at 37 °C in air. After incubation, plates with appropriate number of colonies which were well separated and evenly dispersed were chosen for counting. The number of the colony in oral rinse and dental plaque samples were recorded and expressed as CFU/ml. The selected Candida colonies were subcultured on SDA plates to obtain pure isolates. Candida was speciated and identified based on the followings: colony morphology in CHROMagar and SDA, cell morphology, gram-stain reaction, and result of the API ID 32C system (bioMérieux, France) and RapID-ANA II system (Remel, Lenexa, KS, USA).

Counts of lactobacilli and Candida were expressed as colony forming units per milliliter (CFU/ml) in salivary samples and colony forming units per gram in dental plaque samples.

Study interventions

In the test group, topical fluoride varnish (5% NaF varnish, Duraphat®, Colgate, Colgate-Palmolive Company, New York, USA) was applied; while in the control group, a water-based gel without fluoride was used as placebo (K-Y® Gel, McNEIL-PPC Inc., Fort Washington, USA). A trained clinician applied the fluoride varnish/placebo gel that was dispensed by a dental surgery assistant in single-dose vials with the name and record number of the subjects pre-labelled [14]. All teeth were dried and isolated, and fluoride varnish/placebo gel was applied using a micro-brush to all teeth surfaces. Participants were asked to avoid drinking and eating during the first two hours after application and to avoid eating abrasive food on that day. The dental surgery assistant escorted the patients to leave the clinics after application of the agent, so as to avoid the contact between patients and the examiner or the other patients in this study.

Follow-up visits were arranged every 3 months after baseline for applications of fluoride varnish/placebo gel up to 24 months. Dental condition and oral hygiene condition were recorded at the 12-month and 24-month visits, as well as oral rinse, salivary and dental plaque samples collection, and measurement of the relevant index (pH, buffering capacity and microbiological profiles).

Statistical analysis

Differences in continuous variables between the fluoride and placebo groups were tested by *t*-test or Mann-Whitney *U* test for data which were normally or not normally distributed respectively. Differences in categorical variables between groups were tested by Chi-squared tests or Fisher's exact tests whichever was appropriate. Repeated measures analysis of variance or Friedman test, whichever was appropriate, was performed for evaluating differences among the same continuous variables of three-time point assessments (baseline, 12-month and 24-month). Pearson's correlation or Spearman's rank correlation, whichever was appropriate, was used to explore associations between parameters of interest.

Multivariate analysis of estimation of parameters in occurrence of new caries increments is appropriate for this dataset. The logistic model was applied to predict the occurrence of caries over the 24-month period and to explore the effectiveness of intervention. Potential risk factors associated with development of new caries lesions was assessed by odds ratio through logistic regression analyses. Variables with a *p*-value of 0.10 or below were entered into regression model (Forward selection) for determination of significant factors. The level of significance was set at 5% ($p < 0.05$). Data analysis was processed using SPSS software (version 20.0).

Results

Recruitment and socio-demographic characteristics of participants

The flow of the study is presented in Fig. 1. Among 114 recruited SS patients, 85 patients met the inclusion criteria and received prebaseline treatment. They were randomly allocated into the fluoride group ($N = 43$) and the placebo group ($N = 42$). During the follow-up period, seven patients (3 in the fluoride group and 4 in the placebo group) withdrew. No significant difference was found between the seven drop-outs and the remaining 78 patients (35 pSS and 43 sSS), who were included for data analysis. Out of the 78 patients, 76 (97%) were women and the mean age was 50 years (SD = 9.9). The average duration of diagnosis was 101.3 months (SD = 78.6) (Table 1). More than 85% of the subjects brushed their teeth twice or more per day and used fluoride toothpaste. Approximately 75% of them practised interdental cleaning using dental floss or interdental brush, while only one-third of them used fluoride mouthrinse. There was no significant difference between subjects in fluoride and placebo groups in terms of their regular oral hygiene habits and use of fluoride products ($p > 0.05$), except the frequency of tooth brushing and the use of fluoride toothpaste ($p < 0.05$).There was no statistical significant difference in the type of SS, gender, age, duration since diagnosis, education level or work status between the two groups ($p > 0.05$).

Salivary flow rates, saliva pH, saliva buffering capacity and dental conditions

Mean plaque index scores, DMFS, salivary flow rate and pH of both groups at baseline were shown in Table 1. There was no significant difference in these parameters between the two groups ($p > 0.05$).

The mean salivary pH values over 24 months in fluoride group and placebo group were within the normal range. No statistically significant difference existed between the salivary flow rates, pH value and buffer capacity of the fluoride group and placebo group ($p > 0.05$).

Most subjects developed caries with time in both groups (Table 2). At 12-month, enamel caries accounted for 63.6% of the caries lesions while at 24-month, enamel and dentin caries lesions were equally detected. There was no significant difference in the distribution in enamel lesions, dentin caries lesions and arrested caries lesions between the two groups at 12-month and 24-month visits ($p > 0.05$). The mean number of caries lesions developed in the maxillary and mandibular jaws showed no statistically significant difference ($p > 0.05$). More anterior teeth in the placebo group developed dentin caries lesions than those in the fluoride group ($p < 0.05$), but such difference was not observed in premolars and molars ($p > 0.05$). More distal surfaces in the placebo group developed dentin caries lesions than those in the fluoride group ($p < 0.05$), however the difference was not observed in the other surfaces. The difference in the root caries increments between

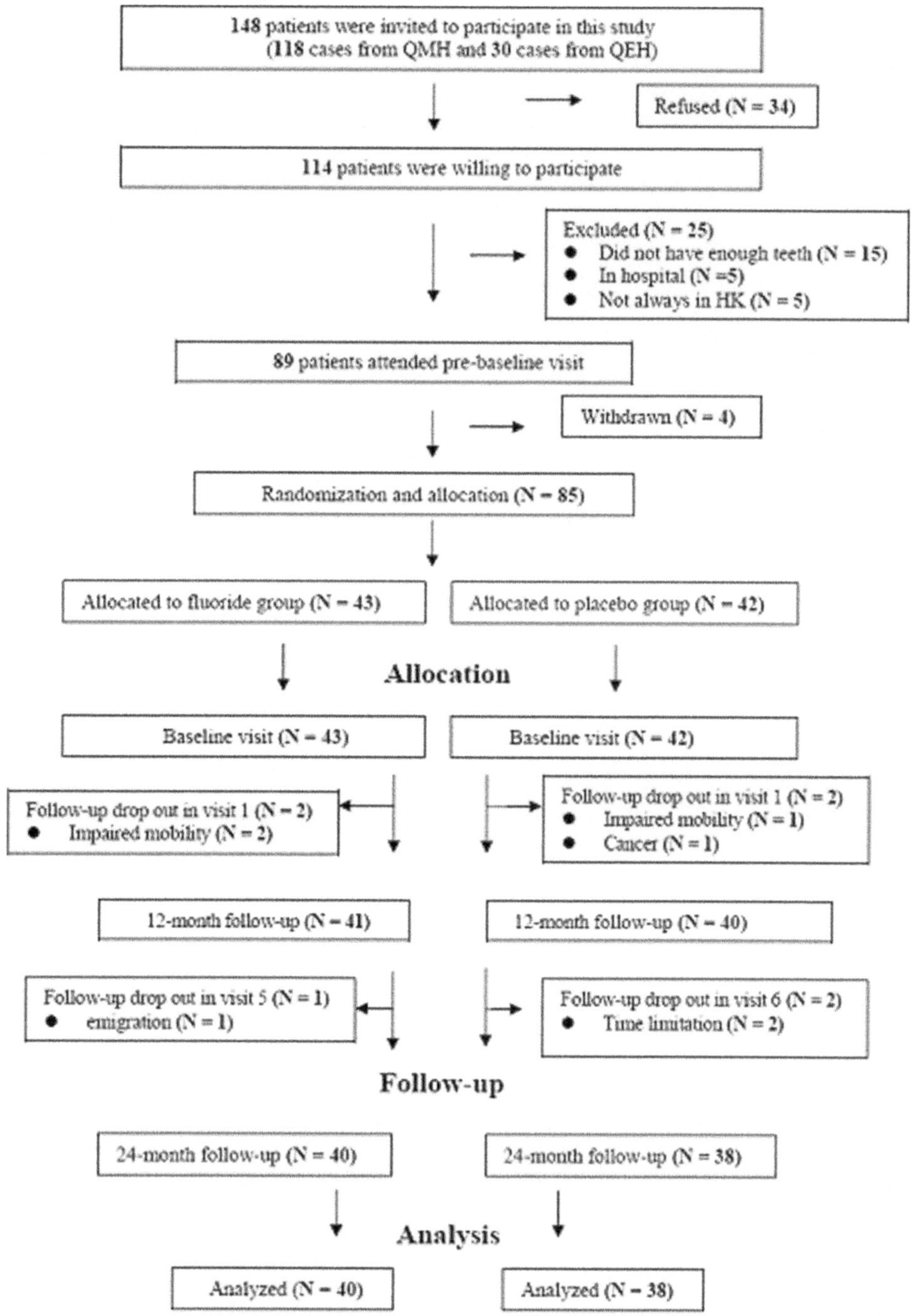

Fig. 1 CONSORT flow diagram of this randomized trial

two groups was not statistically significant ($p > 0.05$). Comparing the difference of the numbers of dentin caries lesions at 24-month, the caries preventive fraction of fluoride varnish in SS patients is 33.3%. Intra-examiner reliability was 0.96 and 0.90 for coronal caries and plaque index respectively.

DMFS at baseline correlated positively to the number of new dentin caries developed at 24-month in the fluoride ($r_s = 0.43$, $p = 0.005$) and the placebo ($r_s = 0.37$, $p = 0.02$) groups. In addition, F-component of DMFS at baseline showed a positive correlation to the number of new dentin caries at 24-month in the fluoride ($r_s = 0.40$, $p = 0.01$) and the placebo ($r_s = 0.36$, $p = 0.03$) groups.

As less than the original estimated sample size was recruited, post-hoc power calculation was conducted. According to the initial sample size determination, 38

Table 1 Socio-demographic features, oral hygiene practice and baseline condition by group

	Fluoride group ($N = 40$)	Placebo group ($N = 38$)	*p*-value
Type of SS (primary: secondary) (%)	45.0 : 55.0	44.7 : 55.3	N.S.
Gender (Female: Male) (%)	97.3 : 2.7	97.4 : 2.6	N.S.
Age at baseline (years)			
Mean (SD)	49.2 (9.1)	50.9 (10.8)	N.S.
Range	29–71	26–75	
Time since diagnosis (months)			
Mean (SD)	117.5 (97.1)	84.2 (48.4)	N.S.
Range	3–425	2–177	
Education level (%)			
Primary school or below	30.0	21.1	N.S.
Secondary school or above	70.0	78.9	
Employed (%)	62.5	44.7	
Oral hygiene practice (%)			
Brushed twice or more per day	100.0	89.5	**0.001**
Practised interdental cleaning	70.0	78.9	N.S.
Daily use of fluoride (%)			
Toothpaste	87.5	100.0	**<0.001**
Mouthrinse	37.5	34.2	N.S.
Three meals or less per day (%)	90.0	89.5	N.S.
Saliva			
Unstimulated whole saliva			
Mean flow rate (SD), range	0.22 (0.24), 0–0.99	0.26 (0.26), 0–1.12	N.S.
Mean pH (SD), range	7.2 (0.4), 6.3–8.3	7.3 (0.5), 6.3–8.5	N.S.
Stimulated whole saliva			N.S.
Mean flow rate (SD), range	0.48 (0.58), 0–2.60	0.51 (0.47), 0–1.73	N.S.
Mean pH (SD), range	7.8 (0.4), 6.8–8.6	7.7 (0.5), 6.5–8.5	N.S.
Dental condition			
Mean number of teeth (SD), range	26.6 (3.0), 18–32	26.7 (3.8), 12–32	N.S.
Mean DMFS (SD), range	45.6 (18.8), 4–78	41.2 (23.1), 1–114	N.S.
Mean DS (SD), range	0.9 (1.1), 0–4	0.9 (0.9), 0–4	N.S.
Mean MS (SD), range	25.0 (13.7), 0–65	25.7 (18.6), 0–94	N.S.
Mean FS (SD), range	19.8 (12.5), 0–54	14.7 (10.6), 0–43	0.06
Mean plaque index (SD) (%)	28 (25), 0–88	33 (26), 4–100	N.S.
Removable partial denture wearers (%)	7.5	13.2	N.S.

N.S. not significant

subjects per group would provide 80% power to detect a preventive fraction of 42.8%, i.e., estimated 24-month mean caries increment of fluoride group would be 2 surfaces (SD = 1.6).

Intra-examiner reliability was 0.96 for coronal caries and 0.90 for plaque index.

Microbiology

The mean counts of lactobacilli and Candida at the various time-points and sites were shown in Table 3. There was no statistically significant difference in the prevalence of species and the mean counts of lactobacilli and Candida between the two groups at baseline and 24-month ($p > 0.05$). Correlations (r_s) between the mean counts of the microbes in the saliva and dental plaque and the mean salivary flow rates and new various lesions were presented in Table 3.

The most predominantly isolated lactobacilli were *L. fermentum*. Others lactobacilli species isolated included *L. acidophilus*, *L. minutis* and *L. casei.*

Table 2 Different types of lesions at the subject and surface levels

	12-month			24-month		
Group	Fluoride group (*N* = 40)	Placebo group (*N* = 38)	*p*-value	Fluoride group (*N* = 40)	Placebo group (*N* = 38)	*p*-value
Number of subjects (%)						
No caries	15 (37.5)	19 (50)	N.S.	11 (27.5)	12 (31.8)	N.S.
Enamel lesion	19 (47.5)	15 (39.4)	N.S.	21 (52.5)	18 (47.4)	N.S.
Dentin lesion	4 (10)	8 (21.1)		13 (32.5)	16 (42.1)	
Arrested lesion	7 (17.5)	5 (13.2)		10 (25.0)	14 (37.5)	
Number of surface						
Enamel lesion						
Sum	41	34	N.S.	64	60	N.S.
Mean (SD)	1.0 (1.5)	0.9 (1.5)		1.6 (2.3)	1.6 (2.5)	
Range	0–6	0–7		0–10	0–11	
Dentin lesion						
Sum	8	35	N.S.	55	78	N.S.
Mean (SD)	0.2 (0.6)	0.9 (2.4)		1.4 (2.6)	2.1 (4.2)	
Range	0–3	0–11		0–11	0–22	
Arrested lesion						
Sum	17	13	N.S.	22	25	N.S.
Mean (SD)	0.4 (1.2)	0.3 (1.2)		0.6 (1.3)	0.7 (1.3)	
Range	0–6	0–6		0–7	0–7	

N.S. not significant

C. albicans was the most frequently isolated Candida species, other Candida species such as *C. dubliniensis*, *C. tropicalis*, *C. glabrata*, *C. sake* and *C. parapsilosis*. More than 10% of patients in both groups had mixed Candida colonization in saliva and dental plaque samples, usually *C. albicans* with another Candida species.

The odds ratio of SS patients receiving fluoride varnish who developed dentin caries was 0.22 (Table 4). The odds ratios per unit increase in the mean number of Candida species in dental plaque and mean UWS pH of dentin caries development were 5.189 (95% CI: 1.307, 20.602) and 0.052 (95% CI: 0.006, 0.414) respectively. Logistic regression analysis revealed that SS patients who received placebo ($p < 0.05$), presented with low UWS pH ($p < 0.01$) and had high baseline DMFS level ($p = 0.050$) were significantly more likely to develop dentin caries when compared to their counterparts.

SS patients who had high UWS buffering capacity ($p < 0.05$) and harbored high level of Candida in the oral rinse samples ($p < 0.05$) were significantly more likely to have caries arrested at 24-month as compared to their counterparts (Table 5). Those with high UWS buffer capacity were five times as likely as those with low or medium UWS buffer capacity to have arrested caries lesions.

Discussion

SS patients who received quarterly applied fluoride varnish developed 32.5% less coronal dentin caries than those who received a placebo, which was similar to the result obtained in a study on hyposalivated patients who self-administered 0.05% NaF mouthrinse 3 times daily [15]. The caries preventive fraction of fluoride varnish in SS patients is similar to that of other groups of subjects [16]. Although subjects in the placebo group developed higher mean new caries lesions than the fluoride group, the differences were not statistically significant. Type II error may be responsible for the apparent lack of difference in caries increments between the two groups as less SS subjects were recruited than estimated. On the contrary, when other confounding factors were controlled, the odds ratio of dentin caries development was significantly lower in the fluoride varnish group than the placebo group. Such contradicting findings imply a lack of clear evidence to support or refute the hypothesis that quarterly applied fluoride varnish can prevent caries development in this group of patients. Nevertheless, it is interesting to note that SS subjects in this study were generally having high dental awareness and their level of oral hygiene was satisfactory. Caries experience as reflected in the number of standing teeth and DMFS is even comparable to some non-SS subjects in other studies [17, 18]. In addition, more than 30 and 50% of them

Table 3 Correlations (r_s) between the mean numbers of species carried, mean counts of *Candida* in the oral rinse samples and dental plaque samples and the mean salivary flow rates and new caries lesions

		Fluoride group ($N = 40$)		Placebo group ($N = 38$)	
Saliva samples					
		Lactobacilli	Candida	Lactobacilli	Candida
Mean counts (×10^4 CFU/ml) (SD)	Baseline	1.6 (4.6)	591.5 (1705.1)	8 (25.8)	184.3 (369.3)
	Over 24-months	6.3 (14.2)	428.3 (828.2)	13.7 (45.6)	291.6 (541.1)
Mean counts					
Correlations (r_s)		Lactobacilli	Candida	Lactobacilli	Candida
Mean salivary flow rates	Unstimulated whole saliva	−0.37*	−0.67**	0.44**	−0.77**
	Stimulated whole saliva	−0.38*	−0.69**	−0.39*	−0.77**
New lesions (over 24 months)	Enamel lesion	−0.03	−0.19	0.17	−0.02
	Dentin lesion	0.40**	0.53**	0.35*	0.56**
	Arrested lesion	0.25	0.44**	0.24	0.32
Dental plaque samples					
		Lactobacilli	Candida	Lactobacilli	Candida
Mean counts (×10^6 CFU/g) (SD)	Baseline	15.8 (62.5)	60.2 (172.9)	1.7 (6.3)	9.5 (20.4)
	Over 24-months	56.6 (178.9)	37.2 (73.5)	119.1 (444.6)	40.9 (164.0)
Mean counts					
Correlations (r_s)		Lactobacilli	Candida	Lactobacilli	Candida
Mean salivary flow rates	Unstimulated whole saliva	0.51**	−0.53**	−0.69**	−0.75**
	Stimulated whole saliva	−0.48**	−0.58**	−0.69**	−0.79**
New lesions (over 24 months)	Enamel lesion	0.11	−0.05	0.04	−0.04
	Dentin lesion	0.44**	0.45**	0.47**	0.48**
	Arrested lesion	0.26	0.38*	0.33*	0.32

* Significant Spearman's correlation $p < 0.05$
** Significant Spearman's correlation $p < 0.01$

presented with normal range of UWS and SWS flow rates respectively. Salivary flow rate, UWS in particular, has been shown to negatively associate with caries development [19].

In this study cohort, both the number of root caries and root caries increment were low. An earlier cross-sectional study of SS patients has revealed a mean decayed or filled root surface of 5.3 which was 10 times as that in the current study cohort [20]. Caries increments in both groups were much lower than the estimated mean annual root caries increment in the general older population [21]. Hence, efficacy of fluoride varnish

Table 4 Final logistic regression model for the occurrence of new dentin caries lesions in SS patients over a 24-month period

		Adjusted		
		Odds ratio	95% confidence interval	
Factors	*P*-value		Lower	Upper
Intervention (Ref. = placebo group)	0.035	0.221	0.054	0.901
Mean number of *Candida* species in the dental plaque samples	0.019	5.189	1.307	20.602
Mean pH of unstimulated whole saliva over 24 months	0.005	0.052	0.006	0.414
DMFS (at baseline)	0.05	1.033	1.000	1.067

Table 5 Final logistic regression model for the occurrence of new arrested caries lesions in SS patients over a 24-month period

		Adjusted		
		Odds ratio	95% confidence interval	
Factors	*P*-value		Lower	Upper
Intervention (Ref. = placebo group)	0.054	0.315	0.097	1.022
Buffering capacity of unstimulated whole saliva at baseline (Ref. = medium and low)	0.017	5.018	1.339	18.804
Mean counts of *Candida* in oral rinse samples over 24 months	0.015	1.002	1.000	1.003

in root caries prevention in SS patients cannot be discerned.

Reduced salivary flow rate leads to changes in some specific components of saliva, including the immunoglobulins (secretory IgA, IgG, and IgM), antibacterial protein (lysozyme, lactoferrin, peroxidases) and the concentrations of electrolytes (sodium, chloride, and phosphate) [17]. In addition, reduced salivary output may hinder mechanical flushing of microorganisms from teeth surfaces [22]. Therefore, antibacterial activity of saliva is decreased and bacteria can flourish in the mouth of SS patients. Despite the fact that salivary pH of most SS subjects in this study was within normal range, a negative correlation between salivary pH and development of new dentin lesions was detected and low UWS pH was found to be a strong predictor of dentin lesions development. Rates of the demineralization and remineralization of dental hard tissues are pH-mediated [23]. At neutral pH (7.0), saliva is supersaturated with calcium phosphate. However, when the pH decreases to a point where the saliva ceases to be supersaturated, the hydroxyapatite crystals begin to dissolve and demineralization occurs. It has been reported that UWS pH in SS patients can be as low as only one tenth of a pH unit above the mean critical pH [17]. A minute drop in pH, hence, can lead to undersaturation of hydroxyapatite that results in either caries lesions or erosive damage to the teeth depending on the origin of the acidic challenge. In addition, acidic oral environment is highly suitable for the survival and proliferation of cariogenic bacteria. Acidic saliva has poor ability to maintain oral homeostasis. When the saliva pH level decreases, the risk of dentin caries development increases.

Buffering capacity of saliva is in fact more critical than its pH value in oral homeostasis [24]. Results of the logistic regression revealed that occurrence of new arrested caries lesions was related to the level of the buffering capacity of UWS. Arrested lesions are the result of remineralization of a demineralized lesion and the buffering capacity of saliva plays a critical role in helping to restore a neutral pH at the tooth surface and to increase the rate of remineralization [25]. Although some studies showed that the salivary bicarbonate and phosphate concentrations of SS patients were lower than those of healthy subjects [17], in this study, more than 80% of SS patients had medium to high salivary buffering capacity, hence enamel and dentin caries lesions in these patients can be remineralized and became arrested lesions.

The oral environment of SS patients does not favor the growth of S. mutans because the saliva pH was higher than the optimal pH that supports its growth. Furthermore, S. mutans and Candida species do not coaggregate well [26]. The high oral prevalence of Candida (55–65%) may prevent the colonization of S. mutans in this study population. The result suggests that fluoride varnish has little effect on the level of lactobacilli in SS patients, which is in agreement with that reported in other studies [27]. Some study found that NaF at one mmol/L could only inhibit the growth of less than half of oral lactobacilli species [28]. The low concentration of fluoride (1.2 mmol/L NaF) in fluoride varnish cannot inhibit the growth of oral lactobacilli. Furthermore, the concentration of fluoride cannot be maintained as it would gradually decline with time after application. An in-vitro study has demonstrated that fluoride varnish could release fluoride for five to 6 months and the mean concentration was about 0.025 mmol/L [29].

In this study, Candida counts were found to be positively correlated to the number of new dentin caries lesions. Candida produces proteolytic enzymes which can break down the organic collagen matrix of dentin [30]. Furthermore, the penetrating power of hyphae from enamel into dentin seems to support that Candida has a crucial role in dental caries development [31]. Mixed colonization of Candida spp. was observed in about 10% of the SS subjects which generally occurs in patients with impaired immunological function [32, 33]. From results of the logistic regression, the more types of Candida spp. detected in dental plaque, the higher likelihood of dentin caries development. Host dental plaque biofilm provided a favorable acidic condition for Candida growth and proliferation, because most yeasts optimally grow at pH 5.5–6 [34]. Hence, patients harboring more Candida species would have a higher risk of demineralization and dissolution of hydroxyapatite.

Nonetheless, the results should be interpreted with caution as one major limitation of this study is the small population size. Only 85 patients were recruited which fell short of the original estimated sample size. Insufficient sample size would lower the statistical power and lead to type II error that might account for the apparent lack of difference in caries increments between the treatment and placebo groups. Furthermore, the length of this study might not be sufficient to fully explore the efficacy of fluoride varnish in caries prevention as caries development is a slow process, despite the fact that SS patients are at high caries risk.

Conclusions

Results of this randomized clinical trial did not provide clear evidence to support or refute that quarterly applications of fluoride varnish can prevent development of dental caries in people with Sjögren's syndrome.

Abbreviations

ADA: American Dental Association; AECG: American-European Consensus Group; CFU: Colony-forming unit; CI: Confidence interval; CO_2: Carbon dioxide; DMFS: Decayed, missing, filled surface; ICDAS: International Caries

Detection and Assessment System; N_2: Nitrogen; NaF: Sodium fluoride; PBS: Phosphate-buffered saline; pH: Potential of hydrogen; PPDH: Prince Philip Dental Hospital; pSS: primary Sjögren's syndrome; QEH: Queen Elizabeth Hospital; QMH: Queen Mary Hospital; r_s: Spearman rank correlation coefficient; SD: Standard deviation; SDA: Sabouraud dextrose agar; SPSS: SS: Sjögren's syndrome; SPSS: Statistical package for social sciences; sSS: Secondary Sjögren's syndrome; SWS: Stimulated whole saliva; UWS: Unstimulated whole saliva; WHO: World Health Organization

Acknowledgements
The authors wish to thank Ms. Samantha Li for her assistance in the statistical analysis of the data.

Funding
This project is supported by General Research Fund of the Research Grants Council of Hong Kong (HKU 769408 M).

Authors' contributions
WX contributed to clinical data acquisition, data analysis and manuscript preparation; KCML contributed to the design of the clinical trial, data analysis and manuscript preparation; ECML contributed to the design of the clinical trial, calibration of examiner, data analysis and revision and advice on the manuscript; MYM and MHL recruited Sjögren's syndrome patients, provided medical assessment and maintenance of the subjects and provided revision and advice on the manuscript. All authors had proofread and approved the manuscript.

Competing interests
The authors declare that they have no competing interests.

Consent for publication
Not applicable.

Ethics approval and consent to participate
This study was approved by the Institutional Review Boards of the University of Hong Kong/Hospital Authority Hong Kong West and Kowloon Central and East Clusters (UW 08-167 and KC/KE-10-0014/ER-2). Each participant was provided with a written informed consent. All the information including personal details and clinical information that have been used for this study were de-identified.

Author details
[1]Dental Care Center, The First Affiliated Hospital of Shantou Medical College, Shantou, China. [2]Prosthodontics, Faculty of Dentistry, The University of Hong Kong, Hong Kong SAR, China. [3]Dental Public Health, Faculty of Dentistry, The University of Hong Kong, Hong Kong SAR, China. [4]Department of Biomedical Sciences, City University of Hong Kong, Hong Kong SAR, China. [5]Department of Medicine, Queen Elizabeth Hospital, Hong Kong SAR, China.

References

1. Seror R, Theander E, Bootsma H, Bowman SJ, Tzioufas A, Gottenberg JE, Ramos-Casals M, Dorner T, Ravaud P, Mariette X, Vitali C. Outcome measures for primary Sjögren's syndrome: a comprehensive review. J Autoimmun. 2014;51:6.
2. Mavragani CP, Moutsopoulos HM. The geoepidemiology of Sjögren's syndrome. Autoimmun Rev. 2010;9:A305–10.
3. Leung KC, McMillan AS, Leung WK, Wong MC, Lau CS, Mok TM. Oral health condition and saliva flow in southern Chinese with Sjögren's syndrome. Int Dent J. 2004;54:159–65.
4. Leung KC, McMillan AS, Cheung BP, Leung WK. Sjögren's syndrome sufferers have increased oral yeast levels despite regular dental care. Oral Dis. 2008;14(2):163–73.
5. Marinho VC. Cochrane reviews of randomized trials of fluoride therapies for preventing dental caries. Eur Arch Paediatr Dent. 2009;10(3):183–91.
6. Zero DT, Brennan MT, Daniels TE, Papas A, Stewart C, Pinto A, Al-Hashimi I, Navazesh M, Rhodus N, Sciubba J, Singh M, Wu AJ, Frantsve-Hawley J, Tracy S, Fox PC, Ford TL, Cohen S, Vivino FB, Hammitt KM. Sjögren's Syndrome Foundation Clinical Practice Guidelines Committee. Clinical practice guidelines for oral management of Sjögren's disease: Dental caries prevention. J Am Dent Assoc. 2016;147(4):295–305.
7. Marinho VC, Worthington HV, Walsh T, Clarkson JE. Fluoride varnishes for preventing dental caries in children and adolescents. Cochrane Database Syst Rev. 2013;7:CD002279.
8. American Dental Association Council on Scientific Affairs. Professionally applied topical fluoride: evidence-based clinical recommendations. J Am Dent Assoc. 2006;137(8):1151–9.
9. Carvalho DM, Salazar M, Oliveira BH, Coutinho ES. Fluoride varnishes and decrease in caries incidence in preschool children: a systematic review. Rev Bras Epidemiol. 2010;13(1):139–49.
10. Vitali C, Bombardieri S, Jonsson R, Moutsopoulos HM, Alexander EL, Carsons SE, Daniels TE, Fox PC, Fox RI, Kassan SS, Pillemer SR, Talal N, Weisman MH. Classification criteria for Sjögren's syndrome: a revised version of the European criteria proposed by the American-European Consensus Group. Ann Rheum Dis. 2002;61(6):554–8.
11. Keech AS. Design techniques to avoid bias. In: KJ K, editor. Introduction to clinical trials research methodology, statistical methods in clinical trials, the ICH GCP guidelines. Hong Kong: The Clinical Trials Centre, Faculty of Medicine, the University of Hong Kong; 1998. p. 238–48.
12. Silness J, Löe H. Periodontal disease in pregnancy II. Correlation between oral hygiene and periodontal condition. Acta Odontol Scand. 1964;22:121–35.
13. Ismail AI, Sohn W, Tellez M, Amaya A, Sen A, Hasson H, Pitts NB. The International Caries Detection and Assessment System (ICDAS): an integrated system for measuring dental caries. Community Dent Oral Epidemiol. 2007;35(3):170–8.
14. Salinas J, Sprinkhuizen SM, Ackerson T, Bernhardt J, Davie C, George MG, Gething S, Kelly AG, Lindsay P, Liu L, Martins SC, Morgan L, Norrving B, Ribbers GM, Silver FL, Smith EE, Williams LS, Schwamm LH. An international standard set of patient-centered outcome measures after stroke. Stroke. 2016;47(1):180–6. doi:10.1161/STROKEAHA.115.010898. Epub 2015 Nov 24.
15. Hay KD, Thomson WM. A clinical trial of the anticaries efficacy of casein derivatives complexed with calcium phosphate in patients with salivary gland dysfunction. Oral Surg Oral Med Oral Pathol Oral Radiol Endod. 2002;93(3):271–5.
16. Marinho VC, Higgins JP, Logan S, Sheiham A. Fluoride gels for preventing dental caries in children and adolescents. Cochrane Database Syst Rev. 2002;2:CD002280. Review.
17. Pedersen AM, Bardow A, Nauntofte B. Salivary changes and dental caries as potential oral markers of autoimmune salivary gland dysfunction in primary Sjögren's syndrome. BMC Clin Pathol. 2005;5(1):4.
18. Najera MP, al-Hashimi I, Plemons JM, Rivera-Hidalgo F, Rees TD, Haghighat N, Wright JM. Prevalence of periodontal disease in patients with Sjögren's syndrome. Oral Surg Oral Med Oral Pathol Oral Radiol Endod. 1997;83:453–7.
19. Spak CJ, Johnson G, Ekstrand J. Caries Incidence, Salivary flow-rate and efficacy of fluoride gel treatment in irradiated patients. Caries Res. 1994;28(5):388–93.
20. Yurtseven N, Gokalp S. Oral sugar clearance and other caries-related factors of stimulated whole saliva in patients with secondary Sjögren's syndrome. Quintessence Int. 2007;38(3):e151–7.
21. Griffin SO, Griffin PM, Swann JL, Zlobin N. Estimating rates of new root caries in older adults. J Dent Res. 2004;83(8):634–8.
22. Stookey GK. The effect of saliva on dental caries. J Am Dent Assoc. 2008;139(Suppl):11S–7S.
23. Hurlbutt M, Novy B, Young D. Dental Caries: A pH-mediated disease. CJDH. 2010;25(1):9–15.
24. Kivela J, Parkkila S, Parkkila AK, Leinonen J, Rajaniemi H. Salivary carbonic anhydrase isoenzyme VI. J Physiol. 1999;520(Pt 2):315–20.
25. Hicks J, Garcia-Godoy F, Flaitz C. Biological factors in dental caries: role of saliva and dental plaque in the dynamic process of demineralization and remineralization (part 1). J Clin Pediatr Dent. 2003;28(1):47–52.
26. Klinke T, Guggenheim B, Klimm W, Thurnheer T. Dental caries in rats associated with Candida albicans. Caries Res. 2011;45(2):100–6.
27. Yoshihara A, Sakuma S, Kobayashi S, Miyazaki H. Antimicrobial effect of fluoride mouthrinse on mutans streptococci and lactobacilli in saliva. Pediatr Dent. 2001;23(2):113–7.

28. del Carmen Ahumada Ostengo M, Wiese B, Nader-Macias ME. Inhibitory effect of sodium fluoride and chlorhexidine on the growth of oral lactobacilli. Can J Microbiol. 2005;51(2):133–40.
29. Castillo JL, Milgrom P, Kharasch E, Izutsu K, Fey M. Evaluation of fluoride release from commercially available fluoride varnishes. J Am Dent Assoc. 2001;132(10):1389–92.
30. Nishimura M, Nikawa H, Yamashiro H, Nishimura H, Hamada T, Embery G. Cell-associated collagenolytic activity by Candida albicans. Mycopathologia. 2002;153(3):125–8.
31. Sen BH, Safavi KE, Spangberg LS. Colonization of Candida albicans on cleaned human dental hard tissues. Arch Oral Biol. 1997;42(7):513–20.
32. Dronda F, Alonso-Sanz M, Laguna F, Chaves F, Martinez-Suarez JV, Rodriguez-Tudela JL, Gonzalez-Lopez A, Valencia E. Mixed oropharyngeal candidiasis due to *Candida albicans* and non-*albicans Candida* strains in HIV-infected patients. Eur J Clin Microbiol Infect Dis. 1996;15(6):446–52.
33. Parisotto TM, King WF, Duque C, Mattos-Graner RO, Steiner-Oliveira C, Nobre-Dos-Santos M, Smith DJ. Immunological and microbiologic changes during caries development in young children. Caries Res. 2011;45:377–85.
34. Kubicek CP, Esser K, Druzhinina IS. Environmental and Microbial Relationships: Springer Science & Business Media. Berlin: Springer; 2007. p. 97.

14

Influence of Invisalign treatment with interproximal enamel reduction (IER) on bone volume for adult crowding: a retrospective three-dimensional cone beam computed tomography study

Andreas Hellak[1,3*], Nicola Schmidt[1], Michael Schauseil[1], Steffen Stein[1], Thomas Drechsler[2] and Heike Maria Korbmacher-Steiner[1]

Abstract

Background: The aim of this study was to use three-dimensional datasets to identify associations between treatment for adult crowding using Invisalign and interproximal enamel reduction (IER) and changes in the bone volume.

Methods: A total of 60 digital cone beam computed tomography (CBCT) scans from 30 patients (28 women, two men; 30 CBCTs pretreatment, 30 posttreatment) were examined retrospectively in order to record bone volume three-dimensionally before and after treatment. The patients' average age was 36.03 ± 9.7 years. The data were collected and analyzed using the computer programs Mimics 15.0 and OsiriX. Differences in bone between T0 and T1 were analyzed with IBM SPSS 21.0 using the Wilcoxon test for paired samples.

Results: Analysis of the orovestibular bone volume showed highly significant changes (bone change P <0. 001) only in the mandible where more expansion of the dental arch was carried out using proclination or protrusion. The bone lamella was thinner buccally and thicker lingually. In general, bone increases in the oral direction were slightly greater than bone losses in the vestibular direction. No significant changes were detected in the maxilla (bone change $P = 0.13$). Significant vertical bone loss in the bone height was detected in both the maxilla and the mandible. The largest bone loss was observed in the vestibular direction in the mandible, at a high level of significance (P <0.001).

Conclusions: Particularly in the mandible, therapeutic reduction of the vertical and sagittal bone volume shows that caution should be used in the treatment of tertiary crowding with proclination and expansion. The cortical walls appear to represent the limits for orthodontic tooth movement, at least in adult female patients.

(Continued on next page)

* Correspondence: hellak@med.uni-marburg.de
[1]Department of Orthodontics, University Hospital Giessen and Marburg, Campus Marburg, Georg-Voigt-Strasse 3, Marburg 35039, Germany
[3]Abt. für Kieferorthopädie, UKGM Standort Marburg, Georg-Voigt-Strasse 3, 35039 Marburg, Germany
Full list of author information is available at the end of the article

(Continued from previous page)
Keywords: Invisalign, Adult crowding, Interproximal enamel reduction (IER), Bone quantity, CBCT, Landmarks, Recessions

Abbreviations: CBCT, Cone beam computed tomography scans; IER, Interproximal enamel reduction

Background

Treatment for adult patients using almost invisible appliances such as aligners is becoming increasingly important [1]. In addition to harmonizing the dental malpositioning, with the consequent improvement of the patient's aesthetic appearance, simultaneous improvement of dental health is also desirable [2].

However, orthodontic treatment for adult crowding has been associated in many reports with recessions and periodontal destruction in the area of the anterior teeth [3–6]. It is known that dental movements cause quantitative changes in the alveolar bone, with osteogenesis and osteoclasis [7–9]. As a result of the two-dimensional imaging that has been conventional to date, quantification of the pretherapeutic and posttherapeutic bone situation is only possible to a limited extent [10]. It is only through modern three-dimensional imaging procedures such as cone beam computed tomography (CBCT) that three-dimensional analysis of bone structures has become possible [11].

There have been no reports in the literature on changes in the bone volume relative to treatment with aligners. The aim of the present study was therefore to investigate whether and to what extent orthodontic treatment with Invisalign aligners leads to changes in the bone volume. Specifically, this raises the following questions:

- How does the bone volume change in the orovestibular direction as a result of Invisalign treatment?
- What changes in the bone height do occur?
- Are there differences in the ways in which the maxilla and mandible respond?
- Does the movement pattern have any effect on bone transformation processes?

Methods

Two CBCT scans (pretherapeutic and posttherapeutic) from a total of 30 patients (28 women, two men) were examined retrospectively. The patients' average age was 36.03 ± 9.7 years. A total of 920 measurements were carried out for orovestibular changes and 480 measurements for bone height. The use of the data was approved by the ethics committee of Marburg University Hospital (ref. no. 34/15).

The following inclusion criteria were used:

- Presence of adult anterior crowding capable of being harmonized using conservative orthodontic space-gaining measures such as protrusion, proclination, expansion and interproximal enamel reduction (IER)
- Permanent dentition
- Successfully completed treatment with Invisalign aligners
- Availability of one CBCT scan each from before and after treatment

The following parameters represented exclusion criteria:

- Extraction of anterior teeth during the course of treatment
- Prosthetic treatment
- Skeletal anomalies
- General medical findings relevant to bone metabolism (e.g., osteoporosis, dysostosis, etc.)
- Periodontal disease and previous periodontal surgery procedures

All of the images were taken with a KaVo 3D eXam CBCT system (KaVo Dental Ltd., Biberach an der Riss, Germany) using a scan with 360° revolution, 26,9 s duration (X-ray source voltage: 120kVp; X-ray source current: 5 mA) and 0.25 mm voxel size. The datasets were collected and evaluated using Mimics 15.0 (Materialise, Leuven, Belgium) with Microsoft Windows 7 and OsiriX (Pixmeo, Bernex, Switzerland) with an Apple OS X operating system.

All of the patients had provided written consent to the use of their data in the study (in accordance with the Helsinki Declaration). The datasets were all analyzed on a semiblinded basis.

Measurement of the orovestibular bone volume

Bone thickness was measured orally and vestibularly at two levels (at the apex and mid of the root length) in the anterior tooth areas of the maxilla and mandible.

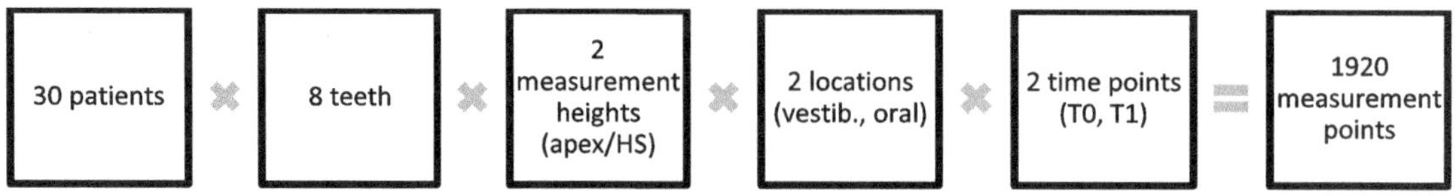

The upper and lower threshold values for the best possible depiction of the skeletal components of the skull were established using the "thresholding" function in Mimics 15.0 (Materialise, Leuven, Belgium).

To be able to carry out the measurements independently of the tooth position, reference planes first had to be created using osseous structures. The reference planes in the maxilla and mandible were created using clearly defined anatomic landmarks. Table 1 and Fig. 1 show the points used to establish the reference planes in the maxilla and mandible. Clearly defined reference points produced the distances shown in Fig. 2a, which were always measured vertically to the alveolar process and parallel to the previously established reference plane in the maxilla or mandible. The following measurement distances resulted:

- Apex–ApexKnoBuk: bone from the apex to the labial boundary of the cortex
- Apex–ApexKnoLing: bone from the apex to the oral boundary of the cortex
- HSbuk–HSKnoBuk: bone from the buccal root contour to the labial boundary of the cortex at the level of the mid of the root length
- Hsling–HSKnoLing: bone from the lingual/palatine root contour to the oral boundary of the cortex at the level of the mid of the root length

Figure 3 shows an example of the way in which the measurement points were set. The red line shows the intersection point with the previously mounted plane. This made it possible for the measurement always to be carried out at the same level.

Measurement of bone height

The distance from the enamel–cement boundary to the crestal alveolar bone on all four anterior teeth in the maxilla and mandible was measured using the OsiriX program (Pixmeo, Bernex, Switzerland).

This method was adopted in a slightly modified form from the retrospective CBCT study by Kim et al. [12].

The most coronal level of the alveolar bone was defined as the crestal bone ridge, independently of whether bone fenestrations were identifiable apical to that level. In the sagittal view, the distance from the crestal bone edge to the enamel–cement boundary was then measured using OsiriX's measurement function. Measurements were carried out parallel to the dental axis both at the buccal root surface and at the lingual root surface (Figs. 2b and 4).

The following measurement distances resulted:

- Vestibular bone height (a): distance between the vestibular crestal bone edge and the enamel–cement boundary
- Oral bone height (b): distance between the oral crestal bone edge and the enamel–cement boundary

Figure 4 shows an example of the way in which the tooth is oriented in order to measure the bone height.

Statistical analyses were carried out using IBM SPSS for Mac, version 21.0 (IBM Corporation, Armonk, New York, USA). The intraoperator correlation for each examination was initially calculated. For further analysis, the normal distribution of the values was checked. Statistical comparison of the values was carried out using the Wilcoxon test. The significance level was set at $P = 0.05$.

Results

A high level of correlation ($r = 0.903$) was noted using Kendall's tau-b test for the examiner's accuracy in measurements of the orovestibular bone thickness. The correlation was highly significant, at the $P < 0.001$ level (two-sided). The Kolmogorov–Smirnov test did not show a normal distribution for measurements of vestibular and oral bone thickness. The Wilcoxon test was

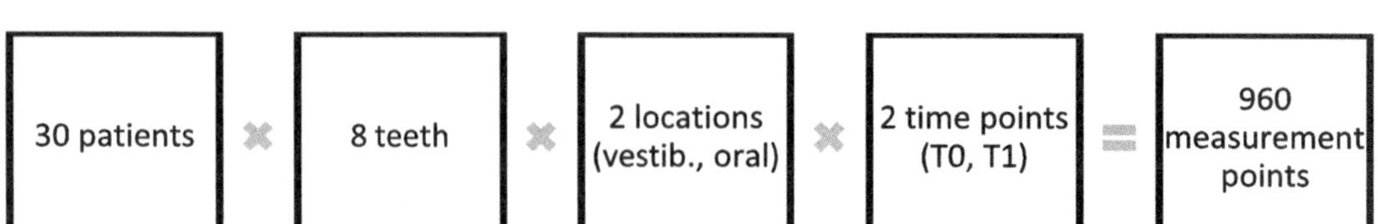

Table 1 Reference points for establishing reference levels in the maxilla and mandible

Reference level	Analysis points	Positioning
Maxillary level	Emartrechts	Deepest point on the right articular tubercle
	Emartlinks	Deepest point on the left articular tubercle
	Nasion	Furthest anterior contour of the frontonasal suture
Mandibular level	MandPlre	Deepest point on the mandible in the area of the mandibular angle on the right
	MandPlli	Deepest point on the mandible in the area of the mandibular angle on the left
	MandPlvorne	Deepest point in the area of the ventral mandible

therefore used for statistical analysis of the bone thickness measurements (Table 2). Clear changes were only observed in the mandible. The sums of the mean differences showed bone losses in the maxilla and slight bone increases in the mandible. An increase in bone was evident at both levels for the mandibular measurement points, while bone loss was evident buccally.

In the statistical analysis, the Wilcoxon test showed highly significant changes in the mandible ($P \leq 0.001$). The results in the maxilla only showed significant differences in the palatine area at the level of the mid of the root length (HSPulpa; $P \leq 0.05$) (Table 2).

Bone height

A high level of intraoperator correlation was also observed for the measurements of bone height (Kendall's tau-b: $r = 0.779$). The correlation was highly significant, at the $P < 0.001$ level (two-sided).

The distance from the enamel–cement boundary to the alveolar crest was measured. Bone loss was indicated by positive values. For clarity, all values in the subsequent analysis of this part of the study were therefore multiplied by −1. This results in negative values for bone losses and positive values for bone increases on the vertical plane.

Significant vertical bone losses were identified in both the maxilla and the mandible (Table 3). This was true both for the buccal and also for the oral measurement points. Vertical bone loss was particularly marked buccally in the mandible ($P < 0.001$). The lingual bone height in the mandible did not show any significant changes ($P = 0.345$).

Tables were prepared to analyze the influence of the movement pattern on the way in which the bone reacted (Tables 4 and 5). When expansion of the dental arch was carried out using proclination/protrusion, the affected teeth were shown in red; in the absence of dental arch expansion, they were shown in green.

Tables 4 and 5 show that protrusion and proclination to expand the dental arch were selected more frequently as a treatment strategy in the area of the mandible. In the mandible 83.3 % of the teeth studied were moved labially, in comparison with only 15 % in the maxilla.

Discussion

Highly significant changes in bone volume in the orovestibular direction were only found in the mandible. A reduction in the vestibular bone lamella and an increase in bone in the lingual area of the mandible were observed. This might possibly be explained by different movement patterns. Bone changes in the direction of the tooth

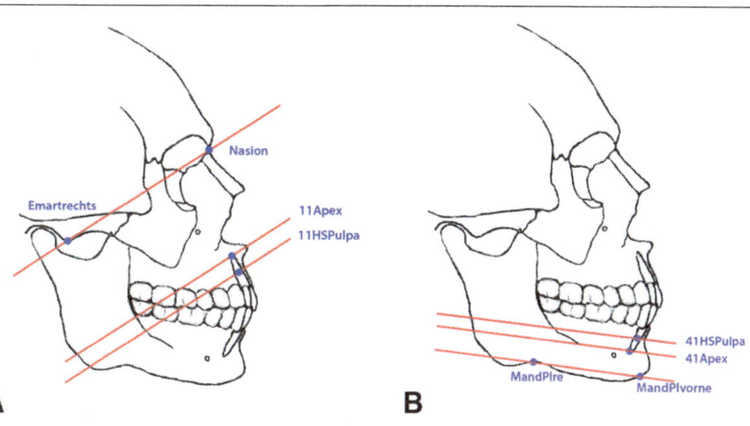

Fig. 1 a+b Two-dimensional illustration of the maxillary and mandibular reference plane. **a** Two-dimensional illustration of the maxillary reference plane, with the reference points "Emartrechts" and "Nasion" and the parallel measurement planes at the level of the apex and center of the root, for tooth 11. **b** Two-dimensional illustration of the mandibular reference plane, with the reference points "MandPlre" and "MandPlvorne" and the measurement planes at the level of the apex and center of the root, for tooth 41

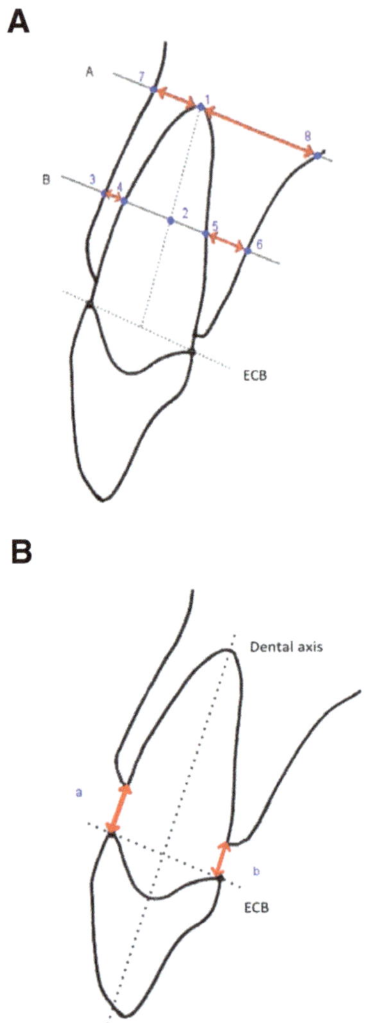

Measurement points and levels

1 Apex

2 HSPulpa

3 HSKnobuk

4 HSbuk

5 HSling

6 HSKnoling

7 ApexKnobuk

8 ApexKnoling

A Plane at apex level

B Plane at the level of the center of the root

a Vestibular bone height

b Oral bone height

Fig. 2 a+b Two-dimensional diagram showing the measurement points. **a** Sketch, Tooth 11 as an example. *ECB* enamel–cement boundary. Two-dimensional diagram showing the measurement points and distances for measuring bone height. **b** Sketch, Tooth 11 as an example. *ECB* enamel–cement boundary

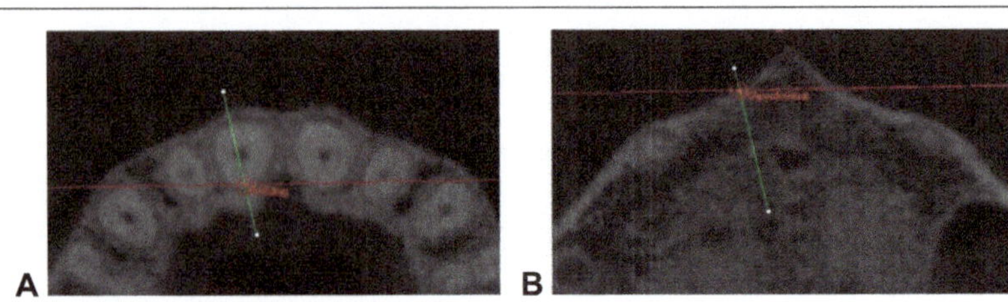

Fig. 3 a+b Setting the reference points. Reference points at the intersection between the transverse and sagittal planes at the corresponding anatomic structure are shown using the example of tooth 11 at the axial plane. **a** "11Hsling" at the lingual root contour at the level of the center of the root. **b** "11ApexKnobuk" at the buccal bone contour at the level of the apex

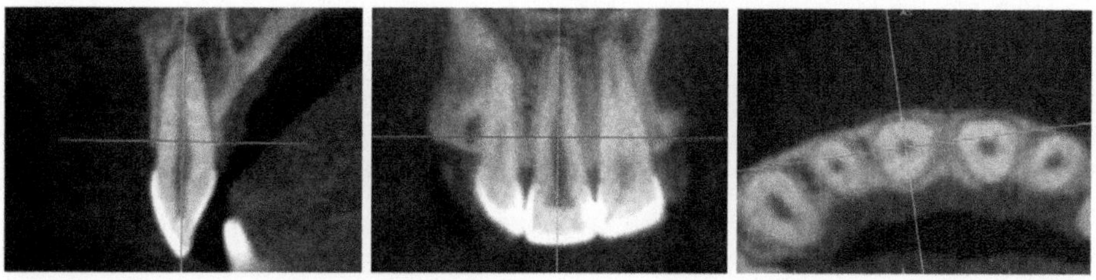

Fig. 4 Measurement of the buccal and lingual bone height. Measurement of the bone height on tooth 11 was carried out parallel to the dental axis both at buccal root surface and at lingual root surface

movement. The present study only included patients with adult crowding. One possible noninvasive treatment for crowding involves expanding the dental arch labially in order to create space for normal positioning of the affected teeth [13]. This method of creating space was used much more often in the mandible. The results of reducing the bone thickness in the direction of the orthodontic tooth movement have been described previously in two-dimensional studies [14–16]. However, only limited visualization of the three-dimensional changes that take place in the bone is possible with two-dimensional images. To date, the specialist literature only includes some three-dimensional studies on this topic [17, 18]. In contrast to the present report, all of the patients included in these studies had been treated with multibracket appliances. In their study, Ahn et al. detected a reduced palatine bone plate and an enlarged buccal bone plate during retraction of the upper incisors using a multibracket appliance [17]. The present study also showed a similar bone reaction to the tooth movement created by the Invisalign aligners.

Overall, the present study showed an increase in bone in the sagittal direction in the mandible, as the bone increase on the lingual side was greater than the bone reduction on the buccal side. This effect was seen particularly clearly at the level of the mid of the root length. This suggests that either increased bone apposition was taking place in the traction zone on the inner side of the lingual bone, or additional bone apposition on the outer side of the lingual alveolar bone. Treatment appears in general to have a slight positive effect on bone remodeling.

With regard to the bone height, vertical bone loss was detected overall. The largest and most significant vertical loss of bone was seen in the vestibular mandible. The reduction in bone height in the direction of the

Table 2 Comparison of differences in the sagittal bone thickness (in mm) between T1 and T0

	Position	Level		n	Min.	Max.	Mean	SD	Wilcoxon test T1–T0	
Maxilla	Buccal	Apex	T1–T0	120	−2.36	4,01	0,04	1,04	Z	−0.063 [a]
									A. significance (two-sided)	*P* = *0.950*
		HSPulpa (HEJ)	T1–T0	120	−1.19	1,36	0,02	0,41	Z	−0.965 [b]
									A. significance (two-sided)	*P* = *0.334*
	Oral	Apex	T1–T0	120	−3.87	2,66	−0.17	1,2	Z	−0.980 [a]
									A. significance (two-sided)	*P* = *0.327*
		HSPulpa (HEJ)	T1–T0	120	−1.94	1,34	−0.11	0,58	Z	−2.069 [a]
									A. significance (two-sided)	*P* = *0.039*
Mandible	Buccal	Apex	T1–T0	120	−2.59	3,6	−0.42	0,86	Z	−5.853 [a]
									A. significance (two-sided)	*P* <*0.001*
		HSPulpa (HEJ)	T1–T0	120	−1.43	0,47	−0.17	0,25	Z	−6.646 [a]
									A. significance (two-sided)	*P* <*0.001*
	Oral	Apex	T1–T0	120	−3.56	2,31	0,48	0,84	Z	−6.630 [b]
									A. significance (two-sided)	*P* <*0.001*
		HSPulpa (HEJ)	T1–T0	120	−0.81	1,97	0,39	0,46	Z	−7.377 [b]
									A. significance (two-sided)	*P* <*0.001*

Wilcoxon test* for statistical analysis
* Wilcoxon signed rank test
[a] Based on positive ranks
[b] Based on negative ranks

Table 3 Comparison of differences in bone height (in mm) between T1 and T0

	Position		n	Min.	Max.	Mean	SD	Wilcoxon test T1–T0	
Maxilla	Buccal	T1–T0	111	−7.85	3,53	−0.24	1,15	Z	−3.058 [a]
								A. significance (two-sided)	*P <0.01*
	Oral	T1–T0	119	−9.80	3,64	−0.57	1,86	Z	−3.287 [a]
								A. significance (two-sided)	*P =0.001*
Mandible	Buccal	T1–T0	120	−9.99	6,4	−2.42	3,37	Z	−6.864 [a]
								A. significance (two-sided)	*P <0.001*
	Oral	T1–T0	120	−6.74	4,65	−0.05	1,63	Z	−0.944 [b]
								A. significance (two-sided)	*P =0.345*

Wilcoxon test* for statistical analysis
* Wilcoxon signed rank test
[a] Based on positive ranks
[b] Based on negative ranks

orthodontic tooth movement is even stronger than the change of the bone thickness in orovestibular direction. Extensive movement in the labial direction should be avoided during treatment planning. In this case other methods of creating space like i.e. IER or extractions should be considered. This is of high importance in respect of orthodontic treatment outcome, since long-term prognosis of tooth movement is only favourable, if the teeth remain firmly embedded in their bony alveolar sockets. Otherwise occurring recessions and a poor periodontal support might jeopardizing the success of orthodontic treatment. Dehiscences and fenestrations were observed on the CBCT scans between T0 and T1 in several cases. The long-term sequelae of this type of alveolar bone loss are as yet unclear. It is also unclear whether this type of damage is permanent or whether neo-osteogenesis is possible after a few months.

Akyalcin et al. [19] noted an increase in the buccal bone thickness after a 3-month retention period. Wainwright [14] reported a slight increase during a 4-month retention period. Follow-up research on the patients included in the present study would be desirable in order to investigate the positive or negative long-term results of Aligner treatment.

When the effects of the treatment in the maxilla and mandible are compared with regard to all the subtopics in the present study, different types of reaction are evident. Highly significant differences between the maxilla and mandible were noted. This is consistent with the findings of previous publications [20]. Movement out of the bony alveolar compartment is associated with bone dehiscences and fenestrations [6]. The size of the symphysis is decisive for the potential movement of the lower incisors. The labiolingual diameter of the bone is smaller in this area than in the maxilla, resulting in a

Table 4 Frequency distribution for planned tooth movement in upper arch

11 apex buk	11 apex ling	11 HS buk	11 HS ling	12 apex buk	12 apex ling	12 HS buk	12 HS ling	21 apex buk	21 apex ling	21 HS buk	21 HS ling	22 apex buk	22 apex ling	22 HS buk	22 HS ling
1,57	-2,19	0,6	-1,13	0,8	-1,73	0,1	-0,91	0,51	-0,74	0,09	-0,43	0,7	-1,92	0,45	-0,78
1,11	-1,29	0,17	-0,61	0,3	-0,21	0,01	-0,02	0,1	-0,57	0,16	-0,61	1,5	-1,18	0	-0,17
0,31	-0,22	0,15	-0,17	0,5	-0,13	-0,17	-0,46	0,86	-0,82	0,64	-0,61	0,07	-0,04	0,1	-0,29
-0,1	-0,06	-0,04	-0,5	-0,38	0,58	0,23	0,07	-0,37	2,66	-0,17	0,09	-0,39	-0,33	-0,32	-0,01
-0,69	0,67	-0,58	0,51	-2,36	2,64	-0,98	1,34	-2,31	2,08	-0,76	1,19	-1,24	0,71	-0,16	1,01
-0,97	-0,05	-0,07	0,66	0,15	-0,74	0,03	-0,56	-1,3	-0,47	-0,79	0,49	-0,8	0,32	0,04	0,03
-0,95	1	-0,3	0,49	0,34	2,58	-0,36	0,84	-1,1	1,22	-0,4	0,75	-1,24	1,88	-0,02	0,78
-0,27	0,3	-0,03	-0,05	-0,03	0,07	-0,11	-0,09	-0,03	0,16	-0,03	0,67	-0,13	0,06	0,42	-0,03
1,26	-2,35	0,92	-1,09	-1,2	0,79	0,22	0,1	2,49	-2,45	0,34	-1,31	-1,01	0,68	0,05	0,62
-1,94	0,98	-0,79	0,9	0	1,59	-1,19	1,16	-0,5	0,41	-0,49	0,07	-0,87	0,35	-0,44	0,51
0,76	-0,59	-0,07	-0,18	-1,16	0,61	-0,58	0,27	0,07	-0,63	-0,15	0,15	-0,66	0,12	-0,36	0,11
-0,67	0,82	-0,49	0,46	-0,71	0,49	0,08	-0,12	-0,24	0,76	0,07	0,14	0	0,08	0,18	0,08
0,25	-0,3	0,03	-0,21	-0,75	0,34	0,06	-0,08	0,02	-0,18	-0,03	0,27	-0,37	0,4	0,37	-0,11
-0,84	0,11	-0,25	0,03	-0,83	0,16	-0,23	0,88	-0,8	-0,19	0,42	-0,38	-0,23	0,48	-0,57	-0,1
0,43	-0,37	0,05	-0,07	-0,44	1	-0,46	0,46	-0,27	0,48	-0,14	0	-0,07	0,78	0,04	0,12
-0,57	0,56	-0,02	-0,52	-0,79	0,61	0,09	0,07	-0,23	0,22	0,01	-0,17	-0,75	0,7	0,09	0,05
0,14	0,5	0,31	-0,93	1,58	-2,09	0,45	-0,61	-0,31	0,81	-0,43	-0,2	-1,37	1,04	0,04	-0,12
-0,36	0,74	-0,19	0,05	-0,91	1,2	-0,73	0,82	-0,17	-0,93	-0,24	-0,37	-1,07	1,06	0,26	0,14
0,21	-0,15	0,03	-0,21	0,7	-0,93	0,24	-0,52	0,81	-0,83	0,68	-0,3	1,46	-1,5	0,69	-0,85
0,78	-0,8	-0,01	-0,47	-0,16	0,02	0,07	0,04	0,88	-0,95	0,21	-0,19	0,74	-0,91	0,36	-0,66
0,76	-1,27	0,39	-0,32	-1,95	1,36	-0,12	0,19	0,69	-0,73	0,28	-0,12	-1,1	0,31	0,13	-0,32
1,01	-1,35	0,32	-0,48	-0,63	0,96	-0,15	0,25	-0,94	0,92	-0,6	0,05	0,18	-0,25	-0,39	0,49
4,01	-3,87	1,36	-0,77	0,7	-1,28	0,27	-0,49	3,14	-3,46	1,01	-1,06	2,01	-1,67	0,54	0
0,11	0,11	0,17	0,1	-0,29	0,27	-0,2	0,25	0,37	-0,03	0,27	0,34	0,19	-0,37	-0,07	-0,35
1,35	-3,18	0,16	-1,94	2,96	-3,61	1,28	-1,71	-0,29	-1,38	-0,37	-0,32	0,75	-1,55	0,81	-1,19
0,47	-0,51	0,09	-0,38	0,56	-0,73	0,19	-0,45	1,07	-1,18	0,06	-0,93	1,76	-2,23	0,09	-1,13
-0,11	-0,33	0,02	-0,29	0,62	-1,22	0,14	0,21	1,18	-1,23	0,11	-0,66	-0,44	0,68	-0,18	0,97
1,34	0,58	0,04	-0,31	0,78	-1,02	-0,08	-0,46	-0,01	0,44	0,26	-0,7	0,24	-0,5	0,08	-0,86
0,31	0,5	0,34	0,15	-0,22	0,61	0,16	-0,12	0,71	-0,65	0,41	-0,17	-0,49	-0,35	0,47	0,16
0,73	-1,88	0,05	-0,3	-1,55	1,25	-0,65	0,32	0,15	0	0,13	-0,03	-1,3	0,88	-0,35	0,28

Red: expansion of the dental arch in the maxilla using proclination/protrusion; green: proclination/protrusion not planned

Table 5 Frequency distribution for planned tooth movement in lower arch

31 apex buk	31 apex ling	31 HS buk	31 HS ling	32 apex buk	32 apex ling	32 HS buk	32 HS ling	41 apex buk	41 apex ling	41 HS buk	41 HS ling	42 apex buk	42 apex ling	42 HS buk	42 HS ling
-0,08	0,62	0,31	0,15	-1	1,15	-0,14	1,12	-1,19	1,5	-0,13	0,69	-0,41	0,48	-0,37	0,74
-0,86	0,61	0	-0,03	0,21	-0,34	0	0,31	-0,31	0,23	-0,08	-0,05	0,06	0,25	0	0,65
-0,31	0,48	0,2	-0,05	-0,7	1,19	-0,64	0,43	-0,38	0,73	-0,01	-0,23	0,21	0,14	-0,12	0,13
-1,76	2,31	0	0,56	0,25	-0,19	-0,36	0,92	-1,53	1,42	0	0,78	-0,39	0,51	0	0,27
-0,15	0,29	0	-0,25	-0,93	0,81	-0,23	0,73	-0,32	0,13	-0,2	0,06	-0,13	0,21	-0,32	0,2
-0,27	0,76	0,12	-0,19	-0,4	0,59	-0,21	0,14	-0,09	0,94	-0,05	0,24	-0,85	1,16	-0,19	0,83
1	0,82	-0,21	0,84	-1,65	1,61	-0,49	0,28	-1,7	1,39	-0,42	0,36	-0,25	0,66	-0,64	1,08
0,12	0	-0,06	0,09	-0,38	0,33	-0,25	0,13	-0,67	0,95	0,1	0,2	-0,27	0,8	-0,2	0,67
-0,22	0,14	-0,23	0,38	-1,18	1,22	0,03	0,69	-1,03	0,91	0	0,44	-1,44	1,44	0,05	1
-1,3	0,8	-0,17	0,69	-0,73	0,86	-0,98	1,06	-2,14	1,5	0	1,1	-1,4	1,76	-1,43	1,97
-0,87	0,98	-0,15	0,24	-0,49	0,62	-0,05	0,13	0,11	-0,05	-0,03	-0,29	-0,3	0,5	-0,2	0,54
-1,08	1,7	0	0,64	0,4	0,05	0	0,89	-1,21	1,35	-0,34	1,18	-0,89	1,05	-0,42	1,1
0,02	-0,03	-0,13	0,13	0,3	-0,15	-0,27	0,29	0,56	-0,44	0	0,21	-0,92	0,4	-0,27	-0,05
-0,6	0,9	-0,17	1,11	-0,06	0,49	-0,2	1,33	-1,28	1,47	-0,43	1,39	0,62	-0,07	-0,2	0,74
-0,1	0,38	0,15	0	-0,91	1,06	-0,29	0,39	-0,41	0,03	0,03	0,2	-0,51	0,77	-0,18	0,76
-1,34	1,59	-0,14	0	0,82	-0,62	0	0	-0,91	1,01	-0,33	0	-0,6	0,9	-0,13	0
-0,42	0,5	-0,1	-0,27	0,28	-0,04	0,1	0,17	-0,32	0,21	-0,3	0,12	-0,37	0,4	-0,17	0,07
-0,83	1,07	-0,47	0,62	-0,56	0,52	-0,49	0,37	-1,67	1,52	-0,06	0,53	-0,4	0,3	-0,11	1,17
-0,42	0,55	-0,63	0,65	-0,53	0,75	-0,45	0,24	-0,64	0,72	-0,32	0,42	0,53	-0,2	-0,85	0,54
-0,97	0,77	-0,34	0,49	0,01	0,01	-0,25	0,52	-0,51	0,44	-0,31	-0,03	0,19	-0,05	-0,2	0,16
-0,57	0,51	-0,25	0,1	-0,85	0,63	-0,33	0,07	-0,01	0,21	0,12	-0,25	-0,36	0,49	0,08	-0,14
-0,86	0,65	0,18	-0,11	0,59	-0,33	0,34	0,09	1,34	-1,52	-0,13	-0,44	-1,29	1,05	-0,09	0,55
0,92	-0,96	-0,09	0	3,17	-3,29	0,39	0	0,6	-0,89	-0,23	0	3,6	-3,56	0,47	-0,81
0,19	-0,35	-0,23	0,19	0,51	-0,49	-0,15	-0,1	-0,36	0,06	0,06	-0,2	0,3	-0,42	0	-0,21
-1,58	-0,11	-0,27	0	-0,43	0,78	-0,18	0	-0,91	1,04	-0,3	0,33	-0,34	0,23	0	0,89
-0,43	0,84	-0,36	0,94	-1,21	1,03	-0,3	0,79	-0,85	0,2	0,18	-0,25	-1,1	0,98	-0,56	1,24
0,25	-0,25	-0,45	0,71	0,13	-0,24	0	0,66	0,99	-0,82	-0,17	0,05	0,34	-0,3	0	0,28
-0,64	0,92	-0,18	0,87	-1,58	1,49	-0,34	1,09	-1,5	1,12	-0,19	0,9	-1,93	-0,05	-0,39	1,03
0,16	0,25	-0,21	0,01	-0,29	0,37	-0,14	0,23	-0,39	0,51	0,1	0,06	0,14	-0,19	-0,12	0,03
-1,4	2,15	-0,17	0,73	-0,62	0,81	0	0,69	-2,59	2,27	-0,27	0,31	-0,67	0,63	0	0,43

Red: expansion of the dental arch in the mandible using proclination/protrusion; green: proclination/protrusion not planned

very thin covering layer of bone on the lower incisors. The limits of the bone are therefore reached more quickly during tooth movements in the mandible. Using CBCT measurements in women, Uysal et al. found that bone sizes in the symphysis were smaller than in men [21]. Ninety-three percent of the patients included in the present study were women.

Another reason for the significant buccal bone loss in the mandible might be that the mandibular incisors generally have a smaller root surface in comparison with the maxillary incisors. In the mandible, the orthodontic force is thus distributed to a smaller periodontal ligament surface. The concentrated pressure on the buccal cortical plate of the lower incisors may therefore be greater and might therefore lead to a more severe reduction in bone thickness vestibularly [22]. The adult crowding was usually earlier and more severe in the mandible than in the maxilla in the present group of patients. More extensive space-creating measures were therefore needed in an area with a smaller bone volume. The risk of dehiscences is accordingly greater.

With regard to the movement pattern, it was found that the pattern planned in the ClinCheck software program had a strong influence on the therapeutically induced bone change (Tables 4 and 5). Excessive expansion of the dental arch should therefore be avoided at all costs.

This retrospective study was based on CBCT scans. Other studies on measuring bone volume have only been carried out using two-dimensional imaging. Gribel et al. compared measurements obtained with CBCT and cephalometric radiography with direct measurements on dry skulls [23]. They found that dental volume tomography with a slice thickness of 0.3 mm was extremely accurate, with a mean deviation of 0.1 mm from direct measurements. For traditional measurements with cephalometric radiography, they observed a large difference of 5 mm and poor intraoperator reliability. Cephalometric radiography is therefore unsuitable for measuring bone thickness. Semenoff et al. investigated the suitability of digitized panoramic radiographs in comparison with bitewing radiographs and dental films for diagnosing alveolar bone resorption [24]. Bone losses can also only be assessed imprecisely on panoramic radiographs, as they were often overestimated [24]. Zachrisson and Alnaes used dental films to study the interdental bone height in patients who had undergone orthodontic treatment [10]. They drew attention to the problem of the absence of a third dimension on all conventional two-dimensional radiographs, making precise assessment of buccal and lingual bone changes impossible.

Only three-dimensional images allow precise assessment of the bone. Hatcher and Aboudara considered that CBCT imaging is indicated in order to measure the buccal bone thickness when expansion is being planned [25]. In a study by Timock et al., CBCT with a voxel size of 0.3 mm (field of view 13 mm) was found to be suitable for measuring the buccal bone height and bone thickness quantitatively with a high degree of precision [26].

Unfortunaly 93 % of the patients included in the present study were women. A study group with a more balanced sex ratio would be desirable. Nevertheless, the publication should help to show data of the context between treatment of adult crowding with aligner and the possible bone change. It would be desirable to get more additional data from other hospitals to this subject. Although CBCT appears to have many advantages, the operator always needs to consider its use carefully for reasons of radiation protection. Considering the ALARA (As Low As Reasonably Achievable) principle CBCT is not indicated as a routine method of imaging periodontal bone support. A CBCT may be indicated in selected cases of infra-bony defects, where clinical and conventional radiographic examinations do not provide the information needed for management. If a CBCT is needed Cook et al. recommend the use of shorter scans and a reduced effective radiation dose for measurements of the buccal alveolar bone height and thickness [27]. Prospective RCTs (randomized controlled trials) would be interesting but could currently not be performed in accordance with the ALARA principle.

Conclusions

Overall, Invisalign treatment for adult crowding with IER showed a dependence of the type of tooth movement and change of bone thickness. Bone changes in the direction of the tooth movement. It appears that the vestibular bone lamella in the mandible is decisive in determining the extent of treatment and the method used to relieve adult crowding, at least in adult female patients. This might help defining the correct indication for different methods of creating space like i.e. IER or extractions.

Acknowledgments
The authors thank Mr. Robertson for editing the manuscript.

Authors' contributions
AH conceived the study together with NS and HMKS, and carried out all experiments and drafted the manuscript. AH and MS performed the statistical analysis. TD treated the patients and SS helped with the collection of the data and made substantial contributions to conception and design. HMKS conceived the study, participated in its design and coordination and helped to draft the manuscript. All authors read and approved the final manuscript.

Competing interests
The authors declare that they have no competing interests.

Consent for publication
Not applicable.

Ethics approval and consent to participate
All research activities relevant for our study have been performed in accordance with the Declaration of Helsinki. This manuscript is involving human data: The use of the data was approved by the ethics committee of Marburg University Hospital (ref. no. 34/15).

Author details
[1]Department of Orthodontics, University Hospital Giessen and Marburg, Campus Marburg, Georg-Voigt-Strasse 3, Marburg 35039, Germany. [2]Private practice, Wiesbaden, Germany. [3]Abt. für Kieferorthopädie, UKGM Standort Marburg, Georg-Voigt-Strasse 3, 35039 Marburg, Germany.

References

1. Meier B, Wiemer KB, Miethke RR. Invisalign—patient profiling. Analysis of a prospective survey. J Orofac Orthop. 2003;64(5):352–8.
2. Nedwed V, Miethke RR. Motivation, acceptance and problems of Invisalign patients. J Orofac Orthop. 2005;66(2):162–73.
3. Fuhrmann R. Dreidimensionale Interpretation parodontaler Läsionen und Remodellationen im Verlauf orthodontischer Behandlungen. Teil III. Fortschr Kieferorthop. 1996;57(4):224–37.
4. Renkema AM, et al. Development of labial gingival recessions in orthodontically treated patients. Am J Orthod Dentofacial Orthop. 2013;143(2): 206–12.
5. Vasconcelos G, et al. Prevalence and severity of vestibular recession in mandibular incisors after orthodontic treatment. Angle Orthod. 2012;82(1): 42–7.
6. Wennström JL. Mucogingival considerations in orthodontic treatment. Semin Orthod. 1996;2(1):46–54.
7. Melsen B. Biological reaction of alveolar bone to orthodontic tooth movement. Angle Orthod. 1999;69(2):151–8.
8. Vardimon AD, Oren E, Ben-Bassat Y. Cortical bone remode- ling/tooth movement ratio during maxillary incisor retraction with tip ver- sus torque movements. Am J Orthod Dentofacial Orthop. 1998;114(5):520–9.
9. Verna C, Zaffe D, Siciliani G. Histomorphometric study of bone reactions during orthodontic tooth movement in rats. Bone. 1999;24(4):371–9.
10. Zachrisson BU, Alnaes L. Periodontal condition in orthodontically treated and untreated individuals. II. Alveolar bone loss: radiographic findings. Angle Orthod. 1974;44(1):48–55.
11. Fuhrmann R. Three-dimensional interpretation of periodontal lesions and remodeling during orthodontic treatment. Part III. J Orofac Orthop. 1996; 57(4):224–37.
12. Kim Y, Park JU, Kook YA. Alveolar bone loss around incisors in surgical skeletal Class III patients. Angle Orthod. 2009;79(4):676–82.
13. Stroud JL, English J, Buschang PH. Enamel thickness of the posterior dentition: its implications for nonextraction treatment. Angle Orthod. 1998; 68(2):141–6.
14. Wainwright WM. Faciolingual tooth movement: its influence on the root and cortical plate. Am J Orthod. 1973;64(3):278–302.
15. Vardimon AD, Robbins D, Brosh T. In-vivo von Mises strains during Invisalign treatment. Am J Orthod Dentofac Orthop. 2010;138(4):399–409.
16. Wehrbein H, Fuhrmann RA, Diedrich PR. Periodontal conditions after facial root tipping and palatal root torque of incisors. Am J Orthod Dentofac Orthop. 1994;106(5):455–62.
17. Ahn HW, Moon SC, Baek SH. Morphometric evaluation of changes in the alveolar bone and roots of the maxillary anterior teeth before and after en masse retraction using cone-beam computed tomography. Angle Orthod. 2013;83(2):212–21.
18. Lund H, Gröndahl K, Gröndahl HG. Cone beam computed tomography for assessment of root length and marginal bone level during orthodontic treatment. Angle Orthod. 2010;80(3):466–73.
19. Akyalcin S, Schaefer JS, English JD, Stephens CR, Winkelmann S. A cone-beam computed tomography evaluation of buccal bone thickness following maxillary expansion. Imaging Sci Dent. 2013;43(2):85–90.
20. Lund H, Gröndahl K, Gröndahl HG. Cone beam computed tomography evaluations of marginal alveolar bone before and after orthodontic treatment combined with premolar extractions. Eur J Oral Sci. 2012;120(3):201–11.
21 Uysal T, Yagci A, Ozer T, Veli I, Ozturk A. Mandibular anterior bony support and incisor crowding: Is there a relationship? Am J Orthod Dentofac Orthop. 2012;142(5):645–53.
22 Sarikaya S, Haydar B, Ciğer S, Ariyürek M. Changes in alveolar bone thickness due to retraction of anterior teeth. Am J Orthod Dentofac Orthop. 2002; 122(1):15–26.
23 Gribel BF, Gribel MN, Frazão DC, McNamara JA, Manzi FR. Accuracy and reliability of craniometric measurements on lateral cephalometry and 3D measurements on CBCT scans. Angle Orthod. 2011;81(1):26–35.
24 Semenoff L, Semenoff TAD, Pedro FLM, Volpato ER, de Machado AM, Borges AH, et al. Are panoramic radiographs reliable to diagnose mild alveolar bone resorption? ISRN Dent. 2011;2011:363578.
25 Hatcher DC, Aboudara CL. Diagnosis goes digital. Am J Orthod Dentofac Orthop. 2004;125(4):512–5.

26 Timock AM, Cook V, McDonald T, Leo MC, Crowe J, Benninger BL, et al. Accuracy and reliability of buccal bone height and thickness measurements from cone-beam computed tomography imaging. Am J Orthod Dentofac Orthop. 2011;140(5):734–44.
27 Cook VC, Timock AM, Crowe JJ, Wang M, Covell Jr DA. Accuracy of alveolar bone measurements from cone beam computed tomography acquired using varying settings. Orthod Craniofac Res. 2015;18(1):127–36.

15

Disk displacement, eccentric condylar position, osteoarthrosis – misnomers for variations of normality? Results and interpretations from an MRI study in two age cohorts

Jens C. Türp[1*], Anna Schlenker[2], Johannes Schröder[3], Marco Essig[4] and Marc Schmitter[5]

Abstract

Background: Clinical decision-making and prognostic statements in individuals with manifest or suspected temporomandibular disorders (TMDs) may involve assessment of (a) the position of articular disc relative to the mandibular condyle, (b) the location of the condyle relative to the temporal joint surfaces, and (c) the depth of the glenoid fossa of the temporomandibular joints (TMJs). The aim of this study was twofold: (1) Determination of the prevalence of these variables in two representative population-based birth cohorts. (2) Reinterpretation of the clinical significance of the findings.

Methods: From existing magnetic resonance imaging (MRI) scans of the TMJs that had been taken in 2005 and 2006 from 72 subjects born between 1930 and 1932 and between 1950 and 1952, respectively, the condylar position at closed jaw was calculated as percentage displacement of the condyle from absolute centricity. By using the criteria introduced by Orsini et al. (Oral Surg Oral Med Oral Pathol Oral Radiol Endod 86:489-97, 1998), a textbook-like disc position at closed jaw was distinguished from an anterior location. TMJ morphology of the temporal joint surfaces was assessed at open jaw by measuring the depth of the glenoid fossa, using the method proposed by Muto et al. (J Oral Maxillofac Surg 52:1269-72, 1994).
Frequency distributions were recorded for the condylar and disc positions at closed jaw.
Student's *t*-test with independent samples was used as test of significance to detect differences of condylar positions between the age cohorts (1930 vs. 1950) and the sexes. The significance levels were set at 5%. First, the results from the measurement of the age cohorts were compared without differentiation of sexes, i.e., age cohort 1930–1932 versus age cohort 1950–1952. Subsequently, the age cohorts were compared by sex, i.e., men in cohort 1930–1932 versus men in cohort 1950–1952, and women in cohort 1930–1932 women men in cohort 1950–1952.
(Continued on next page)

* Correspondence: jens.tuerp@unibas.ch
[1]Department of Reconstructive Dentistry and Temporomandibular Disorders, University Center for Dental Medicine Basel, University of Basel, Basel, Switzerland
Full list of author information is available at the end of the article

(Continued from previous page)

Results: In both cohorts, condylar position was characterized by great variability. About 50% of the condyles were located centrically, while the other half was either in an anterior or in a posterior position. In both female cohorts, a posterior position predominated, whereas a centric position prevailed among men. Around 75% of the discs were positioned textbook-like, while the remaining forth was located anteriorly. Age had no statistically significant influence on condylar or on disc position. Conversely, comparison between the age groups revealed a statistically significant decrease of the depth of the glenoid fossa in both older cohorts. This age-dependent changes may be interpreted as flattening of the temporal joint surfaces.

Conclusions: We call for a re-interpretation of imaging findings because they may insinuate pathology which usually is not present. Instead, anterior or posterior positions of the mandibular condyle as well as an anterior location of the articular disc should be construed as a variation of normalcy. Likewise, flattening of articular surfaces of the TMJs may be considered as normal adaptive responses to increased loading, rather than pathological degenerative changes.

Trial registration: Not applicable.

Keywords: Image interpretation, Mandibular condyle, Medicalization, Medical overuse, Osteoarthritis, Osteoarthrosis, Overdiagnosis, Temporomandibular disorders, Temporomandibular joint disc, Terminology

Background

Many descriptive epidemiological studies from different countries have shown that temporomandibular disorders (TMDs) are mostly prevalent among women in the child-bearing age [1–4]. This is also reflected in the higher degree of TMD-related treatment need among females as compared to males [5, 6].

Conversely, recent findings from a large prospective cohort study (OPPERA) revealed that the incidence rate of clinically verified temporomandibular pain was only marginally greater in women than in men, while there was no difference in the annual rate of TMD pain symptom episodes among the two sexes [7]. In contrast to musculoskeletal complaints located in other parts of the body, e.g. osteoarthritis [8], the incidence and prevalence of TMD symptoms, notably pain located in the masticatory muscles and/or the temporomandibular joints (TMJs), decrease remarkably during menopause and in older age [1, 9, 10].

In individuals with manifest or suspected TMDs, clinical decision-making as well as TMD-related prognostic statements of dentists are primarily based on somatic factors, such as the presence of temporomandibular pain, while psychosocial variables do not appear to play an important role, if any [6]. Traditionally, many dentists have focused on morphological variables to suggest etiological models and/or justify initiation of therapy, including (a) the position of the articular disc relative to the mandibular condyle [11, 12], (b) the location of the mandibular condyle relative to the temporal joint surfaces (glenoid fossa and articular eminence) [13, 14], and (c) the depth of the glenoid (mandibular) fossa, including flattening of the temporal surfaces [15, 16].

In the present investigation, these three anatomical variables were reanalyzed in two population-based birth cohorts to determine the prevalence of these variables and to (re)interpret the clinical significance of the findings. The cohorts were stratified by age and biological sex in order to investigate the possible influence of these two variables.

Methods

Previous work

At the beginning of the 1990s, a representative longitudinal population study of adult development based on two cohorts ($N = 1001$) born between 1930 and 1932 and between 1950 and 1952, respectively, had been initiated in two German urban regions, Heidelberg-Mannheim-Ludwigshafen (Baden-Württemberg/ Rhineland-Palatinate) and Leipzig (Saxonia) [17]. In 2005 and 2006, the participants of our study had been recruited from the two Heidelberg cohorts by asking them to participate in a magnetic resonance imaging (MRI) examination of the TMJs. Seventy-two individuals consented, 33 of whom were from the birth cohort 1930–1932 and 39 from the cohort 1950–1952. Data of two subsamples – "cohort 1930–1932" [73–76 years of age], "cohort 1950–1952" [53–56 years of age]) of the Heidelberg cohort – was selected. The distribution of the 72 participants, stratified by cohort and sex, is summarized in Table 1.

Subsequently, all subjects were examined according to the *Research Diagnostic Criteria for Temporomandibular Disorders* (RDC/TMD) [18]. Three participants reported pain in one TMJ. In five individuals, a reciprocal clicking was noticed during jaw opening, closing, and protrusion, but not upon protrusive opening. No subject had a limitation of mandibular movements.

In the Division of Radiology of the German Cancer Research Center at Heidelberg, contrast agent-enhanced

Table 1 Distribution of the two birth cohorts

	Number	f	m	Non-accessible, jaw closed	Non-accessible, jaw open
Cohort 1930–1932	66	30	36	3	10
Cohort 1950–1952	78	36	42	2	4
Σ TMJs	144	66	78	5	14

N: number of temporomandibular joints (TMJs), separated in TMJs from females (f) and males (m). At closed jaw, 139 TMJs were accessible, while 130 TMJs were accessible at open jaw. In the Cohort 1930–1932, one female participant could not be evaluated both at open and closed jaw

(Magnevist; Schering AG, Berlin, Germany) MRI scans of the TMJs in the sagittal and coronal views were made in open and closed jaw positions. For that purpose, a 1.5 Tesla tomography (Symphony; Siemens, Erlangen, Germany) with TMJ surface coils (12 cm diameter; Siemens) was used. Imaging was carried out with a T1 2D fast low-angle shot (FLASH) sequence. For every individual, 10 scans were produced. The following settings were taken: slice thickness 3 mm, distance factor 20%, flip 30°, field of view 120 mm × 120 mm, time of repetition 208 ms, time of echo 10.2 ms, base resolution 256, phase resolution 80%, band width 70 Hz/Px. The slices were oriented rectangular to the long axis of the condyle. The magnetization-prepared gradient echo technique was chosen to enhance the contrast of the various tissues by acquiring the spins in different relaxation times. This technique optimizes imaging of the cartilage and is both time- and cost-effective. For the depiction of the closed position, the subjects had been instructed to close their jaw habitually with slight tooth contacts. For the stabilization of the open jaw position, a mechanical mouth opener (Burnett BiDirectional TMJ Device, Medrad Inc. Pittsburgh, U.S.A.) was used to fix the open jaw position and, therefore, to reduce blurred images due to mandibular motion.

Current study

The total number of MRIs available for evaluation was 139 at closed and 130 at open jaw positions. Exclusion criteria had been low imaging quality and artifacts (Table 1). For each TMJ, one slice of the sagittal views – namely the slice located in the middle of the long axis of the condyle – was selected from the open and closed positions, respectively, for the assessment of the mandibular condyle and the articular disc. For the purpose of this paper, the coronal views were not considered.

Evaluations of the MRIs and all measurements were carried out with the digitizing software DICOM (Digital Imaging and Communications in Medicine) Works (Version 1.3.5, National Electrical Manufactures Association, Virginia, USA).

Position of the mandibular condyle at closed jaw

The condylar position at closed jaw was calculated as percentage displacement of the condyle from absolute geometric centricity. Both the smallest anterior and posterior distances between mandibular condyle and glenoid fossa (i.e., the narrowest anterior and posterior interarticular widths) were determined [19, 20] (Fig. 1). Then, the individual condylar position (CP) was calculated according to the following formula [19, 20]:

$$CP = \frac{\text{posterior-anterior}}{\text{posterior} + \text{anterior}} \times 100\%$$

The result was interpreted according to the recommendations by Ren et al. [21]:

- 0: absolute centric position of the condyle.
- −12% - +12%: centric position of the condyle
- < −12%: posterior position of the condyle
- > +12%: anterior position of the condyle

Position of the articular disc at closed jaw

Determination of the articular disc position at closed jaw was carried out following the criteria proposed by Orsini et al. [22]. A textbook-like "normal" disc position (e.g.,[23]), with the posterior band located at the top of the condyle (12 o'clock position) (Fig. 2a), was distinguished from an anterior location, where in intercuspal position (formerly: maximum intercuspation) the posterior band of the disc was located anterior to the 12 o'clock position (Fig. 2b).

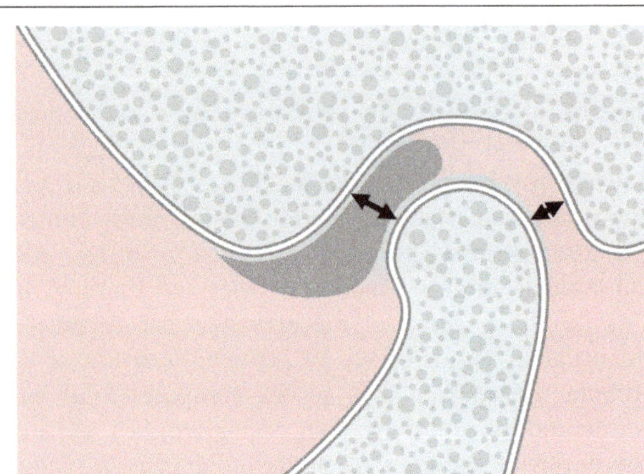

Fig. 1 Evaluation of condylar position at closed jaw: Determination of the smallest anterior and posterior joint spaces

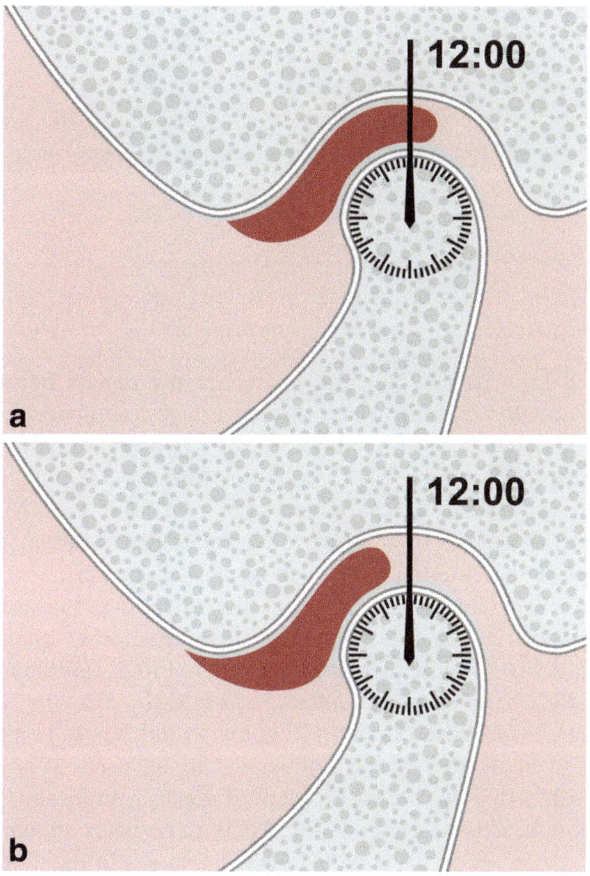

Fig. 2 Evaluation of disc position at closed jaw, based on an imaginary clock located in the condylar head. **a** Textbook-like disc position: The posterior band is located at the 12 o'clock position (at the top of the mandibular condyle). **b** Anterior disc position: The posterior band is located anteriorly of the 12 o'clock position

Depth of the glenoid fossa at open jaw

The depth of the glenoid fossa was assessed during open jaw position by using the method introduced by Muto et al. [24]: A tangent was drawn from the most caudal part of the articular eminence (E) to the apex of the postglenoid spine (S). The distance between E and S, defined as "a", corresponded to the width of the glenoid fossa. Subsequently, a parallel line to SE touching the most superior aspect (F) of the fossa was drawn (P). Finally, a perpendicular line was drawn from SE to P, which was equivalent to the depth (= height) of the fossa "b" (Fig. 3).

Statistical evaluation

The statistical analyses were carried out with SPSS version 21 (Statistical Package for the Social Sciences, Chicago, IL, USA). Frequency distributions were recorded for the condylar and disc positions at closed jaw. Student's *t*-test [25] with independent (unpaired) samples was used as test of significance to detect differences between the age cohorts (1930 vs. 1950) and the sexes. The significance levels were set at 5%. First, the results from the measurement of the age cohorts were compared without differentiation of sexes, i.e., age cohort 1930–1932 versus age cohort 1950–1952. Subsequently, the age cohorts were compared by sex, i.e., men in cohort 1930–1932 versus men in cohort 1950–1952, and women in cohort 1930–1932 versus women in cohort 1950–1952.

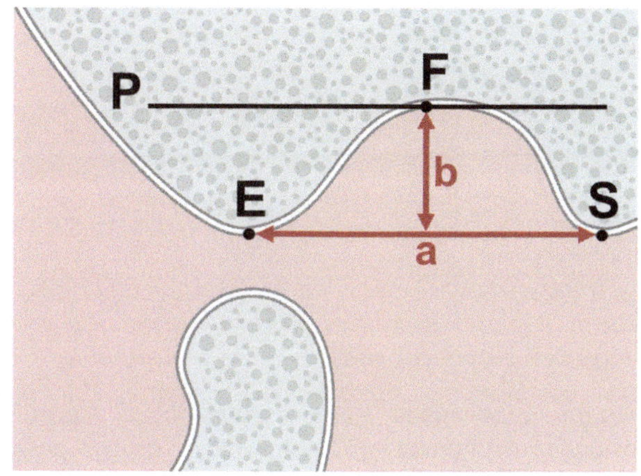

Fig. 3 Points and lines used for measuring glenoid fossa depth. C: highest point of the condyle, E: most caudal part of the articular eminence, F: most superior aspect of the glenoid fossa, S: apex of the postglenoid spine, P: line parallel to the line SE touching F, a: distance from E to S = width of the fossa, b: perpendicular line from SE to P1 = depth of the fossa

Interrater reliability

To assess interrater reliability, the sagittal MRI views of the mandibular condyle and the articular disc of nine participants were evaluated at open and closed jaw positions independently by two authors (A.S. and M.S.) using the above-mentioned computerized digitizing software. The intra-class correlation coefficient [26] was used for the statistical computation. Based on the results of the reliability assessment (see Results: Interrater reliability), it was assumed that the measuring method was reliable. Therefore, the remaining MRIs were assessed by one rater only.

Results

Interrater reliability

Substantial interrater agreement could be reached (ICC: 0.7). Observational discrepancies were discussed until obtaining consensus.

Position of the mandibular condyle at closed jaw

In both cohorts, condylar position was characterized by great variability (Tables 2 and 3). Altogether, 68 of 139 condyles (48.9%) were located centrically, whereas 71 (51.1%) were in an eccentric position. An absolute centric position was a rare exception and was present in less

Table 2 Condylar positions (jaw closed) among women and men, respectively, determined according to the formula $\frac{\text{posterior-anterior}}{\text{posterior+anterior}} \times 100\%$ ($n = 139$). There was no statistical significance in the relationship between the cohorts and the sexes, respectively

	Anterior	Absolutely centric	Centric	Posterior	Σ TMJs
Cohort 1930, women	2 (7%)	2 (7%)	9 (32%)	15 (54%)	28
Cohort 1950, women	3 (8%)	1 (3%)	13 (36%)	18 (50%)	35
Cohort 1930, men	10 (28%)	0	17 (47%)	8 (22%)	35
Cohort 1950, men	10 (24%)	2 (5%)	24 (57%)	5 (12%)	41
Σ TMJs	25 (18.0%)	5 (3.6%)	63 (45.3%)	46 (33.1%)	139

than 4% of individuals. In the female cohorts, a posterior position predominated (52.4%), while a centric position prevailed among men (56.6%). Nevertheless, neither age nor sex had a statistically significant influence on condylar position.

Position of the articular disc at closed jaw

In three-forth of the TMJs, the most frequent position of the articular disc corresponded to the one described in textbooks. With other words, one out of four discs was "anteriorly displaced" (Table 4). The frequency of anteriorly located disc was twice higher in females than in males (22/63 vs. 13/76 = 34.5% vs. 17.1%; $p < 0.05$).

Depth of the glenoid fossa at open jaw

Comparison between the age groups revealed a statistically significant decrease ($p < 0.05$) of the depth of the glenoid fossa in both older cohorts: 6.9 mm (1950) vs. 6.1 mm (1930) among females, 7.8 mm (1950) vs. 6.3 mm (1930) among males (Table 5).

Discussion

Methodology

Our population-based retrospective cohort study was based on imaging data stored in an electronic database. The records were from individuals of a representative population sample. We therefore assume that the participants were representative of that population, hence minimizing selection bias [27]. The typical disadvantages of patient-based retrospective studies, such as recall bias and information bias, did not affect the results because we made anatomical analyses on images, comparable to a histological examination. In our investigation, MRIs were used, which is the gold standard for imaging soft tissues [28]. In the temporomandibular joint area, MRIs are the images of choice to investigate disc position and optimize depiction of the condylar cartilage [29].

Conversely, for the investigation of hard tissues, such as condylar position and osseous changes, other imaging modalities, such as cone-beam computed tomography (CBCT), are more suitable [30, 31]. Yet, in this population-based study, CT scans would not have been allowed by the ethical committee to be used. Without doubt, this is a certain methodological limitation, although, on the other hand, MRIs have been shown to produce highly acceptable osseous changes in the TMJ.

As the slices had been selected identically in each subject, the comparability of the results can be assumed to be valid. Without doubt, the orientation of the slices has an influence on the measurement. Since the orientation was standardized, however, this approach seems to be acceptable. In this context, the shape of the condyle has certainly an impact on the measurement of the condylar position. While the calculated depth of the glenoid fossa based on MRI data might differ from the real anatomical depth, this possible bias is true for all measurements in all subjects and might be acceptable for this reason.

Using the technique FLASH imaging for rapid MRI [32, 33] ensures that acquisition times are reduced to

Table 3 Mean condylar position (jaw closed) among women and men, respectively, calculated according to the formula $\frac{\text{posterior-anterior}}{\text{posterior+anterior}} \times 100\%$ ($n = 139$). There was no statistical significance in the relationship between the cohorts and the sexes, respectively

	Mean	SD	Min	Max
Cohort 1930, women	−20.7	23.5	−100	14.8
Cohort 1950, women	−11.4	19.1	−45.5	40
Cohort 1930, men	1.8	19.5	−40	40.3
Cohort 1950, men	5.1	13.6	−42.3	31.8

Table 4 Distribution of disc positions (jaw closed) among women and men, respectively ($n = 139$). There was no statistical significance in the relationship between the cohorts and the sexes, respectively

	Anterior	Textbook-like	Σ TMJs
Cohort 1930, women	7 (25%)	21 (75%)	28
Cohort 1950, women	15 (42%)	20 (56%)	35
Cohort 1930, men	9 (25%)	26 (72%)	35
Cohort 1950, men	4 (10%)	37 (88%)	41
Σ	35 (25.2%)	104 (74.8%)	139

Table 5 Depth of the glenoid fossa (distance "b") in mm (jaw open) among women and men, respectively ($n = 130$). Statistical significance was reached between the two female and the two male cohorts, respectively

	Mean	SD	Min	Max	*p*
Cohort 1930, women	6.1	1	3.6	7.7	<0.05
Cohort 1950, women	6.9	1.3	4.5	9.4	
Cohort 1930, men	6.3	2.5	3.0	16.5	<0.05
Cohort 1950, men	7.8	2	4.2	15.6	

seconds while spatial resolution is retained. For the purpose of our study, three-dimensional (3D) imaging [34] could not be realized due to unavailability of the existing 3D magnetic resonance scanner and the higher costs due to the longer acquisition time.

Position of the mandibular condyle at closed jaw

We found a nearly 50% chance (71:68) of a deviation from a centric condylar position. These results corroborate findings of two systematic reviews on the position of the mandibular condyles of symptom-free dentate adults during intercuspal position [35, 36]. Stamm et al. [35], who analyzed the results from 49 imaging investigations covering the period until 2001, reported a range of anterior (cranioventral), (con)centric and posterior condylar positions. No statistically significant predominance of any specific condylar position was observed when the results of the six methodically best study articles were considered [35].

In a sequel of the Stamm et al. review, Türp and Walter [36] evaluated the four study reports [37–41] and two overview articles [42, 43] that were published between 2002 and 2012. The results of the four clinical studies attested to the wide interindividual variation. Centric positions were found less frequently than eccentric locations of the condyles. This conclusion stands in contrast to data from a CBCT study in Iran where among individuals without TMD history a centric condylar position was the rule [44].

As in an early investigation report by Pullinger et al. [45], more posterior condylar positions were observed among females and more anterior positions among men. Pullinger et al. [45] raised the question whether this finding could "partially contribute to the greater frequency of TMJ clicking in females". Our study lends support to this hypothesis, because we identified twice as much anterior locations of the disc among women than among men.

Since in TMD patients an apparent association between condylar position and clinical findings worth to be treated is lacking [46], it appears that the often asked question of "the most physiological" or "the most optimum" condylar position in intercuspal position is more of academic interest than of clinical relevance. Instead, a relatively broad range of equally acceptable positions exists [36]. This assertion echoes the conclusion of Hugger et al. [37–41] who after analyzing 136 TMJs on MRIs stated: "Considering the great variability of the condylar position in patients with normal mandibular function and those with functional disorders of the stomatognathic system, the criterion "condyle-fossa relationship" seems more questionable than ever in the context of decision-making with regard to functional normality, adaptation or therapeutic requirements." Hence, by defining "normality" as a "range of results beyond which target disorders become highly probable" [47] we concur with the statement by Pullinger that "non-concentric condyle positions can be compatible with normal function" [48].

Position of the articular disc at closed jaw

Our observation that anterior disc locations are relatively frequent findings, is in concordance with imaging studies from the 1980s [49, 50] and 1990s [51]. More recent investigations have corroborated the assumption that so-called anterior disc displacements are common in normal populations. For example, in a community sample of 1643 individuals in Brazil, the prevalence of disc displacements as diagnosed clinically with the RDC/TMD was around 8% [52]. Not unexpectedly, higher values are found among patients. In a sample of 1603 adult TMD patients in Spain, the prevalence of the RDC/TMD diagnosis "disc displacement with reduction" was around 40% in each TMJ [53]. Among 520 consecutive TMD patients in Italy, RDC/TMD diagnoses of disc displacement were found in 42% of cases [54]. The values from the two European studies are close to those found in our investigation. TMJ sounds are widespread even among children and adolescents, as was recently reported in a systematic review which considered 17,051 individuals: a prevalence of 10% (95% confidence interval: 7.97–12.28) was calculated [55].

In the past, anterior disc displacements with reduction had been construed as the beginning of a cascade-like development leading to more severe TMJ pathology requiring therapy [56]. In the 1980s, Rasmussen [57] as well as Wilkes [58] proposed staging criteria for a progressive development of TMJ problems. While Rasmussen [57] differentiated six phases, Wilkes [58] distinguished five stages. Taking clinical, radiographic, and surgical findings into consideration, Wilkes postulated that a reciprocal TMJ clicking would eventually progress to pain of increasing frequency and intensity, leading to late stages of "chronicity" and "chronic restriction of [mandibular] motion" [58]. Yet, epidemiological population-based studies have challenged this view [59–61], which has also been corroborated by clinical findings among patient samples:

In a recent cross-sectional multicenter study involving 614 cases with at least one TMD diagnosis, the association between TMJ intra-articular status (representing a transition from normal joint structure to TMJ disc displacement with or without reduction to degenerative joint disease) and patient-reported TMD impact (pain intensity, mandibular dysfunction, pain-related disability) was neither statistically significant nor clinically relevant [62]. In fact, the authors found no association between the intraarticular status of the TMJs and TMJ arthralgia or mandibular function [62]. Of course, these statements do not discard the possibility that a subset of individuals does indeed progress from clicking to osteoarthrosis; nonetheless, this is more an exception than the rule [48].

Accordingly, pain-free TMJ clicking (popping, snapping) during opening and/or closing [63], i.e. anterior disc displacement with reduction, may be interpreted as a "normal anatomical variant" presenting as subclinical symptom and/or sign that does not warrant further diagnosis or therapy [64] – as opposed to the alternative interpretation of an "abnormal joint pathology" [65]. The same applies to a pain-free disc displacement without reduction, which, in the absence of pain and/or mandibular dysfunction, should not be interpreted as a sign of pathology.

Although the line separating normal variation from pathological disorder is ill-defined, we agree with Ohrbach and Greene [64] that (a) pain associated with masticatory muscles or TMJs and/or (2) limitations of jaw movements (mostly restricted jaw opening), e.g. mandibular dysfunction, are those clinical symptoms and signs that require therapy, at least in most cases. Hence, *painful* TMJ clicking would warrant pain management, but irrespective of the presence of the clicking sound.

Imaging findings do not contribute to the clinical decision-making process because pain cannot be depicted on radiographs, whereas knowledge about the exact position of the articular disc appears to be unnecessary because there is no need for a therapeutic manipulation of the disc position. With other words: It is unnecessary to "confirm" a TMD-related diagnosis by sophisticated imaging. Instead, the principle of ALARA ("As Low As Reasonably Acceptable") or ALADA ("As Low As Diagnostically Acceptable") should be strictly observed [66].

Depth of the glenoid fossa at open jaw

The age-dependent changes observed in our study may be interpreted as flattening of the temporal joint surfaces, particularly of the posterior slope of the articular eminence. Radiographic observations, such as flattening of the mandibular condyles or the articular eminence, are common among asymptomatic individuals [67, 68] as well as among patients with TMJ pain [69]. These morphological alterations may begin at early age: In a Chinese investigation, 711 of 4883 TMD patients (14.6%) aged between 11 and 30 years showed radiographic signs of TMJ osteoarthrosis [70]. The incidence of such osseous alterations continues with increasing age [71–73], probably as the consequence of long-term adverse loading of the intraarticular tissues [74], for example due to bruxism, while the role of loss of occlusal support on such morphological changes remains controversial [75].

Erosion with articular surface flattening is commonly interpreted as a sign of osteoarthrosis [76]. In the general population, the prevalence of TMJ osteoarthrosis lies between 2.4% [77] and 3.6% [78], whereas among patient populations with TMDs the estimated prevalence is 5.5% (based on seven studies representing 3,055 joints) [79]. In the joints of the human body, osseous changes, osteoarthritic pain, and impaired function generally increase with age [8, 80].

In contrast, the clinical symptoms of the typical TMD patient – a women between 18 und 50 year suffering from masticatory muscle pain – decrease remarkably during menopause and in older age groups [1]. Schmitter et al., for instance, found that among thirty 73 to 75 years old individuals drawn from a representative sample signs of TMJ osteoarthrosis were detected on gadolinium-enhanced MR images in 21 subjects (70%); yet, only one person (3.3%) reported TMJ arthralgia [9]. De Leeuw et al. [81] reported that 30 years after initial diagnosis of osteoarthrosis and internal derangement *clinical signs* were scarce and did hardly differ from those of asymptomatic controls, despite the fact that radiographic signs, such as flattening, were significantly more prevalent in former patients than in controls.

These findings support a statement of De Boever and Carlsson made more than two decades ago [82]. They noted that "many patients are unaware of the deviation in form and the case history is often negative for pain or acute dysfunction", because "it may well be a remodeling due to changed function", leading to pain-free adaptive changes of the osseous structures of the TMJ [83]. Therefore, TMJs with signs of osteoarthrosis are not necessarily associated with more symptoms of TMDs than TMJs without osteoarthrosis [84, 85]. On the other hand, clinical signs and symptoms of TMJ osteoarthritis are poorly correlated with osseous changes depicted with computed tomography [86] or CBCT [30]. Indeed, for a long time it has been known that on the basis of radiographic findings it is difficult to differentiate between osteoarthrosis and adaptive remodeling [87]. Thus, an irregular morphology of the TMJ, such loss of the rounded contour of the surface of the mandibular condyle and/or the posterior slope of the articular eminence, has been considered an indeterminate finding for DJD,

Table 6 Suggested new description of three traditional imaging and clinical findings

Traditional description	Suggested new description
Condylar displacement (eccentric condylar position)	(Anterior, posterior) condylar position
Anterior disc displacement	Anterior disc position
Osteoarthrosis	Adaptive remodeling (due to increased mechanical loading)

which may represent a precursor to osteoarthrosis, but also variation of normalcy, a sign of aging, and/or adaptive remodeling [63, 88]. Indeed, since the classical papers by Sandstedt more than 120 years ago [89–91], it is part of the general knowledge of the dental community that continuous compression may lead to bone resorption, while traction (pull) may cause deposition of new bone (bone apposition). Therefore, we argue that repetitive mechanical load by compressive forces that exceeds the adaptive capacity of the TMJ may result in resorption of bone and flattening of formerly roundish joint surfaces of the mandibular condyle and the articular eminence [92, 93]. From a biological standpoint of plausibility, this would allow for a greater distribution of mechanical forces acting on the joint, for example during bruxing episodes, and could be interpreted as a bony adaptation [94].

Conclusions

Based on the results of our investigation and following the arguments put forth in the discussion, we call for a re-interpretation of the significance and labeling of imaging findings and derived diagnoses because they may insinuate pathology which usually does not exist. Therefore, as far as the mandibular condyles are concerned, expressions such as "condylar displacement" or "eccentric position" for describing of a non-centric condylar position should be avoided. Besides, it may evoke negative cognitions among patients. This interjection also applies to the prevalent diagnoses "anterior disc displacement" and "degenerative joint disease"/"TMJ osteoarthrosis". In most cases, these conditions are chance findings in the course of a clinical or imaging examination, with no disadvantageous outcomes for the individual. Two decades ago, relabeling of the expression "disc displacement" (in favor of "disc position") had been already suggested [95]. We would like to extend our proposal by considering condylar position and TMJ morphology as well (Table 6). By doing so, we intend to protect non-patients against medicalization, overdiagnosis, and unnecessary therapy.

Abbreviations

cm: Centimeter; CP: Condylar position; DC/TMD: Diagnostic Criteria for Temporomandibular Disorders; DJD: Degenerative joint disease; Hz/Px: Herz/Pixel [Bandwidth]; mm: Millimeter; MRI: Magnetic resonance imaging; ms: Millisecond; OPPERA: Orofacial Pain: Prospective Evaluation and Risk Assessment; RDC/TMD: Research Diagnostic Criteria for Temporomandibular Disorders; TMD: Temporomandibular disorders; TMJ: Temporomandibular joint

Acknowledgements

We would like to thank Mrs. Tine Ade, graphic designer, for preparing the figures. We also appreciate the thorough and very helpful suggestions of the reviewers. Their insightful and constructive comments have helped us improve and strengthen our manuscript.
Finally, we would like to express our gratitude to the Ministry of Science, Research, and Arts of the State of Baden-Württemberg, Germany; to the Federal Ministry for Family Affairs, Senior Citizens, Women, and Youth of the Federal Republic of Germany; and to the Dietmar Hopp Stiftung (Foundation), Germany.

Authors' contributions

JCT reinterpreted the data, drafted and wrote the manuscript. AS analyzed the MRIs, carried out the statistical analyses, and contributed to the manuscript. JS designed the study and recruited the patients. ME examined the subjects and analyzed the MRIs. MS designed the study, interpreted the data, and contributed to the manuscript. All authors read and approved the final manuscript.

Competing interests

The authors declare that they have no competing interests.

Ethics approval and consent to participate

Ethics approval was granted by the Ethics Committee of the Medical Faculty of the University of Heidelberg (approval number 181/2005). Written informed consent to participate in the investigation was obtained from each study participant.

Author details

[1]Department of Reconstructive Dentistry and Temporomandibular Disorders, University Center for Dental Medicine Basel, University of Basel, Basel, Switzerland. [2]Department of Prosthodontics, University of Heidelberg, Heidelberg, Germany. [3]Section of Geriatric Psychiatry, University of Heidelberg, Heidelberg, Germany. [4]Department of Radiology, University of Manitoba, Faculty of Medicine, Winnepeg, Canada. [5]Department of Prosthodontics, Dental School of the University of Würzburg, Würzburg, Germany.

References

1. Howard JA. Temporomandibular joint disorders, facial pain, and dental problems in performing artists. In: Sataloff RT, Brandfonbrener AG, Lederman RJ, editors. Textbook of performing arts medicine. New York: Raven; 1991. p. 111–69.
2. Al-Jundi MA, John MT, Setz JM, Szentpétery A, Kuss O. Meta-analysis of treatment need for temporomandibular disorders in adult nonpatients. J Orofacial Pain. 2008;22:97–107.
3. Visscher CM, Ligthart L, Schuller AA, Lobbezoo F, de Jongh A, van Houtem CM, Boomsma DI. Comorbid disorders and sociodemographic variables in temporomandibular pain in the general Dutch population. J Oral Facial Pain Headache. 2015;29:51–9.
4. Kim TY, Shin JS, Lee J, Lee YJ, Kim MR, Ahn YJ, Park KB, Hwang DS, Ha IH. Gender difference in associations between chronic temporomandibular disorders and general quality of life in Koreans: a cross-sectional study. PLoS One. 2015;10:e0145002.
5. Kuttila M, Niemi PM, Kuttila S, Alanen P, Le Bell Y. TMD treatment need in relation to age, gender, stress, and diagnostic subgroup. J Orofac Pain. 1998; 12:67–74.

6. Yekkalam N, Wanman A. Factors associated with clinical decision-making in relation to treatment need for temporomandibular disorders. Acta Odontol Scand. 2016;74:134–41.
7. Slade GD, Sanders AE, Bair E, Brownstein N, Dampier D, Knott C, Fillingim R, Maixner WO, Smith S, Greenspan J, et al. Preclinical episodes of orofacial pain symptoms and their association with health care behaviors in the OPPERA prospective cohort study. Pain. 2013;154:750–60.
8. Neogi T, Zhang Y. Epidemiology of osteoarthritis. Rheum Dis Clin North Am. 2013;39:1–19.
9. Schmitter M, Essig M, Seneadza V, Balke Z, Schröder J, Rammelsberg P. Prevalence of clinical and radiographic signs of osteoarthrosis of the temporomandibular joint in an older persons community. Dentomaxillofac Radiol. 2010;39:231–4.
10. Levitt SR, McKinney MW. Validating the TMJ scale in a national sample of 10,000 patients: demographic and epidemiologic characteristics. J Orofac Pain. 1994;8:25–35.
11. McCarty WL, Farrar WB. Surgery for internal derangements of the temporomandibular joint. J Prosthet Dent. 1979;42:191–6.
12. Liu MQ, Chen HM, Yap AU, Fu KY. Condylar remodeling accompanying splint therapy: a cone-beam computerized tomography study of patients with temporomandibular joint disk displacement. Oral Surg Oral Med Oral Pathol Oral Radiol. 2012;114:259–65.
13. Weinberg LA. Practical evaluation of the lateral temporomandibular joint radiograph. J Prosthet Dent. 1984;51:676–85.
14. Endo M, Terajima M, Goto TK, Tokumori K, Takahashi I. Three-dimensional analysis of the temporomandibular joint and fossa-condyle relationship. Orthodontics (Chic). 2011;12:210–21.
15. Tanaka T, Morimoto Y, Tanaka Y, Kobayashi S, Okumura Y, Kito S, Okabe S, Ohba T. Radiographic examination of the mandibular (glenoid) fossa in ancient and modern man. Oral Dis. 2004;10:369–77.
16. Paknahad M, Shahidi S, Akhlaghian M, Abolvardi M. Is mandibular fossa morphology and articular eminence inclination associated with temporomandibular dysfunction? J Dent (Shiraz). 2016;17:134–41.
17. Martin P, Grünendahl M, Schmitt M. Persönlichkeit, kognitive Leistungsfähigkeit und Gesundheit in Ost und West: Ergebnisse der Interdisziplinären Längsschnittstudie des Erwachsenenalters (ILSE). [Personality, cognitive ability and health in East and West Germany: results of an interdisciplinary longitudinal study of aging]. Z Gerontol Geriatr. 2000;33:111–23.
18. Dworkin SF, LeResche L. Research diagnostic criteria for temporomandibular disorders: review, criteria, examinations and specifications, critique. J Craniomandib Disord Facial Oral Pain. 1992;6:301–55.
19. Pullinger A, Hollender L. Assessment of mandibular condyle position: a comparison of transcranial radiographs and linear tomograms. Oral Surg Oral Med Oral Pathol. 1985;60:329–34.
20. Pullinger A, Hollender L. Variation in condyle-fossa relationships according to different methods of evaluation in tomograms. Oral Surg Oral Med Oral Pathol. 1986;62:719–27.
21. Ren YF, Isberg A, Westesson PL. Condyle position in the temporomandibular joint. Comparison between asymptomatic volunteers with normal disk position and patients with disk displacement. Oral Surg Oral Med Oral Pathol Oral Radiol Endod. 1995;80:101–7.
22. Orsini MG, Kuboki T, Terada S, Matsuka Y, Yamashita A, Clark GT. Diagnostic value of 4 criteria to interpret temporomandibular joint normal disk position on magnetic resonance images. Oral Surg Oral Med Oral Pathol Oral Radiol Endod. 1998;86:489–97.
23. Bermejo-Fenoll A. Anatomy of the temporomandibular joint and masticatory muscles. In: Manfredini D, editor. Current concepts on temporomandibular disorders. London: Quintessence; 2010. p. 3–24. here: 5–7.
24. Muto T, Kohara M, Kanazawa M, Kawakami J. The position of the mandibular condyle at maximal mouth opening in normal subjects. J Oral Maxillofac Surg. 1994;52:1269–72.
25. Student. The probable error of a mean. Biometrika. 1908;6:1–25.
26. Koch GG. Intraclass correlation coefficient. In: Kotz S, Johnson NL, editors. Encyclopedia of Statistical Sciences. New York: Wiley; 1982. p. 213–7.
27. Sedgwick P. Retrospective cohort studies: advantages and disadvantages. BMJ. 2014;348:g1072.
28. Torres MG, Crusoe-Rebello IM, Rosario M, Albuquerque MC, Campos PS. Morphometric features of the mandibular condyle and association with disk abnormalities. Oral Surg Oral Med Oral Pathol Oral Radiol. 2016;121:566–72.
29. Abe S, Kawano F, Kohge K, Kawaoka T, Ueda K, Hattori-Hara E, Mori H, Kuroda S, Tanaka E. Stress analysis in human temporomandibular joint affected by anterior disc displacement during prolonged clenching. J Oral Rehabil. 2013;40:239–46.
30. Cömert Kiliç S, Kiliç N, Sümbüllü MA. Temporomandibular joint osteoarthritis: cone beam computed tomography findings, clinical features, and correlations. Int J Oral Maxillofac Surg. 2015;44:1268–74.
31. Larheim TA, Abrahamsson AK, Kristensen M, Arvidsson LZ. Temporomandibular joint diagnostics using CBCT. Dentomaxillofac Radiol. 2015;44:20140235.
32. Haase A, Frahm J, Matthaei D, Hänicke W, Merboldt KD. FLASH imaging: rapid NMR imaging using low flip-angle pulses. J Magn Reson. 1986;67:258–66.
33. Haase A. FLASH MR, imaging: a success story since 25 years. J Magn Reson. 2011;213:542–3.
34. Frahm J, Haase A, Matthaei D. Rapid three-dimensional MR imaging using the FLASH technique. J Comput Assist Tomogr. 1986;10:363–8.
35. Stamm T, Hohoff A, Van Meegen A, Meyer U. On the three-dimensional physiological position of the temporomandibular joint. J Orofac Orthop. 2004;65:280–9.
36. Türp JC, Walther M. The anteroposterior condylar position in maximum intercuspation in the dentate adult. J Craniomand Funct. 2014;6:9–20.
37. Incesu L, Taşkaya-Yilmaz N, Öğütcen-Toller M, Uzun E. Relationship of condylar position to disc position and morphology. Eur J Radiol. 2004;51:269–73.
38. Menezes AV, de Almeida SM, Boscolo FN, Haiter-Neto F, Ambrosano GM, Manzi FR. Comparison of transcranial radiograph and magnetic resonance imaging in the evaluation of mandibular condyle position. Dentomaxillofac Radiol. 2008;37:293–9.
39. Mupparapu M, Chow I, Uppal A. Hard tissue structural changes in TMJ morphology prior to orthodontic therapy: a complex motion tomographic study. Quintessence Int. 2011;42:427–34.
40. Almăşan OC, Hedeşiu M, Baciuţ G, Leucuţa DC, Băciuţ M. Disk and joint morphology variations on coronal and sagittal MRI in temporomandibular joint disorders. Clin Oral Investig. 2012;17:1243–50.
41. Hugger A, Sons T, Kordaß B, Assheuer J, Stüttgen U. Analyse der Kondylenposition im sagittalen Kernspintomogramm [Analysis of the condylar position in the sagittal magnetic resonance tomogram]. Dtsch Zahnärztl Z. 1999;54:380–3.
42. Gonzalez B. The not-so-controversial issue of condylar position. Int J Orthod Milwaukee. 2007;18:17–26.
43. Rinchuse DJ, Kandasamy S. Centric relation: A historical and contemporary orthodontic perspective. J Am Dent Assoc. 2006;137:494–501.
44. Dalili Z, Khaki N, Kia SJ, Salamat F. Assessing joint space and condylar position in the people with normal function of temporomandibular joint with cone-beam computed tomography. Dent Res J (Isfahan). 2012;9:607–12.
45. Pullinger AG, Hollender L, Solberg WK, Petersson A. A tomographic study of mandibular condyle position in an asymptomatic population. J Prosthet Dent. 1985;53:706–13.
46. Paknahad M, Shahidi S, Iranpour S, Mirhadi S. Cone-Beam computed tomographic assessment of mandibular condylar position in patients with temporomandibular joint dysfunction and in healthy subjects. Int J Dent. 2015;2015:301796.
47. Straus SE, Richardson WS, Glasziou P, Haynes RB. Evidence-Based Medicine. How to Practice and Teach EBM. 3rd ed. Edinburgh: Churchill Livingstone; 2005. here: 69.
48. Pullinger A. Establishing better biological models to understand occlusion. I: TM joint anatomic relationships. J Oral Rehabil. 2013;40:296–318.
49. Wiesel SW, Tsourmas N, Feffer HL, Citrin CM, Patronas N. A study of computer-assisted tomography I The incidence of positive CAT scans in an asymptomatic group of patients. Spine. 1984;9:549–51.
50. Westesson P-L, Eriksson L, Kurita K. Reliability of a negative clinical temporomandibular joint examination: prevalence of disk displacement in asymptomatic temporomandibular joints. Oral Surg Oral Med Oral Pathol. 1989;68:551–4.
51. Katzberg RW, Westesson PL, Tallents RH, Drake CM. Anatomic disorders of the temporomandibular joint disc in asymptomatic subjects. J Oral Maxillofac Surg. 1996;54:147–53.
52. Progiante PS, Pattussi MP, Lawrence HP, Goya S, Grossi PK, Grossi ML. Prevalence of temporomandibular disorders in an adult Brazilian community population using the Research Diagnostic Criteria (Axes I and II) for Temporomandibular Disorders (The Maringá Study). Int J Prosthodont. 2015;28:600–9.
53. Blanco-Hungría A, Blanco-Aguilera A, Blanco-Aguilera E, Serrano-Del-Rosal R, Biedma-Velázquez L, Rodríguez-Torronteras A, Segura-Saint-Gerons R.

Prevalence of the different Axis I clinical subtypes in a sample of patients with orofacial pain and temporomandibular disorders in the Andalusian Healthcare Service. Med Oral Patol Oral Cir Bucal. 2016;21:e169–77.
54. Manfredini D, Arveda N, Guarda-Nardini L, Segu M, Collesano V. Distribution of diagnoses in a population of patients with temporomandibular disorders. Oral Surg Oral Med Oral Pathol Oral Radiol. 2012;114:e35–41.
55. da Silva CG, Pachêco-Pereira C, Porporatti AL, Savi MG, Peres MA, Flores-Mir C, Canto GL. Prevalence of clinical signs of intra-articular temporomandibular disorders in children and adolescents: A systematic review and meta-analysis. J Am Dent Assoc. 2016;147:10–8. e8.
56. Rammelsberg P, Pospiech P, Heumann C, Toutenburg H. Ätiologische Faktoren für Diskusverlagerungen im Kiefergelenk [Etiologic factors for disc displacement in the temporomandibular joint.]. Dtsch Zahnärztl Z. 1996;51:211–8.
57. Rasmussen OC. Description of population and progress of symptoms in a longitudinal study of temporomandibular arthropathy. Scand J Dent Res. 1981;89:196–203.
58. Wilkes CH. Internal derangements of the temporomandibular joint. Pathological variations. Arch Otolaryngol Head Neck Surg. 1989;115:469–77.
59. Könönen M, Waltimo A, Nyström M. Does clicking in adolescence lead to painful temporomandibular joint locking? Lancet. 1996;347:1080–1.
60. Torii K. Longitudinal course of temporomandibular joint sounds in Japanese children and adolescents. Head Face Med. 2011;7:17.
61. Egermark I, Carlsson GE, Magnusson T. A 20-year longitudinal study of subjective symptoms of temporomandibular disorders from childhood to adulthood. Acta Odontol Scand. 2001;59:40–8.
62. Chantaracherd P, John MT, Hodges JS, Schiffman EL. Temporomandibular joint disorders' impact on pain, function, and disability. J Dent Res. 2015;94:79S–86.
63. de Leeuw R, Klasser GD. Orofacial pain: guidelines for assessment, diagnosis, and management. 5th ed. Chicago: Quintessence; 2013. here: 139–43.
64. Ohrbach R, Greene C. Temporomandibular joint diagnosis: striking a balance between the sufficiency of clinical assessment and the need for imaging. Oral Surg Oral Med Oral Pathol Oral Radiol. 2013;116:124–5.
65. Rohlin M, Westesson PL, Eriksson L. The correlation of temporomandibular joint sounds with joint morphology in fifty-five autopsy specimens. J Oral Maxillofac Surg. 1985;43:194–200.
66. Berkhout WE. Het ALARA-principe. Achtergronden en toepassing in de praktijk. [The ALARA-principle. Backgrounds and enforcement in dental practices.]. Ned Tijdschr Tandheelkd. 2015;122:263–70.
67. Muir CB, Goss AN. The radiologic morphology of asymptomatic temporomandibular joints. Oral Surg Oral Med Oral Pathol. 1990;70:349–54.
68. Brooks SL, Westesson PL, Eriksson L, Hansson LG, Barsotti JB. Prevalence of osseous changes in the temporomandibular joint of asymptomatic persons without internal derangement. Oral Surg Oral Med Oral Pathol. 1992;73:118–22.
69. Muir CB, Goss AN. The radiologic morphology of painful temporomandibular joints. Oral Surg Oral Med Oral Pathol. 1990;70:355–9.
70. Zhao YP, Zhang ZY, Wu YT, Zhang WL, Ma XC. Investigation of the clinical and radiographic features of osteoarthrosis of the temporomandibular joints in adolescents and young adults. Oral Surg Oral Med Oral Pathol Oral Radiol Endod. 2011;111:e27–34.
71. Ishibashi H, Takenoshita Y, Ishibashi K, Oka M. Age-related changes in the human mandibular condyle: a morphologic, radiologic, and histologic study. J Oral Maxillofac Surg. 1995;53:1016–23. discussion 23–4.
72. Widmalm SE, Westesson PL, Kim IK, Pereira Jr FJ, Lundh H, Tasaki MM. Temporomandibular joint pathosis related to sex, age, and dentition in autopsy material. Oral Surg Oral Med Oral Pathol. 1994;78:416–25.
73. Pereira Jr FJ, Lundh H, Westesson PL. Morphologic changes in the temporomandibular joint in different age groups. An autopsy investigation. Oral Surg Oral Med Oral Pathol. 1994;78:279–87.
74. Hansson TL. Pathological aspects of arthritides and derangements. In: Sarnat BG, Laskin DM, editors. The temporomandibular joint: a biological basis for clinical practice. 4th ed. Philadelphia: Saunders; 1992. p. 165–82. here: 171.
75. Magnusson C, Nilsson M, Magnusson T. Degenerative changes of the temporomandibular joint. Relationship to ethnicity, sex and occlusal supporting zones based on a skull material. Acta Odontol Scand. 2012;70:207–12.
76. de Leeuw R, Boering G, Stegenga B, de Bont LG. Radiographic signs of temporomandibular joint osteoarthrosis and internal derangement 30 years after nonsurgical treatment. Oral Surg Oral Med Oral Pathol Oral Radiol Endod. 1995;79:382–92.
77. Rantala MA, Ahlberg J, Suvinen TI, Savolainen A, Könönen M. Symptoms, signs, and clinical diagnoses according to the research diagnostic criteria for temporomandibular disorders among Finnish multiprofessional media personnel. J Orofac Pain. 2003;17:311–6.
78. Abrahamsson C, Ekberg E, Henrikson T, Nilner M, Sunzel B, Bondemark L. TMD in consecutive patients referred for orthognathic surgery. Angle Orthod. 2009;79:621–7.
79. Manfredini D, Guarda-Nardini L, Winocur E, Piccotti F, Ahlberg J, Lobbezoo F. Research diagnostic criteria for temporomandibular disorders: a systematic review of axis I epidemiologic findings. Oral Surg Oral Med Oral Pathol Oral Radiol Endod. 2011;112:453–62.
80. Johnson VL, Hunter DJ. The epidemiology of osteoarthritis. Best Pract Res Clin Rheumatol. 2014;28:5–15.
81. de Leeuw R, Boering G, van der Kuijl B, Stegenga B. Hard and soft tissue imaging of the temporomandibular joint 30 years after diagnosis of osteoarthrosis and internal derangement. J Oral Maxillofac Surg. 1996;54:1270–80.
82. De Boever JA, Carlsson GE. Etiology and differential diagnosis. In: Zarb GA, Carlsson GE, Sessle BE, Mohl ND, editors. Temporomandibular Joint and Masticatory Muscle Disorders. Copenhagen: Munksgaard - Mosby; 1994. p. 171–87. here: 183–184.
83. Okeson JP. Bell's oral and facial pain. 7th ed. Chicago: Quintessence; 2014. here: 348.
84. Wiberg B, Wänman A. Signs of osteoarthrosis of the temporomandibular joints in young patients: a clinical and radiographic study. Oral Surg Oral Med Oral Pathol Oral Radiol Endod. 1998;86:158–64.
85. Lee JY, Kim DJ, Lee SG, Chung JW. A longitudinal study on the osteoarthritic change of the temporomandibular joint based on 1-year follow-up computed tomography. J Craniomaxillofac Surg. 2012;40:e223–8.
86. Kim K, Wojczynska A, Lee JY. The incidence of osteoarthritic change on computed tomography of Korean temporomandibular disorder patients diagnosed by RDC/TMD; a retrospective study. Acta Odontol Scand. 2016;74:337-42.
87. Haskin CL, Milam SB, Cameron IL. Pathogenesis of degenerative joint disease in the human temporomandibular joint. Crit Rev Oral Biol Med. 1995;6:248–77.
88. Milano V, Desiate A, Bellino R, Garofalo T. Magnetic resonance imaging of temporomandibular disorders: classification, prevalence and interpretation of disc displacement and deformation. Dentomaxillofac Radiol. 2000;29:352–61.
89. Sandstedt C. Einige Beiträge zur Theorie der Zahnregulierung [Some contributions to the theory of the regualtion of teeth]. Nordisk Tandlak Tidskr. 1904;5:236–56.
90. Sandstedt C. Einige Beiträge zur Theorie der Zahnregulierung [Some contributions to the theory of the regualtion of teeth]. Nordisk Tandlak Tidskr. 1905;6:1–25. 141–68.
91. Bister D, Meikle MC. Re-examination of 'Einige Beiträge zur Theorie der Zahnregulierung' (Some contributions to the theory of the regulation of teeth) published in 1904–1905 by Carl Sandstedt. Eur J Orthod. 2013;35:160–8.
92. Mongini F. Dental abrasion as a factor in remodeling of the mandibular condyle. Acta Anat. 1975;92:292–300.
93. Yamada K, Tsuruta A, Hanada K, Hayashi T. Morphology of the articular eminence in temporomandibular joints and condylar bone change. J Oral Rehabil. 2004;31:438–44.
94. Nishio C, Tanimoto K, Hirose M, Horiuchi S, Kuroda S, Tanne K, Tanaka E. Stress analysis in the mandibular condyle during prolonged clenching: a theoretical approach with the finite element method. Proc Inst Mech Eng H. 2009;223:739–48.
95. Türp JC. Diskusverlagerungen neu überdacht [Disc displacements revisited]. Dtsch Zahnärztl Z. 1998;53:369–73.

16

Three/four-dimensional (3D/4D) microscopic imaging and processing in clinical dental research

Ping Ye[1,2*], Hong Yu[3] and Mojgan Houshmandi[1]

Abstract

Background: Confocal laser scanning microscope (CLSM) has been widely employed in our laboratory for structural and functional analysis of clinical dental specimens and live cell imaging of cultured oral epithelial cells.

Methods: In this vitro study, a Fluoview 1000 (Olympus) confocal system was utilised to study thick sections of carious lesions (40–100 μm) and periodontal disease tissue samples (20–40 μm) by 2D Z stacking imaging and 3-dimentional (3D) reconstruction. Four-dimensional (4D) imaging when including time or position points was used for live cells to assess penetration/localisation/co-localization of oral pathogen proteins and therapeutic drugs.

Results: Three-dimensional (3D) reconstruction revealed latent features of carious hard tissues (strongly expressed amelogenin proteins in dentin tubules), and soft tissues (increased glial markers GFAP and S100B in pulp components). We also found the oral microbial specific pathogens, *Porphyromonas gingivalis* to be widely localised inside the periodontal pocket epithelial tissues as detected by 3D reconstruction from a series of 2D sections from periodontal disease tissue samples. 4D live cell imaging showed the diffusion patterns of fluorescent molecules in response to a bacterial virulence factor, the pathogen (gingipain haemagglutinin) domain that attacked epithelial integrity. This technology also showed uptake of a novel porphyrin-linked metronidazole antibiotic into epithelial cells to kill intracellular oral pathogen, *P. gingivalis*.

Conclusions: Three/four-dimensional (3D/4D) imaging and processing in confocal microscopy is of great interest and benefit to clinical dental researchers.

Keywords: 3D reconstruction, 4D imaging, Live cell imaging, Carious lesion, Periodontitis, *Porphyromonas gingivalis*

Abbreviations: 3D, Three dimension (XYZ); 4D, Four dimension (XYZT or XYZP); CLSM, Confocal laser scanning microscope; EDTA, Ethylenediaminetetraacetic acid; GFAP, Glial fibrillary acidic protein; *P. gingivalis*, *Porphyromonas gingivalis*; PBS, Phosphate-buffered saline; S100B, S100 calcium-binding protein B; XYZP, 3D (XYZ) plus position points; XYZT, 3D (XYZ) plus time lapse

Background

Confocal laser scanning microscope (CLSM) has been developed and improved enormously over the past 10 years. This powerful technology has several advantages over conventional epi-fluorescence microscopy, including improved performance in contrast and free out-of-focus blur for thin or thick specimens [1], excellent high resolution and analysis of fluorescent labelled thick specimens without physical sectioning [1, 2], capacity for complex three-dimensional (XYZ) architecture called 3D reconstruction [2], and 4D imaging and processing on live cells when including time (XYZT) or position (XYZP) points [3], and even 5D imaging when including numerous channels [3]. These images have volumetric and texture details and it is impossible to obtain such details with conventional microscopes.

The technology enables to capture thin optical sections from thick specimens with controllable depth of field to produce 2D z-stack images through a three-dimensional

* Correspondence: p.ye@sydney.edu.au
[1]Institute of Dental Research, Oral Health, Westmead Hospital, Westmead, Australia
[2]Affiliation of Faculty of Dentistry, the University of Sydney, Sydney, Australia
Full list of author information is available at the end of the article

(3D) object with accurate information, allowing 3D reconstructions to be generated with the digital data from 2D z-stack images. Processing turns 2D images into a 3D image [1, 2], revealing latent features of specimens from carious lesions and inflamed gingival tissues.

Confocal microscopy is a widely applied tool for studying the functions and activities of live cells through a time-change, dye diffusion, and concentration of fluorescent-labeled substances, and also studying for the cellular functions of drug applicants. For live cell imaging, confocal optics provides a major improvement in dimensional resolution and real time [4].

Most microscopic samples are essentially transparent, and the depths of fields of focused samples are exceptionally narrow. Therefore, another advantage of confocal laser scanning microscope (CLSM) is the capacity to distinguish between different depths of a sample, which is free of out-of-focus blur for thin or thick specimens [1]. This process can provide good quality high resolution images for publishing.

In this vitro study, overviews of four applications for 3D/4D microscopic imaging and processing in clinical dental research were introduced. We utilised the Fluoview 1000 Olympus confocal system to study 3D reconstruction for thick sections (up to 100 μm) of dental pulp, 3D reconstruction for oral pathogens in periodontitis tissues, 4D imaging and processing of live cells including time (XYZT) or position (XYZP) to assess proteins of oral pathogen, and confocal microscopy application in drug development.

Methods

Carious teeth

The detailed processing of teeth has been described in the previous paper [5]. Briefly, healthy ($n = 15$) and carious teeth ($n = 37$) were obtained with approval of the Ethics Committee of Sydney West Local Health Service and informed consent from patients, aged from 20 to 45 years. The half tooth contained the pulp was fixed in 1 % paraformaldehyde in PBS (phosphate-buffered saline) for 3 h, then washed in PBS and EDTA (ethylenediaminetetraacetic acid, pH 7.0) for 5 or 6 days, changed EDTA each day and equilibrated in 30 % sucrose (*w/v*) for 3 to 5 days at 4 °C. A diamond disc (Thin-Flex, Abrasive Technology, Chicago, IL) was used to trim enamel and the majority of dentin. Samples were cooled down with ample water. Specimens were in cryo-embedding matrix -Tissue Freezing Medium (Triangle Biomedical Sciences, Durham, NC) for quick chill (5 min), and frozen in liquid nitrogen. Sections of 40–100 μm were prepared and stored at −80 °C until required.

Gingival tissues

The detailed processing of gingival tissue specimens has been described in the previous paper [6]. Briefly, obtained gingival tissues were approved by the Ethics Committee of Sydney Dental Hospital and informed consent from adult participants ($n = 26$) in the periodontal clinics. All patients had detailed clinical records and radiographs with no systemic disease and no periodontal therapy for the past 3 years. Tissues were grouped by clinical and histological criteria as clinically healthy gingival sites and paired periodontitis sites. Gingival tissues were snap-frozen in isopentane, cooled in liquid nitrogen, and 20–40 μm sections prepared for study.

Oral epithelial cell culture for live/fixed cell imaging

The H413 epithelial cell line original from a human oral squamous cell carcinoma [7] exhibits stratified epithelial cell morphology and high CD24 marker expression in culture. Cell clonal lines of H413 were constructed using a limit dilution method as described previously [8]. H413 colone-1 cells were cultured in Joklik modification's minimum essential medium (Sigma-Aldrich), supplemented with penicillin/streptomycin (100 IU/ml, Sigma) and 10 % fetal calf serum (FCS, CSL Limited, Victoria, Australia) at 37 °C in 5 % CO_2 [9]. Cultures were collected with trypsin replacement - triple express (Invitrogen, Australia) in PBS and sub-cultured every 3 days.

To further confirm biological function, live cell imaging was performed to determine intracellular versus paracellular pathways of movement of labeled dextran. Cloned H413-1 cells ($2 \times 10^5/cm^2$) were cultured in 8-well slide chambers (ibidi, cat 80826, Germany), 300 μl per well. Confluence was achieved within 48 h. A haemolytic gingipain adhesin domain K2 (100 pM) from *Porphyromonas gingivalis* [10] or a gingipain haemagglutinin subdomain named Ka 100 pM (constructed in our laboratory, unpublished) was added and each well was simultaneously supplemented with a low molecular weight dextran Alexa Fluor 647 (10 kDa, Invitrogen, Australia) at 1:50 dilution from a stock solution of 1 mg/ml in medium.

For drug development assay, oral pathogen *P.gingivalis* strain ATCC 33277 at MOI (multiplicity of infection) 100 cells per one epithelial cell [11] was added to confluent H413 clone-1 epithelial monolayers for 1.5 h at 37 °C in 5 % CO_2. Monolayers were washed twice with Dulbecco's phosphate-buffered saline (DPBS) [12]. Gentamycin (300 μg/ml, Sigma) and metronidazole (200 μg/ml, Sigma) were added to kill adherent *P.gingivalis* on the cell surface (extracellular bacteria, [12]). After an additional 1 h incubation and washing off antibiotics, we added a porphyrin-linked metronidazole adduct (40 μM) developed in our laboratory (auto-fluorescence in red, [13]) to cell culture up to additional 1.5 h. Then *P.*

gingivalis was targeted by mouse monoclonal antibody IIB2 (5 μm/ml) [14] at various time points. For live cells, nuclei were stained with NucBlue (Invitrogen, Australia). For fixed cells, the secondary antibody was goat anti-mouse conjugated with Alexa Fluor 488 (Life Technologies, USA).

Immunostaining for frozen sections

Frozen sections including teeth and gingival tissues were fixed in 4 % paraformaldehyde in PBS for 30 min at room temperature. Slides were washed with PBS and placed in glycine-PBS for 10 min, then washed in PBS and incubated in PBS containing 0.2 % Tween-20 and 10 % goat serum for 1 h at room temperature. Sections were washed in PBS and incubated with primary antibodies: polyclonal rabbit anti-human GFAP (5 μg/ml, Dako), polyclonal rabbit anti-human S100 (4 μg/ml, reacts strongly with human S100B, Dako), polyclonal rabbit anti-human amelogenin (5 mg/ml, Abcam, UK), and mouse monoclonal antibody IIB2 (5 μm/ml) [14] to *P. gingivalis* bacteria, for 1 h at room temperature. For controls, rabbit or mouse IgG (Dakocytomation) was served as the primary antibody. Sections were washed 3 times in PBS and then incubated with secondary antibodies: goat anti-rabbit or mouse IgG conjugated with Alexa Fluor 488 or 594 (Life Technologies, USA) for 1 h at room temperature. Slides were mounted in Prolong gold anti-fade reagent with DAPI (Molecular Probes, Invitrogen).

Confocal laser scanning microscopy

An Olympus Fluoview (FV) 1000 was used to capture confocal images under multi lasers (405 nm, 473 nm, 633 nm) and NTT electronic Optiλ (559 nm). Visual observation under the objective lens [Olympus 40X/1.30/0.20 (WD) Oil UPLSAPO] was performed. The cells were selected at random and adjusted focus before image acquisition.

For 3D reconstruction imaging on thick teeth and gingival tissue sections, the fundamental step was in staining of the preparations. An appropriate stained section showed the same intensity from the top to the bottom of the stack. Over-stained or under-stained sections would greatly reduce imaging clarity of thick teeth and gingival tissues. Z-stack imaging was performed with a 40X objective using up to three corresponding lasers (405 nm, 473 nm and 559 nm). Briefly, the procedure was to set up step size between 0.5 and 1.5 μm depending on the thickness of samples, and then consecutive cross-section images (XYZ) were acquired from the top to the bottom. After acquisition, projection of z-stack images was displayed using the click Z mode. 3D reconstruction and display of cubic imaging were built up by 3D Olympus Fluoview software. It was essential for 3D reconstructions achieved identical to any z-stack preparation [15].

For 4D (3D time lapse) imaging on live cells, chamber slides with stained samples were operated in the microscope stage incubation chamber (with temperature controller at 37 °C and CO_2 controller at 5 % of CO_2) [16]. Time-lapse imaging was performed over a period of hours with a 40X objective using the time-lapse function of confocal microscopy Auto Imaging System. Two corresponding lasers (405 nm and 633 nm) were selected. Combined z-stack and time-lapse functions were used in the present study to swiftly capture the images [16]. Serial images were taken at regular time points to capture the dynamics.

All fluorescence images captured with confocal acquisition software (FV10-ASW 1.7) were stored as Olympus Image Format (OIF) for signal analysis and exported images as TIF files.

Imaging analysis

Three-dimensional (3D) reconstruction images were processed using Olympus Fluoview (FV) software (4.2 viewer, Japan) or Image J software (version 1.50). Co-localization image analysis was as described in reference papers [17, 18] or by using recently developed advanced software: Huygens Professional (https://svi.nl/HuygensProfessional).

Results

Three-dimensional reconstruction for thick carious lesions

Specimens used in this study were soft pulp tissues connected with hard dentin tissues (Fig. 1a). 2D images with an overlay of the differential interference contrast (DIC) channel image of a healthy control tooth were displayed scant expression of GFAP and S100B (Fig. 1b). For comparison, a matched set of 2D images from a carious tooth was shown in Fig. 1c. Figure 1d showed projection of 2D stack images from a carious tooth (Fig. 1c) using frozen (40–100 μm) sections, 40–50 images of 0.8–1.5 μm step size acquired as z-stacks by confocal laser scanning microscopy. Three-dimensional (3D) imaging from 2D z-stack images (Fig. 1d) was reconstructed and viewed using confocal software (4.2 viewer, Japan) (Fig. 1e). A 3D movie in the Additional file 1: Movie 1 revealed latent features of glial cell markers GFAP (green) and S100B (red) from thick specimens.

Another example was distribution of amelogenin protein (green) expressed in carious adult human teeth although not detected in healthy adult human teeth. Figure 2a showed 2D images of a healthy control tooth displaying trace expression of amelogenin protein considered as background staining compared to isotype control antibody staining (data not shown). An overlay image using the DIC (differential interference contrast) channel showed anatomical structure and orientation of the tooth. For comparison, a matched set of 2D images from a tooth with a carious lesion was shown (Fig. 2b).

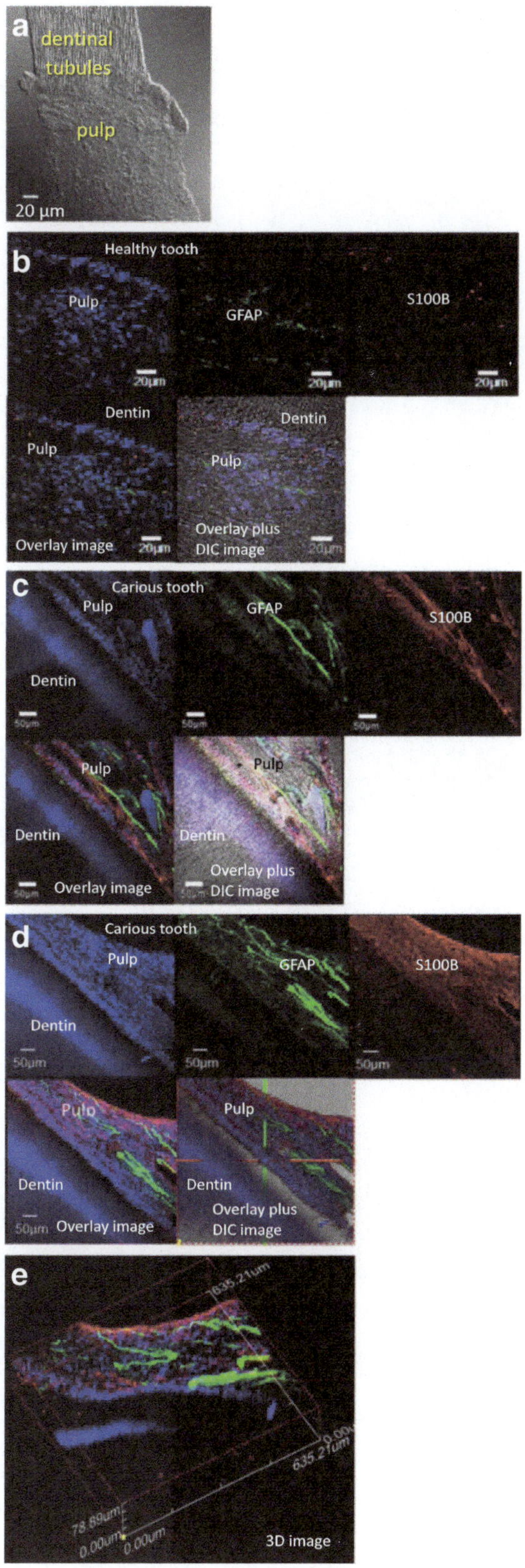

Fig. 1 **a** Differential interference contrast (DIC) image displayed the anatomical structure of hard tissue dentin connected with soft pulp tissue from a tooth. **b** 2D images of a healthy control tooth showed scant expression of glial markers GFAP (*green*), S100B (*red*) and the overlay image with DIC channel to show the tooth orientation. **c** A matched set of 2D images showed increased expression of glial markers GFAP (*green*), S100B (*red*) and the overlay image with DIC channel for the orientation of an adult carious tooth. **d** Projection of 2D z-stack images of an adult carious tooth. **e** A 3D image generated by 2D z-stack data (**d**) from a thick carious specimen (78.89 µm)

Figure 2c showed strong expression of amelogenin protein in pulp cells (odontoblasts) and in dentinal tubules in the projection of 2D z-stack images, Fig. 2d and e displayed 3D images built from 2D z-stack images (Fig. 2c), and a 3D movie was shown in the Additional file 1: Movie 2.

Three-dimensional reconstruction for detection of an oral pathogen in periodontitis tissues

Using 3D reconstruction to analyse oral microbial biofilm structure, we found one of the specific pathogens *P. gingivalis* to be widely localised inside the periodontal pocket epithelial tissues from a series of 2D-stack images from periodontal disease tissue samples (Fig. 3b) compared to clinically healthy gingiva where the pathogens were only located on the gingival surface (Fig. 3a). The image in Fig. 3c showed a cross cutting section by confocal software, contained *P. gingivalis* (red) inside pocket epithelium. The 3D cross cutting section movie was shown in the Additional file 1: Movie 3.

Four-dimensional imaging and processing on live cells to assess oral pathogen proteins

Confocal microscopy used on live cells through time-change, dye diffusion, and concentration of fluorescent-labeled substances. In this study, we added the oral pathogen protein domain K2 from *P. gingivalis* constructed in our laboratory [10] to confluent gingival epithelial monolayers from cell culture, then added fluorescent dye (dextran Alexa Fluor 647) to measure the diffusion patterns of fluorescent molecules in response to this bacterial virulence factor, which attacked epithelial integrity. Figure 4a showed a model of paracellular movement of the labelled dextran (red) for cells challenged with K2 at 15 and 30 min observation times. Figure 4b and c showed 2D z-stacking time lapse images in the beginning (T = 15 min) and end of the exposure time-lapse period (T = 1.5 h) for cells challenged with K2. Figure 4d showed 3D reconstruction time lapse image (XYZT, 4D) when including time points, and a 4D movie was shown in the Additional file 1: Movie 4.

Another example of 4D image processing including position points (XYZP). Figure 4e showed 2D z-stack

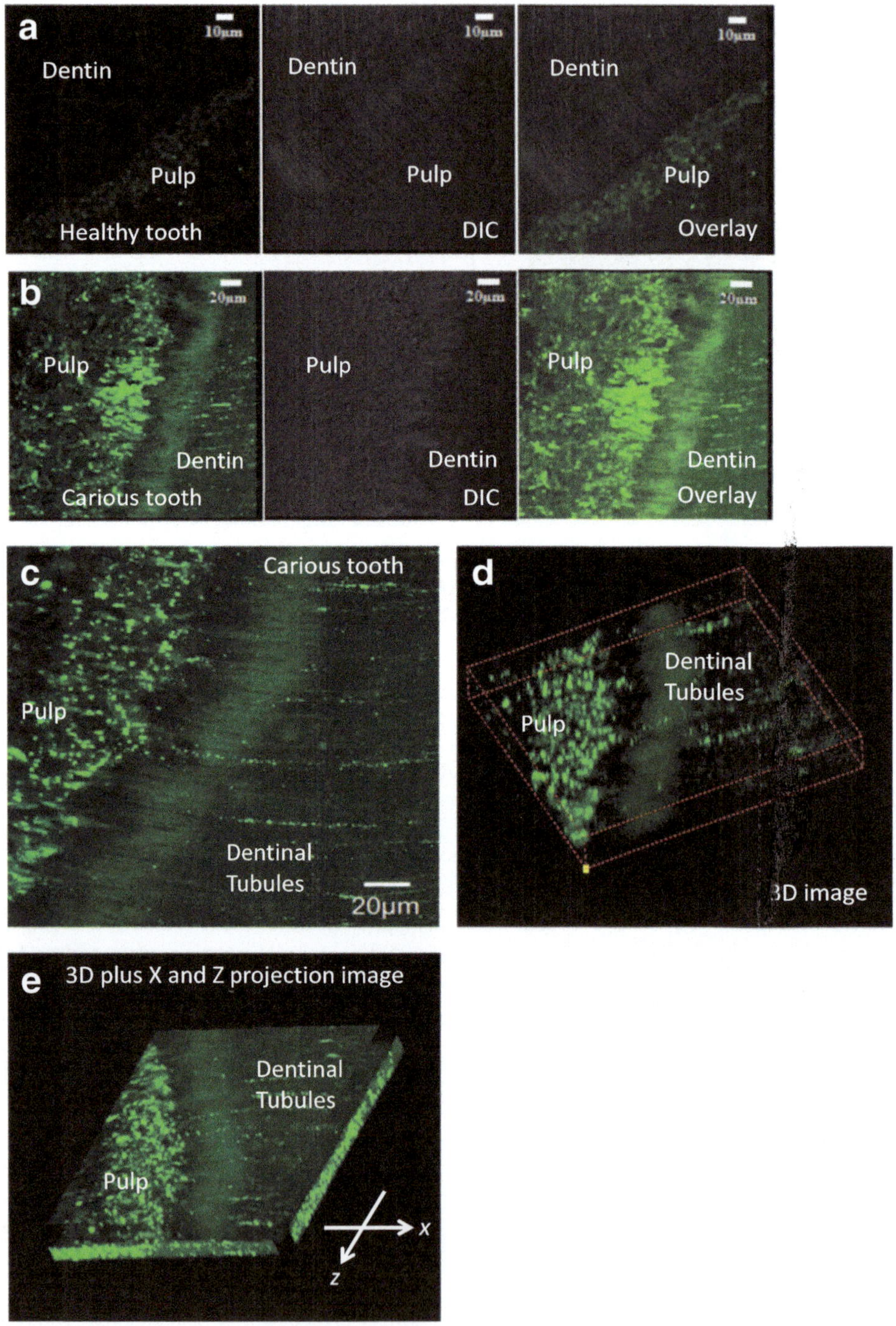

Fig. 2 Another example of amelogenin protein strongly re-expressed in newly differentiated pulp cells (odontoblasts) and distributed in dentinal tubules under the lesion site. **a** 2D images of a healthy control tooth, **b** a matched set of 2D images was from an adult carious lesion. **c** Projection of 2D z-stack images from a carious tooth, **d** a 3D reconstruction image from (**c**), **e** a 3D image plus x and z axes projection

image in which *P. gingivalis* proteins Ka (green) penetrated into nuclei (red) after 30 min on live cells. One of the cells was picked from 2D z-stack images to build up a 3D image (XYZ Plus position point, Fig. 4f). A 4D movie was shown in the Additional file 1: Movie 5.

Confocal laser scanning microscopy in drug development

Using confocal microscopy, it was possible to identify the penetration/localization/co-localisation of a porphyrin-linked metronidazole antibiotic and *P. gingivalis* bacteria. The porphyrin adducts exhibiting autofluorescence in the red range of wavelengths (600–

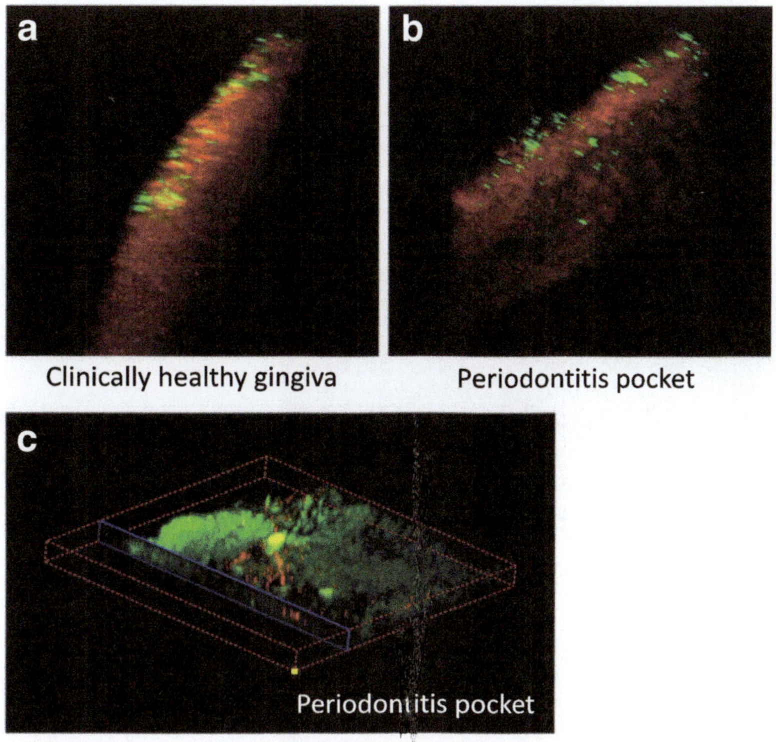

Fig. 3 Example of 3D reconstruction to analyse oral microbial biofilm structure. One of the specific pathogens *P. gingivalis* (*green colour*) was found to be widely localised on the surface of clinically healthy gingiva (**a**), but inside the periodontal pocket epithelial tissue from a series of 2D z-stack images (**b**) and one of 3D cross cutting sections, *P. gingivalis* (*red colour*) (**c**)

650 nm), penetrated into the cells and localized within the cytoplasm (Fig. 5a). Immuno-stained *P. gingivalis* potent gingipain-RgpA was shown in Fig. 5b–d in green fluorescence, also localized within cytoplasm. This modified drug could kill oral intracellular pathogens *P. gingivalis* with a time course at 30 min (Fig. 5b), 1 h (Fig. 5c) and 1.5 h (Fig. 5d).

Discussion

Why do we need confocal microscopy as a visual tool for clinical dental research? As noted previously, confocal microscopy has several advantages particularly for 3D visualization on thick specimens to reveal latent features of cell and tissue structures. The present study demonstrates that latent patterns of the increased glial cell markers GFAP and S100B on carious teeth lesions can be revealed through 3D reconstruction from thick specimens. The increased abundance of these markers in carious teeth lesions indicates a response to initial microbial invasion of dentin [5]. In the current study, 3D reconstruction also reveals strong expression of amelogenin protein in pulp cells (odontoblasts) and in dentinal tubules from adult human teeth with carious lesions. In a normal condition, this amelogenin protein is only appeared during tooth embryonic development including expression in tooth enamel, dentin, and pulp cells (odontoblasts) [19]. When tooth becomes mature, amelogenin is absent in dentin and pulp cells (odontoblasts). However, in injured or carious teeth amelogenin protein is highly re-presented in newly differentiated pulp cells (odontoblasts) and allotted in the dentinal tubules under the adult carious teeth [19] corresponding to our findings.

Dental researchers face major issues when cutting thin sections of soft pulp tissues connected with hard dentin tissues. Therefore, we utilise the advantage of analysis of fluorescent labeled thick specimens without physical sectioning for carious teeth and thick gingival tissues.

Confocal laser scanning microscopy (CLSM) is a useful method to study the interface of bacteria within biofilms and inflamed gingival tissues. Images obtained from CLSM are free of out-of-focus blur. CLSM-based imaging platform has been widely used for analysis of oral bacterial pathogens or biofilm structures on gingival tissues [20–23]. The images shown in the present study illustrate that 3D visualization is a promising method for representative analysis of oral bacterial pathogens or biofilm components [20].

In the present confocal microscopy study, using 4D (3D time lapse) imaging and processing on live cells we demonstrate that time-lapse imaging is a powerful technique for analysis of dynamic cellular events and

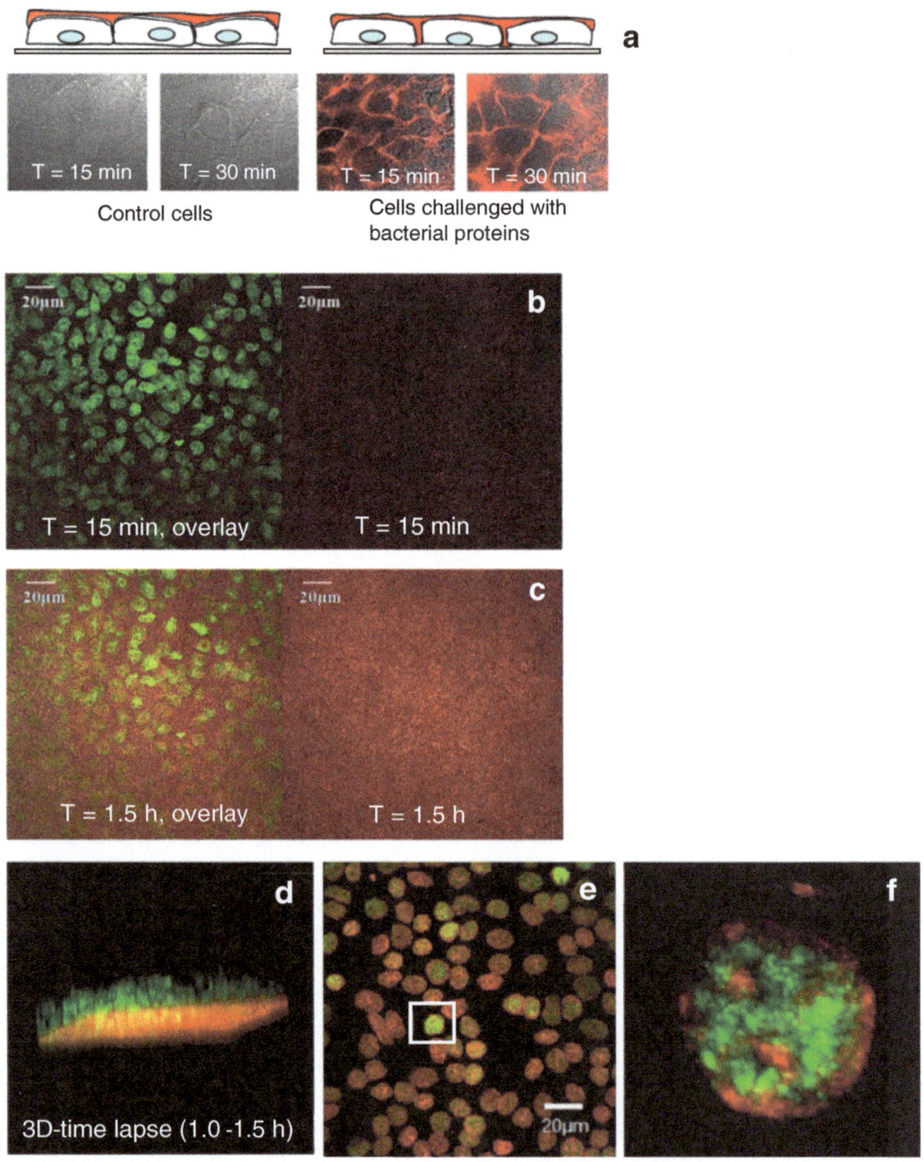

Fig. 4 **a** A model of adding oral pathogen *P. gingivalis* proteins K2 and fluorescent dye (Alexa Fluor dextran 647, *red colour*) to confluent gingival epithelial monolayers, to track pathological changes of epithelial integrity at a time course. Paracellular pathway of movement of the labelled dextran (*red*) was shown at 15 and 30 min observation times. **b** and **c** 2D z-stacking images in the beginning (T = 15 min) and end of the exposure time-lapse period (T = 1.5 h): left panels were the overlay images of cells (*green nuclei*) with far-red dye channel; right panels were far-red dye channel only. **d** 3D reconstruction time lapse images from (**b-c**) on live cells challenged with bacterial protein (K2) (*green colour*: cell nuclei; *red colour*: dye). **e** Another example of projection of 2D z-stack imaging plus a position point. **f** A 3D reconstruction image with a position point (**e**) on live cells challenged with *P. gingivalis* bacterial protein (Ka) at 30 min (*green colour*: Ka protein; *red colour*: nuclei)

morphology in real time and real space. There are two issues that researchers need to be aware of while performing experiments on live cells. Firstly, how to choose the right dye? The excitation (absorption, short wavelength) and emission (long wavelength) spectra of the Alexa Fluor series cover the visible spectrum and extend to the invisible infrared [24]. The closer to infrared wavelengths, the less damage to live cells [25], therefore, the far-red dye of Alexa Fluor 647 was chosen in the current study.

Secondly, illumination by fluorophores can cause photo bleaching and cell damage, hence there is a need to raise the speed of image acquisition by confocal microscopy. However the confocal microscopy has a limitation of raising an acquisition speed, which can result in a low resolution of image [26]. This image resolution can be improved by the use of DeltaVision super-resolution microscope (GE Healthcare, Japan). DeltaVision microscopy can offer better performance at high magnification (100 times), absolutely high resolution and

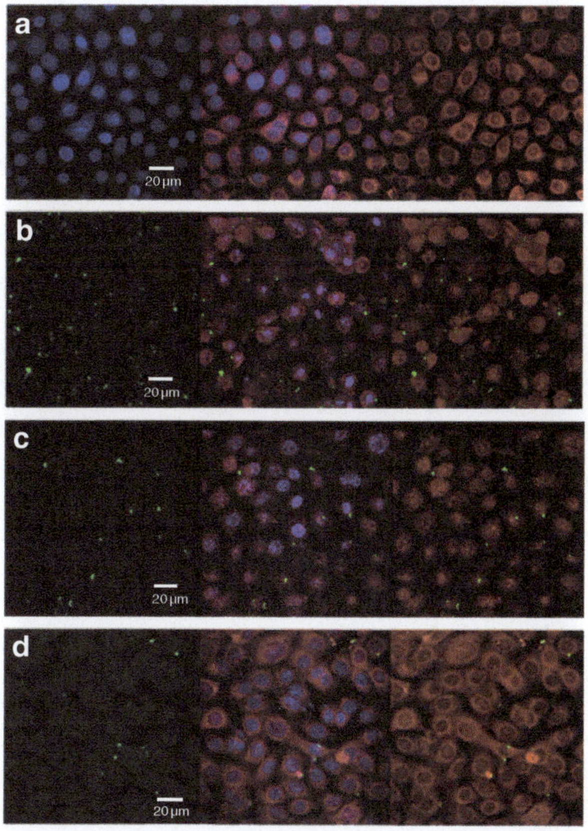

Fig. 5 a A pathogen-specific antimicrobial compound (a porphyrin-linked metronidazole) developed in our laboratory [13] which can target intracellular oral pathogens *P.gingivalis* displayed in red auto-fluorescence. Left: nuclei staining with DAPI (*blue channel*), middle: an overlay image of drug (*red channel*) with nuclei (*blue channel*), and right image was drug only (*red channel*). Images showed that this modified drug penetrated into the cells and localized within the cytoplasm (*red*) to kill oral intracellular pathogens *P. gingivalis* (*green*) with a time course at 30 min (**b**), 1 h (**c**) and 1.5 h (**d**). From (**b–d**), left panels showed green colour bacteria *P. gingivalis*; middle panels showed the overlay images of cells' nuclei (*blue channel*), *P.gingivalis* (*green channel*) and drug (*red channel*); right panels showed the overlay images of *P.gingivalis* (*green channel*) and drug (*red channel*) only

contrast through de-convolution of images, especially on live cell imaging where faster image acquisition, lower excitation power, and less photo bleaching and cell damage [27, 28]. This is a key consideration which can be improved by DeltaVision microscopy in the future study on live cells [27, 28].

Using confocal microscopy in the present drug development study, has determined that a novel porphyrin-linked metronidazole antibiotic can penetrate into epithelial cells to kill intracellular oral pathogens. However, researchers need to be aware of that an overlap in fluorescence does not necessarily demonstrate co-localization of two colours (probes) in the same cellular structure [17]. Therefore the co-distribution of two colours (probes) in fluorescence microscope images can be evaluated quantitatively and statistically on either co-localisation or two colours' ratio change using Huygens professional software (https://svi.nl/HuygensProfessional). For the images shown in Fig. 5, we could explain it as the ratio change of two colours which bacterial spots in green were decreasing with a time lapse comparing to drugs in red colour.

Conclusions

Confocal laser scanning microscope is a valuable tool in dental research, particularly for probing thick specimens of carious teeth, formation of microbial biofilms on gingival tissues, tracing pathological changes in live cells and studying the cellular effects of drug candidates. Future developments of powerful microscopy will be of great interest and benefit in clinical dental research.

Acknowledgements
We would like to thank Professor Neil Hunter and Ms Mary Simonian for their technical and laboratory supports.

Funding
There was no finding obtained for this study.

Authors' contributions
PY participated in the experimental design and data analysis, and contributed to the draft of manuscript. HY provided confocal microscopy support for the study. MH performed immunohistology work and data analysis. The authors reviewed and approved the final manuscript.

Competing interests
The authors declare that they have no competing interests.

Consent for publication
Not applicable, as this manuscript does not contain any individual persons' identifying information.

Ethics approval and consent to participate
Ethical approvals for data and sample collection from the patients have been obtained by Ethics Committees of the Sydney Dental Hospital and the Sydney West Area Health Service. All data and samples from the patients were collected following informed written consent. All the information including personal details, images and videos of patients' teeth and gingival tissues that have been used for this study were de-identified.

Author details
[1]Institute of Dental Research, Oral Health, Westmead Hospital, Westmead, Australia. [2]Affiliation of Faculty of Dentistry, the University of Sydney, Sydney, Australia. [3]Microscopy Laboratory, Westmead Institute for Medical Research, Westmead, Australia.

References

1. Shotton D, White N. Confocal scanning microscopy: three-dimensional biological imaging. Trends Biochem Sci. 1989;14:435–9.
2. Wright SJ, Schatten G. Confocal fluorescence microscopy and three-dimensional reconstruction. J Electron Microsc Tech. 1991;18:2–10.
3. Roux P, Münter S, Frischknecht F, Herbomel P, Shorte SL. Focusing light on infection in four dimensions. Cell Microbiol. 2004;6:333–43.
4. Zemanová L, Schenk A, Valler MJ, Nienhaus GU, Heilker R. Confocal optics microscopy for biochemical and cellular high-throughput screening. Drug Discov Today. 2003;8:1085–93.
5. Houshmandi M, Ye P, Hunter N. Glial network responses to polymicrobial invasion of dentin. Caries Res. 2014;48:534–48.
6. Guo W, Ye P, Yu H, Liu Z, Yang P, Hunter N. CD24 activates the NLRP3 inflammasome through c-Src kinase activity in a model of the lining epithelium of inflamed periodontal tissues. Immun Inflamm Dis. 2014;2:239–53.
7. Prime SS, Nixon SV, Crane IJ, Stone A, Matthews JB, Maitland NJ, Remnant L, Powell SK, et al. The behaviour of human oral squamous cell carcinoma in cell culture. J Pathol. 1990;160:259–69.
8. Ye P, Nadkarni MA, Hunter N. Regulation of Ecadherin and TGF-beta3 expression by CD24 in cultured oral epithelial cells. Biochem Biophys Res Commun. 2006;349:229–35.
9. Swierenga SH, MacManus JP. Preparation of low calcium growth medium suitable for determination of tumorigenicity of cultured cells. J Tissue Culture Methods. 1982;7:1–3.
10. Li N, Yun P, Nadkarni MA, Ghadikolaee NB, Nguyen KA, Lee M, Hunter N, Collyer CA. Structure determination and analysis of a haemolytic gingipain adhesin domain from Porphyromonas gingivalis. Mol Microbiol. 2010;76:861–73.
11. Ye P, Harty D, Commandeur Z, Hunter N. Binding of Streptococcus gordonii to oral epithelial monolayers increases paracellular barrier function. Microb Pathog. 2013;56:53–9.
12. Nisapakultorn K, Ross KF, Herzberg MC. Calprotectin expression in vitro by oral epithelial cells confers resistance to infection by *Porphyromonas gingivalis*. Infect Immun. 2001;69:4242–7.
13. Yap BC, Simpkins GL, Collyer CA, Hunter N, Crossley MJ. Porphyrin-linked nitroimidazole antibiotics targeting Porphyromonas gingivalis. Org Biomol Chem. 2009;7:2855–63.
14. DeCarlo AA, Paramaesvaran M, Yun PL, Collyer C, Hunter N. Porphyrin-mediated binding to hemoglobin by the HA2 domain of cysteine proteinases (gingipains) and hemagglutinins from the periodontal pathogen Porphyromonas gingivalis. J Bacteriol. 1999;181:3784–91.
15. Kopecky BJ, Duncan JS, Elliott KL, Fritzsch B. Three-dimensional reconstructions from optical sections of thick mouse inner ears using confocal microscopy. J Microsc. 2012;248:292–8.
16. Attik GN, Gritsch K, Colon P, Grosgogeat B. Confocal time lapse imaging as an efficient method for the cytocompatibility evaluation of dental composites. J Vis Exp. 2014;93:e51949.
17. Dunn KW, Kamocka MM, McDonald JH. A practical guide to evaluating colocalization in biological microscopy. Am J Physiol Cell Physiol. 2011;300:C723–42.
18. Costes SV, Daelemans D, Cho EH, Dobbin Z, Pavlakis G, Lockett S. Automatic and Quantitative Measurement of Protein-Protein Colocalization in Live Cells. Biophys J. 2004;86:3993–4003.
19. Mitsiadis TA, Filatova A, Papaccio G, Goldberg M, About I, Papagerakis P. Distribution of the amelogenin protein in developing, injured and carious human teeth. Front Physiol. 2014;5:477.
20. Karygianni L, Follo M, Hellwig E, Burghardt D, Wolkewitz M, Anderson A, Al-Ahmad A. Microscope-Based Imaging Platform for Large-Scale Analysis of Oral Biofilms. Appl Environ Microbiol. 2012;78:8703–11.
21. Thurnheer T, Belibasakis GN, Bostanci N. Colonisation of gingival epithelia by subgingival biofilms in vitro: Role of "red complex" bacteria. Arch Oral Biol. 2014;59:977–86.
22. Rudney JD, Chen R, Sedgewick GJ. Intracellular *Actinobacillus actinomycetemcomitans* and *Porphyromonas gingivalis* in Buccal Epithelial Cells Collected from Human Subjects. Infect Immun. 2001;69:2700–7.
23. Zhang B, Elmabsout AA, Khalaf H, Basic VT, Jayaprakash K, Kruse R, Bengtsson T, Sirsjö A. The periodontal pathogen *Porphyromonas gingivalis* changes the gene expression in vascular smooth muscle cells involving the TGFbeta/Notch signalling pathway and increased cell proliferation. BMC Genomics. 2013;14:770.
24. Sowell J, Strekowski L, Patonay G. DNA and protein applications of near-infrared dyes. J Biomed Opt. 2002;7:571–5.
25. Dempsey GT. A user's guide to localization-based super-resolution fluorescence imaging. Methods Cell Biol. 2013;114:561–92.
26. Laurent M, Johannin G, Gilbert N, Lucas L, Cassio D, Petit PX, Fleury A. Power and limits of laser scanning confocal microscopy. Biol Cell. 1994;80:229–40.
27. Schermelleh L, Heintzmann R, Leonhardt H. A guide to super-resolution fluorescence microscopy. J Cell Biol. 2010;190:165–75.
28. Ball G, Parton RM, Hamilton RS, Davis I. A cell biologist's guide to high resolution imaging. Methods Enzymol. 2012;504:29–55.

17

Association between Low blood lead levels and increased risk of dental caries in children

Young-Suk Kim[1], Mina Ha[2*], Ho-Jang Kwon[2], Hae-Young Kim[3] and Youn-Hee Choi[4]

Abstract

Background: The objective of this study was to examine the association between low blood lead levels of <5 μg/dL and the development of dental caries among children.

Methods: The Children's Health and Environment Research (CHEER) group recruited a cohort of 7,059 school-aged children from six Korean cities. The final study populations in the permanent and deciduous teeth groups were 1,564 and 1,241 children, respectively, after excluding 4 children with blood lead levels of >5 μg/dL. Compared with the children who did not have dental caries, the risk of having dental caries according to blood lead level was estimated by using the zero-inflated negative binomial model.

Results: The geometric mean (geometric standard deviation, maximum) blood lead level was 1.53 μg/dL (1.57, 4.89 μg/dL), and 74.4% of children had a level of <2 μg/dL. Blood lead level was significantly higher in the children with than in those without deciduous dental caries (1.59 vs. 1.51 μg/dL), similarly with permanent dental caries (1.65 vs. 1.51 μg/dL). After adjustment for covariates, deciduous teeth surfaces that were decayed and filled increased significantly with increasing blood lead levels in a dose-dependent manner (prevalence ratio, 1.14; 95% confidence interval: 1.02–1.27). However, the risk of having dental caries in permanent teeth was not linearly associated with the increase in blood lead level.

Conclusions: In the sum of decayed and filled surfaces, we found a significant increase in risk of dental caries of the deciduous teeth with an increase in blood lead levels (<5 μg/dL) but found no statistical significance in the association with decayed and filled surfaces of caries separately.

Keywords: Blood lead, Children, Dental caries, Deciduous dentition

Background

Dental caries is a chronic disease that progresses slowly in most people [1] and is one of the most prevalent diseases in children worldwide. The prevalence of dental caries among Korean children was 30.4% in 8-year-olds in deciduous teeth and 57.3% in 12-year-olds in permanent teeth in 2012 [2]. In China, the prevalence of dental caries in 2013 was 52% in children aged 5–6 years and 41% in those aged 12–13 years [3]. The proportion of children between the ages of 5 and 17 years who had untreated dental caries was approximately 20.1% in the United States [4].

Dental caries is a complex disease, and several microbial, genetic, immunological, behavioral, and environmental factors contribute to its risk and severity [1]. Dental caries occurs from a series of interactions over time between bacteria, which produce acid, and host factors, including teeth and saliva [1]. Endogenous bacteria produce organic acid that decreases plaque pH, which leads to demineralization of the tooth surface [5, 6]. A destroyed tooth structure requires restoration and maintenance throughout life; therefore, the burden of dental caries continues for a lifetime [1]. Furthermore, it is influenced by various systemic diseases such as asthma [7, 8] and diabetes mellitus [9].

* Correspondence: minaha@dku.edu
[2]Department of Preventive Medicine, Dankook University College of Medicine, 119 Dandae-ro, Dongnam-gu, Cheonan, Chungnam 31116, Republic of Korea
Full list of author information is available at the end of the article

Lead has been used extensively by humans for a long period and spread to the environment widely [10]. In most developed countries, concerted efforts have been made to reduce lead levels in the environment in recent years, although in developing countries, lead is still a significant public health problem [11]. Susceptible populations, including children and pregnant women, may be more affected than non-susceptible populations by environmental lead. The mean blood lead levels were 1.34, 1.26, and 1.14 μg/dL in Korean children aged 3–5, 6–11, and 12–18 years, respectively, from 2012 to 2014 [12], which were higher than the 0.838 and 0.680 μg/dL in US children aged 6–11 and 12–19 years, respectively, from 2009 to 2010 [13]. Higher lead levels in bone and blood are a risk factor of systemic diseases such as ischemic heart disease [14] and hypertension [15]. In addition, blood lead levels affect neurological and neurobehavioral development, as well as oral health.

Each 1-μg/dL increase in blood lead level results in a decrease of 0.87 intelligence quotient (IQ) points; in the range of <10 μg/dL, an increase of 1 μg/dL results in a 1.37 decrease in IQ measured with the Stanford-Binet Intelligence Scale [16]. In an animal study, exposure of less-mature enamel to lead resulted in decreased hardness in comparison with the enamel of control animals [17]. In addition, epidemiological studies have reported an association between lead exposure and dental caries in children [18–22].

However, the blood lead levels in the previous studies were relatively higher (≥2 μg/dL) than those reported recently in children in Korea and other developed countries. The aim of this study was to examine the association between blood lead concentration and dental caries in Korean children with a blood lead level of ≤5 μg/dL, the reference value recently proposed by the US Centers for Disease Control and Prevention (CDC) [23].

Methods

Study population

The present study was conducted as a part of the Children's Health and Environment Research (CHEER) study, which was a cohort study conducted from 2005 to 2010 to investigate the association between environmental exposure and health in school-aged children recruited from urban, rural, and industrial areas within Korea [24]. Children underwent oral examinations from 2008 to 2010 in four cities: Seoul (urban area), Daegu (urban area), Cheonan (rural area), and Busan (industrialized area) at a cross-sectional time frame. After excluding 63 children whose blood lead concentrations were not measured and 4 children who had a blood lead level of >5 μg/dL, the final numbers of subjects in the present study were 1,564 and 1,241 for analysis of permanent and deciduous teeth, respectively. The study protocol was reviewed and approved by the institutional review board of the Dankook University College of Medicine, and all the participants' parents or guardians were provided written informed consent before participation. This study has been conducted in full accordance with the World Medical Association Declaration of Helsinki.

Oral examinations

Oral examinations were performed based on the oral examination guidelines for epidemiological investigation established by the World Health Organization [25]. Two dentists examined the children's oral status, and a trained dental hygienist recorded the oral index. The oral examination instruments used included a front surface mouth mirror and a double-ended Shepherd's hook and Orban explorer. Dental caries was defined by the number of decayed surfaces (ds), filled surfaces (fs), and the sum of decayed and filled surfaces (dfs) for deciduous teeth, and by the number of decayed surfaces (DS), filled surfaces (FS), and the sum of decayed and filled surfaces and missing teeth due to dental caries (DMFS) for permanent teeth.

Blood lead measurement

To measure blood lead concentrations, 3–5 ml of whole blood was drawn from each child by using a syringe and then sealed in a heparin-containing tube. The blood lead levels were determined by using atomic absorption spectrophotometry (Spectral AA-800 Zeeman Correction, Varian, Australia) at a commercial laboratory. The limit of quantification (LOQ) was 0.030 μg/dL.

Potential confounders and covariates

To estimate the risk of dental caries in association with blood lead level, potential confounding factors or covariates were considered. Information on basic demographic variables was obtained from a questionnaire survey, including sex (male or female), age (≤9, 10, 11, and ≥12 years), and mother's educational level (≤12 and >12 years), and monthly household income (<2000, 2000–2990, 3000–3990, and ≥4000 10^3 KRW). Urinary cotinine level was measured by using a gas chromatograph-mass selective detector (Perkin Elmer, Clarus 600 T, Waltham, USA), and the limit of detection (LOD) of urinary cotinine was 0.396 μg/dL. We categorized the cotinine level in urine for the analysis as ≤3 or >3 μg/g.

Lead interrupts the absorption of calcium and iron in the human body [10]. Nutritional status of calcium and iron can influence an individual's susceptibility to lead toxicity [26]. However, blood lead levels were not associated with calcium and iron concentrations in the subjects of the present study. Therefore, calcium and iron concentrations were not included in the multivariate models.

Statistical analysis

The Kruskal-Wallis or Wilcoxon rank sum tests were applied to assess differences in geometric mean blood lead level according to sociodemographic characteristics. The adjusted mean blood lead levels for dental caries-positive and dental caries-negative statuses were calculated by using the least square mean estimation in the corresponding multiple linear regression model. Based on a previous study [27], among the Poisson, negative binomial, and zero-inflated Poisson models, the zero-inflated negative binomial model (ZINB) was reported to be the best-fitted model for the dental caries study because of excess zero of caries in children. Therefore, we used the ZINB model adjusted for the above-mentioned potential confounders and covariates. The risk (prevalence ratio) and 95% confidence interval (CI) for having dental caries in deciduous and permanent teeth were estimated. The analyses were conducted by using R version 3.1.1 (R Foundation for Statistical Computing, Vienna, Austria) [28], with a significance level of 0.05. Moreover, Stata 12.1 (Stata Corp LP, College Station, TX, USA) was used to apply the ZINB model.

Results

In the deciduous teeth group, about 42% of the children had more than one decayed surface (ds) and 73% of the children had more than one filled surface (fs) due to dental caries. Most (81.7%) of the children had more than one dfs in the deciduous teeth group. The number of ds was significantly higher among the males than among the females ($p = 0.05$), but fs and dfs were not significantly different between the sexes in the deciduous teeth group. Geographically, ds, fs, and dfs were significantly higher in the industrial areas than in the urban or rural areas in the deciduous teeth group. The number of ds was significantly higher in the children with less-educated parents, single parents, and lower household income. The prevalence rates of DS, FS, and DMFS were 16.3%, 33.4%, and 44.6%, respectively, in the permanent teeth group. The prevalence rates of FS and DMFS, but not DS, were significantly higher in the females than in the males. As in the deciduous teeth group, DS rate was significantly higher in the children with less-educated parents, single parents, and lower household incomes (Table 1).

The geometric mean blood lead levels (geometric standard deviation) in the children was 1.53 (1.57) μg/dL. The highest, median, and lowest blood lead levels were 4.89, 1.58, and 0.11 μg/dL, respectively. In our study, 25.6% ($n = 400$) of the children had blood lead levels of >2.0 μg/dL.

The least square mean blood lead level adjusted for potential confounding factors was significantly higher in the children with than in those without decayed surfaces in both deciduous and permanent teeth: 1.59 μg/dL (95% CI: 1.53–1.65 μg/dL) versus 1.51 μg/dL (1.46–1.56 μg/dL) for deciduous teeth ($p = 0.01$); and 1.65 μg/dL (1.56–1.75 μg/dL) versus 1.51 μg/dL (1.47–1.55 μg/dL) for permanent teeth ($p = 0.001$). However, the blood lead levels were not different between the children with filled surfaces, missing teeth, or both and those with neither filled surfaces nor missing teeth in both deciduous and permanent teeth (Fig. 1).

The prevalence ratio and 95% CI of the risk of having dfs increased with increasing blood lead concentrations in a dose-dependent manner (1.14, 1.02–1.27). However, permanent teeth were negatively associated with higher blood lead levels (0.83, 0.69-0.99; Table 2).

Discussion

The results of this study show a significant increased risk of dental caries with increasing blood lead level among children with blood lead levels of <5 μg/dL, particularly for deciduous tooth surfaces, which exhibited a linear relationship.

The mean blood lead concentration in our study subjects (GM, 1.53 μg/dL; maximum, 4.89 μg/dL) was lower than those in previous reports of a significant association between blood lead and dental caries. The mean blood lead levels in these reports were between 2.1 (0.10 μmol/L) and 2.8 μg/dL (0.14 μmol/L) [18], specifically 10.7 μg/dL [19], 2.3 μg/dL [20], 7.2 μg/dL [21], and 4.6 μg/dL [22]. All these blood lead levels were higher than those in the present study (<5 μg/dL), which was recommended recently as the reference value by the US CDC to protect children [23].

The significant relationship in deciduous teeth is consistent with all of the above-mentioned epidemiological studies [19–22], except one study that reported a significant association in permanent teeth [18]. One possible explanation for the difference is that the subjects in the previous study (2–17 years old) [18] were older than those in other studies, including the present study, in which sufficient time for development of caries (DMFS) in permanent teeth was allowed. A recent study using the ZINB model also showed a significant association between blood lead and dfs, which is consistent with our findings [27].

We also found significantly higher blood lead levels in the children with decayed tooth surfaces but found no significant differences between the children with and those without filled or both decayed and filled surfaces in both deciduous and permanent teeth. The decayed

Table 1 Frequency of dental caries according to general characteristics of study subjects

Characteristics	Deciduous teeth				Permanent teeth			
	N	ds (≥1)	fs (≥1)	dfs (≥1)	N	DS (≥1)	FS (≥1)	DMFS (≥1)
		%	%	%		%	%	%
All	1,241	41.9	72.8	81.7	1,564	16.3	33.4	44.6
Gender								
Boy	646	44.6	74.6	83.1	806	14.9	31.0	41.1
Girl	595	39.0	70.8	80.2	758	17.8	36.0	48.4
p-value		*0.05*	*0.14*	*0.20*		*0.14*	*0.04*	*0.004*
Age (years)								
≤ 9	933	42.3	74.3	81.9	963	13.4	29.7	39.6
10	62	37.1	64.5	77.4	92	16.3	34.8	44.6
11	177	43.5	70.1	83.1	300	22.0	39.3	53.0
≥ 12	69	36.2	66.7	79.7	209	21.5	41.6	56.0
Mean (SD)	9.8 (1.1)				10.2 (1.3)			
p-value		*0.62*	*0.16*	*0.76*		*0.001*	*0.001*	*<0.0001*
Living area								
Urban (Seoul,Daegu)	757	38.6	73.4	80.6	986	14.4	35.0	44.1
Industrial (Busan)	216	54.2	78.7	88.4	226	21.7	39.4	55.8
Rural (Cheonan)	268	41.4	66.0	79.5	352	18.2	25.3	38.9
p-value		*0.0002*	*0.01*	*0.02*		*0.02*	*0.001*	*0.0003*
Educational level of father (years)								
≤ 12	436	48.4	73.2	83.5	572	19.6	34.1	48.6
> 12	641	36.5	73.3	80.2	774	11.8	31.5	38.9
Unknown	164	45.7	69.5	82.9	218	23.9	38.5	54.6
p-value		*0.01*	*0.92*	*0.94*		*<0.0001*	*0.56*	*0.05*
Educational level of mother (years)								
≤ 12	583	44.6	73.2	82.5	745	19.9	33.3	47.2
> 12	496	36.9	73.4	80.2	599	9.8	32.1	38.1
Unknown	162	47.5	69.1	83.3	220	21.8	37.7	53.6
p-value		*0.19*	*0.99*	*0.97*		*<0.0001*	*0.30*	*0.004*
Parental marital status								
Single	147	52.4	71.4	85.7	200	27.0	33.5	52.5
Couple	1,039	39.6	73.1	80.8	1286	14.0	33.1	42.8
Unknown	55	58.2	70.9	87.3	78	26.9	38.5	55.1
p-value		*0.03*	*0.98*	*0.40*		*<0.0001*	*0.84*	*0.08*
Household income (1,000KRW)								
< 2000	248	48.4	71.4	84.7	343	25.4	33.8	51.6
2000–2990	367	41.1	70.0	79.0	452	16.2	35.2	45.4
3000–3990	255	43.5	73.3	81.6	318	12.9	33.0	42.5
≥ 4000	280	35.0	76.8	81.4	333	9.9	32.1	38.7
Unknown	91	44.0	73.6	85.7	118	17.8	30.5	44.1
p-value		*0.02*	*0.27*	*0.37*		*0.05*	*0.83*	*0.01*
Urinary cotinine concentration (ug/g cr.)								
≤ 3.0	585	40.9	72.1	81.4	761	16.0	33.2	44.0
> 3.0	346	45.1	76.3	82.7	382	16.8	30.9	41.4

Table 1 Frequency of dental caries according to general characteristics of study subjects *(Continued)*

Unknown	310	40.3	70.0	81.3	421	16.4	36.1	48.7
Mean (SD)	2.15 (3.21)				1.93 (3.24)			
p-value		*0.23*	*0.19*	*0.68*		*0.82*	*0.46*	*0.43*

p-value calculated by x^2 - test excluding unknown category
ds decayed surfaces for deciduous tooth, *fs* filled surfaces because of caries for deciduous tooth, *dfs* the sum of decayed and filled surfaces for deciduous tooth. *DS* decayed surfaces for permanent tooth, *FS* filled surfaces because of caries for permanent tooth, *DMFS* the sum of decayed, filled surfaces and missing because of caries for permanent tooth

surfaces reflect currently extant and not-yet-treated caries, while filled surfaces are developed and treated caries, and reflect the availability of oral health-care services. Therefore, decayed surfaces might be a better indicator of current lead exposure related dental caries.

For permanent dental caries, DMFS showed a significant negative association with blood lead level. Unlike deciduous teeth, which are temporary for a certain period and soon replaced by permanent teeth, permanent teeth might have attracted more attention from parents and received more care services. Therefore, the higher prevalence of DMFS in permanent tooth than caries in deciduous tooth is more influenced by other factors such as social and health-care conditions rather than causal risk factors such as lead exposure. In this case, the reverse causality between blood lead level and permanent dental caries might be a more plausible explanation considering the cross-sectional design of the present study. As lead level has been reported to be higher in those with lower socioeconomic position (SEP) in this population [29], children with higher SEP, well-treated caries, and more DMFS showed lower blood lead level.

Although the adjusted mean blood lead level was significantly higher in the children with than in those without dental caries both in deciduous and permanent teeth, the significant increase in the risk of having dental caries was found only in deciduous teeth in the present study. The difference might be due in part to the different statistical models for estimating adjusted mean and risk of having caries. However, an important thing might be the susceptibility to lead toxicity in caries development because younger children have deciduous teeth rather than permanent teeth.

A previous study [22] reported a sex-related difference in the association between blood lead and dental caries; that is, a relationship existed only in males. We thus

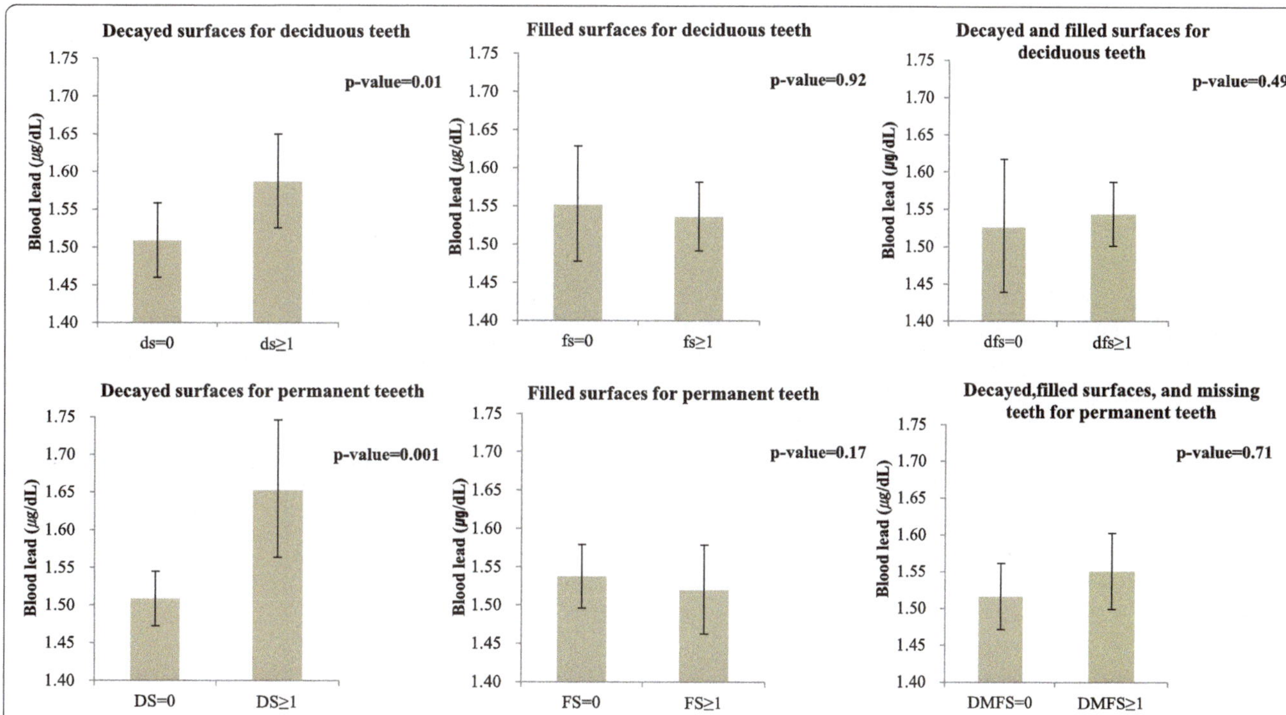

Fig. 1 Blood lead concentration according to dental caries status. Blood lead concentrations were estimated with the least-square mean by using log-transformed and exponential function, adjusted for gender, age, educational level of mother, and urinary cotinine

Table 2 Association between blood lead concentration and dental caries in deciduous and permanent teeth

		Crude model		Adjusted model[a]		
For Blood lead level (ug/dL)	N(≥1)	Prevalence Ratio	95% CI	Prevalence Ratio	95% CI	Model fit (*p*-value)*
Deciduous teeth						
ds	520	1.15	0.96–1.36	1.16	0.91–1.49	22.86 (0.0018)
fs	903	1.08	0.98–1.20	1.11	0.98–1.25	25.70 (0.0006)
dfs	1,014	1.09	1.00–1.19	1.14	1.02–1.27	35.09 (<.0001)
Permanent teeth						
DS	255	0.77	0.62–0.97	0.69	0.45–1.07	9.87 (0.1960)
FS	523	0.89	0.81–0.99	0.87	0.73–1.04	16.25 (0.0229)
DMFS	698	0.86	0.78–0.95	0.83	0.69–0.99	14.56 (0.0421)

Prevalence ratio and 95% Confidence Intervals (CI) estimated using zero inflated negative binomial (ZINB) model
ds decayed surfaces for deciduous tooth, *fs* filled surfaces because of caries for deciduous tooth, *dfs* the sum of decayed and filled surfaces for deciduous tooth. *DS* decayed surfaces for permanent tooth, *FS* filled surfaces because of caries for permanent tooth, *DMFS* the sum of decayed, filled surfaces and missing because of caries for permanent tooth
*Chi-square difference values for likelihood ratio test
[a]ZINB model adjusted for gender, age (categorical), household income (categorical), and urinary cotinine level (categorical)

reanalyzed the data with regard to sex. However, we could not reproduce the finding of the previous study and found no significant difference between the sexes (prevalence ratio [95% CI] for dfs: 1.11 [1.00–1.23] in males and 1.07 [0.94–1.22] in females, p value for multiplicative interaction for sex = 0.60).

Lead is initially distributed to soft tissues such as the kidney and liver, and then redistributed to bone and hair [10]. Lead is absorbed into the teeth and delays the mineralization of enamel [19]. In blood, lead has a half-life of up to 30 days and is excreted into the urine; it can be stored in bone for >20 years [30]. Persistent release of lead from bone into the blood can delay tooth calcification, in which the mineralization process continues even after oral tooth eruption. Dental caries can be prevented by regular brushing and water fluoridation. However, lead may bind to fluoride ions in saliva and plaque, and thereby reduce the ability of fluoride to remineralize enamel after an acid challenge [31].

This study has several limitations. First, lead exposure at the time of enamel formation is the mechanism most relevant to a causal lead-caries association [18]. This is a cross-sectional study, so we could not provide evidence that the teeth were influenced by blood lead level during the period of ontogeny or after mineralization. To identify a causal relationship between blood lead level and dental caries, a cohort study that measures lead exposure in pregnant women and then observes their infants is warranted. Next, we did not include calcium and iron intakes in our multivariate models as covariates that influence bone and teeth growth. However, the present results may not be confounded by these factors because blood lead levels were not correlated with calcium or iron concentrations in the present study.

In conclusion, we found a linear dose–response association between low blood lead levels (<5 μg/dL) and the development of caries in deciduous teeth.

Conclusions

This study showed an association between low blood lead levels (<5 μg/dL) and development of dental caries in deciduous teeth but not in permanent teeth. These results suggest that blood lead level is a risk factor for the development of dental caries in deciduous dentition.

Abbreviations

CDC: Centers for disease control and prevention; CHEER: Children's Health and Environment Research; CI: Confidence interval; dfs: The sum of decayed and filled surfaces for deciduous teeth; DMFS: The sum of decayed and filled surfaces and missing teeth due to dental caries for permanent teeth; ds: The number of decayed surfaces for deciduous teeth; DS: The number of decayed surfaces for permanent teeth; FS: The number of filled surfaces for permanent teeth; fs: The number of filled surfaces for deciduous teeth; IQ: Intelligence quotient; LOD: Limit of detection; LOQ: Limit of quantification; SEP: Socioeconomic position; ZINB: Zero-inflated negative binomial model

Acknowledgements

We would like to thank Professors Yun-Chul Hong, Chul Gab Lee, Jong-Han Leem, Joon Sakong, Dongmug Kang, and Su Young Kim for their dedication to the CHEER data collection.

Funding

This study was financially supported by the National Institute of Environmental Research and Korean Ministry of Environment and by a grant (15162MFDS045) from Ministry of Food and Drug Safety. The funding bodies did not play any role in the design of the study and collection, analysis, and interpretation of data and in writing the manuscript.

Authors' contributions

YSK analyzed data and drafted the manuscript. MH revised the manuscript and contributed to conception, design and interpretation of the study. HJK and YHC participated in the design of the study and collection of the data.

HYK contributed to statistical analysis. All the authors have given their approval to the final version of the article.

Competing interests
The authors declare that they have no competing interests.

Consent for publication
Not applicable.

Ethics approval and consent to participate
The study protocol was reviewed and approved by the Institutional Review Board of the Dankook University College of Medicine and all participants' parents or guardians provided written informed consent before participation.

Author details
[1]Department of Dental Hygiene, U1 University, Yeongdong, Korea. [2]Department of Preventive Medicine, Dankook University College of Medicine, 119 Dandae-ro, Dongnam-gu, Cheonan, Chungnam 31116, Republic of Korea. [3]Department of Health Policy and Management, College of Health Science, and Department of Health Science, Graduate School, Korea University, Seoul, Korea. [4]Department of Preventive Dentistry, School of Dentistry, Kyungpook National University, Daegu, Korea.

References
1. Selwitz RH, Ismail AI, Pitts NB. Dental caries. Lancet. 2007;369:51–9.
2. Korean National Oral Health Survey. Korean center of disease center. 2012. http://knhanes.cdc.go.kr. Accessed 21 Feb 2014.
3. Prasai Dixit L, Shakya A, Shrestha M, Shrestha A. Dental caries prevalence, oral health knowledge and practice among indigenous Chepang school children of Nepal. BMC Oral Health. 2013;13:20.
4. Chi DL, Masterson EE, Carle AC, Mancl LA, Coldwell SE. Socioeconomic status, food security, and dental caries in US children: mediation analyses of data from the National Health and Nutrition Examination Survey, 2007–2008. Am J Public Health. 2014;104:860–4.
5. Caufield PW, Griffen AL. Dental caries. An infectious and transmissible disease. Pediatr Clin North Am. 2000;47:1001–19.
6. Featherstone JD. The science and practice of caries prevention. J Am Dent Assoc. 2000;131(7):887–99.
7. Reddy DK, Hegde AM, Munshi AK. Dental caries status of children with bronchial asthma. J Clin Pediatr Dent. 2003;27:293–5.
8. Stensson M, Wendt LK, Koch G, Oldaeus G, Birkhed D. Oral health in preschool children with asthma. Int J Paediatr Dent. 2008;18:243–50.
9. Miralles L, Silvestre FJ, Hernández-Mijares A, Bautista D, Llambes F, Grau D. Dental caries in type 1 diabetics: influence of systemic factors of the disease upon the development of dental caries. Med Oral Patol Oral Cir Bucal. 2006; 11:E256–60.
10. Klaassen CD. Casarett and Doull's toxicology the basic science of poisons. 7th ed. New York: McGrew-Hill; 2007. p. 943–4.
11. Tong S, Schirnding YEV, Prapamontol T. Environmental lead exposure: a public health problem of global dimensions. Bull World Health Organ. 2000;78:1068–77.
12. Burm E, Song I, Ha M, Kim YM, Lee KJ, Kim HC, et al. Representative levels of blood lead, mercury, and urinary cadmium in youth: Korean Environmental Health Survey in Children and Adolescents (KorEHS-C), 2012–2014. Int J Hyg Environ Health. 2016;219(4–5):412–8.
13. CDC. Forth national report on human exposure to environmental chemical. 2009. http://www.cdc.gov. Accessed 27 Feb 2014.
14. Jain NB, Potula V, Schwartz J, Vokonas PS, Sparrow D, Wright RO, et al. Lead levels and ischemic heart disease in a prospective study of middle-aged and elderly men: the VA Normative Aging Study. Environ Health Perspect. 2007;115:871–5.
15. Hu H, Aro A, Payton M, Korrick S, Sparrow D, Weiss ST, et al. The relationship of bone and blood lead to hypertension. The Normative Aging Study. JAMA. 1996;275:1171–6.
16. Canfield RL, Henderson Jr CR, Cory-Slechta DA, Cox C, Jusko TA, Lanphear BP. Intellectual impairment in children with blood lead concentrations below 10 microg per deciliter. N Engl J Med. 2003;348:1517–26.
17. Gerlach RF, Cury JA, Krug FJ, Line SR. Effect of lead on dental enamel formation. Toxicology. 2002;175:27–34.
18. Moss ME, Lanphear BP, Auinger P. Association of dental caries and blood lead levels. JAMA. 1999;281:2294–8.
19. Campbell JR, Moss ME, Raubertas RF. The association between caries and childhood lead exposure. Environ Health Perspect. 2000;108:1099–102.
20. Gemmel A, Tavares M, Alperin S, Soncini J, Daniel D, Dunn J, et al. Blood lead level and dental caries in school-age children. Environ Health Perspect. 2002;110:A625–30.
21. Youravong N, Chongsuvivatwong V, Geater AF, Dahlén G, Teanpaisan R. Lead associated caries development in children living in a lead contaminated area, Thailand. Sci Total Environ. 2006;361:88–96.
22. Martin MD, Benton T, Bernardo M, Woods JS, Townes BD, Luis H, et al. The association of dental caries with blood lead in children when adjusted for IQ and neurobehavioral performance. Sci Total Environ. 2007;377:159–64.
23. Centers for Disease Control and Prevention. Advisory Committee on Childhood Lead Poisoning Prevention (ACCLPP). 2012. Available at: http://www.cdc.gov/nceh/lead/acclpp/acclpp_main.htm. Accessed 18 June 2014.
24. Ha M, Kwon HJ, Lim MH, Jee YK, Hong YC, Leem JH, et al. Low blood levels of lead and mercury and symptoms of attention deficit hyperactivity in children: a report of the children's health and environment research (CHEER). Neurotoxicology. 2009;30:31–6.
25. World Health Organization. Oral health surveys; basic methods. 4th ed. Geneva: WHO; 1997.
26. Mahaffey KR. Nutrition and lead: strategies for public health. Environ Health Perspect. 1995;103:191–6.
27. Wiener RC, Long DL, Jurevic RJ. Blood levels of the heavy metal, lead, and caries in children aged 24–72 months: NHANES III. Caries Res. 2015;49(1):26–33.
28. R Development Core Team. R: a language and environment for statistical computing. 10th ed. Vienna: R Foundation for Statistical Computing; 2011. http://www.r-project.org/. ISBN 3-900051-07-0.
29. Lim S, Ha M, Hwang SS, Son M, Kwon HJ. Disparities in Children's blood lead and mercury levels according to community and individual socioeconomic positions. Int J Environ Res Public Health. 2015;12(6):6232–48.
30. Rosin A. The long-term consequences of exposure to lead. 1st Med Assoc J. 2009;11:689–94.
31. Rao GS. Dietary intake and bioavailability of fluoride. Annu Rev Nutr. 1984;4: 115–36.

18

Knowledge of caries risk factors/indicators among Japanese and Irish adult patients with different socio-economic profiles

Makiko Nishi[1*], Máiréad Harding[1], Virginia Kelleher[1], Helen Whelton[2] and Finbarr Allen[3]

Abstract

Background: A previous study has shown deficient knowledge of caries risk factors/indicators in a Japanese adult population regarded to have a high interest in preventive dentistry. No prior research has investigated caries risk knowledge in an Irish adult population. We hypothesise there may be *unexpected* differences or similarities in knowledge across countries with similar levels of economic development when comparing groups with different socio-economic and cultural profiles. Understanding what influences knowledge is important for the development of effective and efficient caries prevention strategies. The current paper aims to describe the knowledge of caries risk factors/indicators in two groups with different socio-economic profiles from two culturally distinct countries.

Methods: Cross-sectional surveys of adult dental patients were carried out in Japan and in the Republic of Ireland (RoI) using similar self-administered paper questionnaires. Patients were asked to identify caries risk factors/indicators from eight (Japan) or ten (RoI) listed items. The Japanese study involved 482 patients (aged ≥20 years) from 52 dental members of a nationwide web-based initiative Promoting Scientific Assessment in Prevention of Tooth Decay and Gum Disease (PSAP). The Irish study involved 159 patients (aged 20–69 years) accessing state-provided ('medical card') dental services from eight dental practices in County Cork. The two samples were compared.

Results: A higher proportion of Irish respondents identified 'Not visiting the dentist for check-up and cleaning' (OR 2.655; 99% CI 1.550, 4.547) and 'Not using fluoride' (OR 1.714; 99% CI 1.049, 2.802) than did Japanese respondents. A lower proportion of Irish respondents identified 'A reduced amount of saliva' (OR 0.262; 99% CI 0.159, 0.433) than Japanese respondents. Similarly shown in both studies were a persistent belief that 'Not brushing teeth properly' is a caries risk factor and a lack of knowledge on saliva buffering capacity as a caries risk factor.

Conclusions: Deficiencies in knowledge which should be addressed: among the Japanese group, of dental check-up/cleaning visits and of fluoride use for caries prevention; among the Irish group, of saliva quantity as a caries risk factor. In addition, in both groups, we need to inform patients of the defensive role of saliva.

Keywords: Dental caries, Risk factors, Knowledge, Fluorides, Saliva, Cross-cultural comparison, Japan, Ireland, Socioeconomic factors, Social determinants of health

* Correspondence: makikonishi@hotmail.com
[1]Oral Health Services Research Centre, University College Cork, Wilton, Cork, Ireland
Full list of author information is available at the end of the article

Background

Dental caries has complex causes involving the interplay of host (saliva and teeth), microflora (plaque) and substrate (diet) factors [1]. A recent Japanese study of patients regarded to have a high interest in preventive dentistry revealed that knowledge among the public of these multiple factors is still lacking [2]; respondents were asked to identify caries risk factors/indicators from eight listed items (plus "Other") associated with these host, microflora, substrate factors and showed that the percentage of respondents identifying the caries risk factors/indicators correctly ranged from 2.0 to 36.8%. Since these respondents were considered to be more knowledgeable regarding caries prevention compared to the average Japanese person, this deficiency in knowledge of caries risk factors/indicators may be due to country-specific circumstances.

A prime example would be knowledge of fluoride; many studies have consistently shown a low level of knowledge about fluoride among the Japanese public [3, 4], although it has long been considered as the single most effective factor for the prevention of dental caries [5]. This may be attributed to the low availability over recent decades of fluoride-containing products in Japan compared to Western countries. Until 1994, only 46% of toothpaste on the Japanese market was fluoridated [6]; it was not until 2005 that this market share hit 88% [7]. On the other hand, the Republic of Ireland (RoI), which has a similar scale of per capita Gross Domestic Product (GDP) and health expenditure to Japan [8], has a long history of water fluoridation dating back to the 1960's [9]. Furthermore, the fluoridation debate in RoI involves the public and is quite active.

Despite having similar scales of per capita health expenditure, Japan and RoI have fundamentally different public policies on oral health. The Japanese health insurance system is universal health care that reimburses for sickness but not preventive care. In RoI, there are two dental treatment schemes: the Dental Treatment Benefit Scheme (DTBS) for employers and employees paying social insurance (Pay-Related Social Insurance (PRSI)) contributions and the Dental Treatment Services Scheme (DTSS) for medical-card holders who are means-tested. Both schemes pay for preventive care in the form of an annual oral examination in addition to covering some treatment costs. For medical card holders, treatment is limited to two fillings per calendar year, any extractions required and emergency dental treatment.

Cross-country comparisons allow us to inspect how differences in the social context of countries shape social determinants of health [10]. When comparing two countries with similar levels of economic development, such as Japan and RoI, the natural expectation is that the health-conscious population of one country would be more knowledgeable health-wise than the economically disadvantaged population of the second country. We hypothesise that there may be *unexpected* differences or similarities in knowledge between these two disparate groups across two economically similar countries. If our hypothesis holds, it becomes important to explore how a country's social/cultural profile shapes its social determinants of health and influences knowledge of caries risk. Understanding the influences on caries risk knowledge within a country is important for the development of effective and efficient strategies (especially population-based prevention strategies) for caries prevention.

The current paper aims to explore the knowledge of caries risk factors/indicators across two economically similar but culturally distinct countries by comparing two groups with different socio-economic profiles.

Methods

Two cross-sectional surveys were carried out, one in Japan, the other in RoI, using similar questionnaires on caries risk factors/indicators.

The Japanese study

The Japanese study targeted a population deemed to have a high interest in preventive dentistry, in order to investigate the current status of caries risk knowledge among potential opinion leaders [11] of personalised caries prevention programmes (i.e., based on each individual's caries risk assessment) [2]. Participants were patients of fee-paying dentist members of the nationwide web-based initiative *Promoting Scientific Assessment in Prevention of Tooth Decay and Gum Disease* (PSAP) [12], ≥20 years of age and not dental professionals (dentist, dental hygienist, dental assistant, dental technician). The PSAP, located in Tokyo, administered the Japanese study. Detailed data collection and data management procedures are described elsewhere [2]. All fee-paying dentist members of the PSAP were asked to distribute the paper questionnaires together with stamped, addressed (to the PSAP) return envelopes, to their patients on a first-come basis. The number of patient questionnaires issued to each PSAP dentist was limited to 20, as we did not wish to over-burden the dentists with the survey. A total of 2780 paper questionnaires were issued. Respondents who were dental professionals (dentist, dental hygienist, dental assistant, dental technician), <20 years of age or did not answer all socio-demographic factors (age, gender, whether dental professional or not) were excluded. Recruitment and questionnaire collection were conducted over a two-year period from May 2013 to May 2015. The ethics committee of the Japanese Society for Oral Health approved this study (No. 24–4).

The Irish study

The self-administered questionnaire survey was carried out on Irish adults aged 19–70 years who had 20 or more teeth as part of a randomised controlled clinical study among economically disadvantaged people. As a proxy for low socioeconomic status, we selected medical-card holders, who are entitled to free General Practitioner (GP) care and other services [13]. Medical-card eligibility is based on the applicant's financial means. Approximately four out of ten Irish people were covered by a medical card in 2014 [14]. Recruitment was through eight dental practitioners in Cork, RoI. A sample size of $n = 200$ (including dropouts) was calculated for the randomised controlled clinical study. At the baseline examination, the dentists distributed the paper questionnaire and 3-day food diary with a stamped addressed return envelope to their patient. The respondents posted their completed questionnaire and food diary to the Oral Health Services Research Centre (OHSRC). After assessing their baseline data (clinical examination and 3-day food diary), we sent a €20 voucher to each respondent as a gesture of thanks. The questionnaire was anonymous but contained the respondent's mobile phone number through which they could be identified; the food diary which was sent with the questionnaire contained the respondent's name and phone number. Those who were <20 years of age were excluded, in accordance with the age criteria of the Japanese study (≥20 years). Recruitment was carried out over seven months between February and September 2015. Collection of questionnaires continued until November 2015. Ethical approval was given by the Clinical Research Ethics Committee of the Cork Teaching Hospitals (ECM 4 (r) 12/08/14).

Questionnaires

To allow comparison between different cultures, the self-administered paper questionnaires for the two study groups contained similar questions. English language versions of the questionnaires are provided as additional files (see Additional files 1 and 2). The Japanese study questionnaire was developed first; it was pre-piloted in English, piloted in Japanese and then further refined after piloting [2]. Among the listed risk factors/indicators, 'Not visiting the dentist for a dental maintenance programme (check-ups and cleaning)' may be regarded as a controversial risk indicator, as some dentists continue to perform unnecessary restorative intervention to early caries lesions during or after a routine check-up [15]. This may be detrimental because repetitive restorations (the 'drill, fill and bill' philosophy) result in a shorter tooth life span [16]. Hence, the statement 'The more I visit the dentist for check-ups, the more teeth, I think, are drilled' was included in the Japanese study and respondents were asked whether they agreed or not. The Irish questionnaire included a similar but, in keeping with the Irish context, less explicitly worded statement; thus, to avoid misinterpretation, the current study excluded the Irish statement. "Low saliva buffering capacity" was simplified with non-technical language (Japanese study: *Low quality of saliva*; Irish study: *Having saliva (spit) that does not have the right composition to protect against decay*). For the sake of simplicity, the questionnaires avoided technical language in favour of layman's terms such as 'bad' or 'weak' even though such terminology might be prone to subjective interpretations. Translations between Japanese and English were carried out by MN (Japanese and English speaker) and VK (English speaker). Based on the Japanese study questionnaire written in English, three dentists (MN, MH and FA), one economist (VK) and the project manager developed the Irish study questionnaire and assessed its face validity. Regarding the Japanese study questionnaire, face validity was assessed by two non-dental Japanese speakers, one dental office worker and one dentist. Table 1 shows the corresponding questions in both study questionnaires analysed by this paper. Both studies were conducted according to the principles outlined in the Declaration of Helsinki. Respondents completed the questionnaires at home to avoid undue influence from the dental practice on their answers. All patients provided written informed consent.

Data analysis

Respondent characteristics including age, gender, age by gender and attendance for check-up and tooth cleaning were summarised for Japanese patients of PSAP dentists and for Irish medical-card patients from dental practices in Cork. We set two age groups (20–39, 40+ years), as the age distribution was different in the two studies. For the Japanese data, Stata's Survey data analysis method, with the dentist specified as the primary sampling unit (PSU), was employed to adjust standard errors used in the calculation of 95% confidence intervals (CIs) for intra-class correlation among responses from patients who attended the same dentist. This adjustment was not made to the 95% confidence intervals for the Irish data, due to the small number of dentists and low response level from patients of some dentists. Results are presented by age group for both study groups. Percentage frequencies and 95% CI's are given for the questions on knowledge of caries risk factors/indicators and for respondents choosing seven caries risk factors/indicators. Means and 95% CI's are presented for total number of identified risk factor/indicator excluding diet item(s). Percentage frequencies are shown for patients' opinions on the statement 'The more I visit the dentist for check-ups, the more teeth, I think, are drilled.' (in the Japanese study only).

The questions on diet were not included in the comparison analysis as these were framed differently in the two studies, and were compared between age groups

Table 1 Correspondence table of questions on caries risk/indicator knowledge and other items

Question category	Japanese study[a]		Irish study
Caries risk	Generally speaking, what do you think is (are) the reason(s) for susceptibility (risk) of getting tooth-decay? Please choose all that apply.	d	Generally speaking, which of the following do you think would increase the risk of developing dental decay? Please choose all that apply.
	Not brushing your teeth properly		Not brushing your teeth properly
	Bad eating habit	e	Consuming too much sugary foods and drinks
			Consuming sugary foods and drinks too often
			Consuming sugary foods and drinks just before bedtime
	Having naturally 'weak teeth'		Having naturally "weak teeth"
	Not visiting the dentist for a dental maintenance programme (check-ups and cleaning)	d	Not visiting the dentist for check-up and cleaning
	Not using fluoride		Not using fluoride
	Having particular bacteria in the mouth that contribute to the development of dental decay		Having particular bacteria in the mouth that contribute to the development of dental decay
	Low saliva flow rate	d	Having a reduced amount of saliva (spit) in the mouth
	Low quality of saliva[c]	d	Having saliva (spit) that does not have the right composition to protect against decay[c]
	Other (please specify):		Other (please specify):
Opinion	How strongly do you agree with these statements?		
	The more I visit the dentist for check-ups, the more teeth, I think, are drilled. (Strongly agree, Somewhat agree, Neither agree nor disagree, Somewhat disagree, Strongly disagree)		
Attendance for check-up and cleaning	Do you go to the dentist for a dental maintenance programme (check-ups and cleaning)? Yes, No		Do you go to the dentist for a dental maintenance programme (check-ups and cleaning)? Yes, No
Gender	Male, Female		Male, Female[b]
Age	19 or younger than 19, 20–29, 30–39, 40–49, 50–59, 60 or older than 60	d	Age at informed consent was calculated with the date of birth[b].
Dental professionals	Are you a dental professional (dentist, dental hygienist, dental assistant and dental technician)? Yes, No		

English language versions of the questionnaires are provided as additional files (see Additional files 1 and 2)
[a]The original questionnaire was in Japanese
[b]Information was derived from the case report form which the dentist filled in
[c]Wording used for low saliva buffering capacity
[d]The questions were slightly different between the Japanese and Irish studies
[e]The question was different between the Japanese and Irish studies

only. A logistic regression model was fitted to each of the binary variables of the risk indicators list common to both countries, with country, age and their interaction as predictors. A linear regression was fitted to the data with total number of identified risk factors/indicators excluding diet item(s) as dependent variable and country, age group and their interaction as predictors. A backward elimination process was performed for both types of regression until only significant terms remained in the model. An adjustment to standard errors was not made in these analyses due to the small number of dentists in the Irish study. The Mann-Whitney test was employed to compare ordinal responses between two age groups. Missing data were excluded from the analysis. We utilised the IBM SPSS Statistics Version 22 (SPSS Inc., Chicago, IL), R 3.2.3 (R Core Team, 2015 [17]) and the Survey Data Analysis procedure in Stata 12.1 (Stata Corp, College Station, TX). Two-sided significance level was set at 0.05, but the focus was on results showing a significance level less than 0.01, due to multiple testing.

Results

Characteristics of the samples

The paper questionnaires were distributed by 52 dentists in Japan and eight dentists in RoI (Table 2). For the Japanese study, it is unknown how many paper questionnaires out of 2780 issued by the PSAP were distributed by the PSAP dentists to their patients. In total, 482 questionnaires were returned and met the inclusion criteria (Fig. 1). For the Irish study, 191 questionnaires were distributed by the eight dentists; 159

Table 2 Number of dentists and respondents per dentist

		Japanese study	Irish study
Number of dentists		$n = 52$	$n = 8$
Respondents per dentist			
	min.	1	1
	avg.	9.3	19.9
	s.d.	5.1	26.5
	max.	18	83
Number of respondents		$n = 482$	$n = 159$
Gender (%)	Male	30.9	32.1
	Female	69.1	67.9
Age (%)	20–29	8.1	22.0
	30–39	19.9	33.3
	40–49	23.4	24.5
	50–59	19.7	13.2
	60+	28.8	6.9
Gender & Age			
Males		$n = 149$	$n = 51$
Age (%)	20–29	7.4	25.5
	30–39	16.8	25.5
	40–49	15.4	27.5
	50–59	22.8	15.7
	60+	37.6	5.9
Females		$n = 333$	$n = 108$
Age (%)	20–29	8.4	20.4
	30–39	21.3	37.0
	40–49	27.0	23.1
	50–59	18.3	12.0
	60+	24.9	7.4
Attendance for check-up and cleaning (%)		$n = 481$	$n = 156$
	Yes	91.5	69.2
	No	8.5	30.8

The table shows number of dentists and respondents per dentist; respondents by gender, age group and attendance for check-up and cleaning in the Japanese and Irish studies

were returned and met the inclusion criteria (Fig. 1). Gender distributions were similar between the Japanese and Irish studies: the male to female ratio was 3 to 7. Age distributions were rather different: the Irish study had more young respondents than the Japanese study. Check-up and tooth cleaning attendance in the Japanese study was quite high (91.5%) compared to the Irish study (69.2%).

Knowledge of caries risk factors/indicators

The results of fitting the binary logistic model to each of the risk factors/indicators are presented in Table 3. In both studies, common tendencies were observed: more than 90% in both age groups identified 'Not brushing your teeth properly'; saliva buffering capacity was the least identified caries risk factor. The major differences were that 'Not visiting the dentist for check-up and cleaning' (OR 2.655; 99% CI 1.550, 4.547; $p < 0.001$) and 'Not using fluoride' (OR 1.714; 99% CI 1.049, 2.802; $p = 0.005$) were identified more frequently by the medical-card patients in RoI than by the potential opinion leaders in Japan. 'Having a reduced amount of saliva (spit) in the mouth' (OR 0.262; 99% CI 0.159, 0.433; $p < 0.001$) was identified in the Japanese study much more frequently than in the Irish study.

Respondents had the opportunity to list other caries risk factors/indicators not included in the tick box options. In the Japanese study, heredity [18], smoking [19], crooked teeth [20] and caregivers at high caries risk [21] were listed under the 'Other' category and considered as correct and different from the listed alternatives. In the Irish study, smoking [19] and substance abuse [22] were specified under 'Other' and considered as correct risk factors. The percentages of respondents choosing seven items including "Other" with a correctly specified caries risk factor/indicator and excluding the diet items were higher in the younger age group (11.9%) than the older age group (9.8%) in the Japanese study. The Irish study showed the opposite tendency with the younger age group scoring lower (9.1%) and older age group higher (12.7%). The number of chosen caries risk factors/indicators was higher in the 20–39 age group (mean = 3.87, sd = 1.76) of the Japanese study and in the 40+ age group (mean = 3.71, sd = 1.62) of the Irish study (Table 4). The results of fitting the linear model to the variable *total number correct* showed that neither age nor country were associated with total number of identified risk factor/indicator excluding diet item(s) (Table 4).

Agreement with the statement on dental visit for check-up

Table 5 presents the percentage of Japanese respondents agreeing with the statement 'The more I visit the dentist for check-ups, the more teeth are drilled' by age group. Only a minority of respondents agreed with the statement (12.6% in the 20–39 age group; 9.9% in the 40+ age group). Number of respondents with missing data was 13; all 13 (100%) were in the 40+ age group, 11 (84.6%) were female and 11 (84.6%) attended for check-up and professional cleaning. The Mann-Whitney test showed that the ordinal responses to the statement were similar for younger (Median = 3) and older (Median = 3) age groups (U = 22593, $p = 0.969$).

Discussion

To the best of our knowledge, this is the first study to compare two populations from different countries on their knowledge of caries risk. It is a unique comparison,

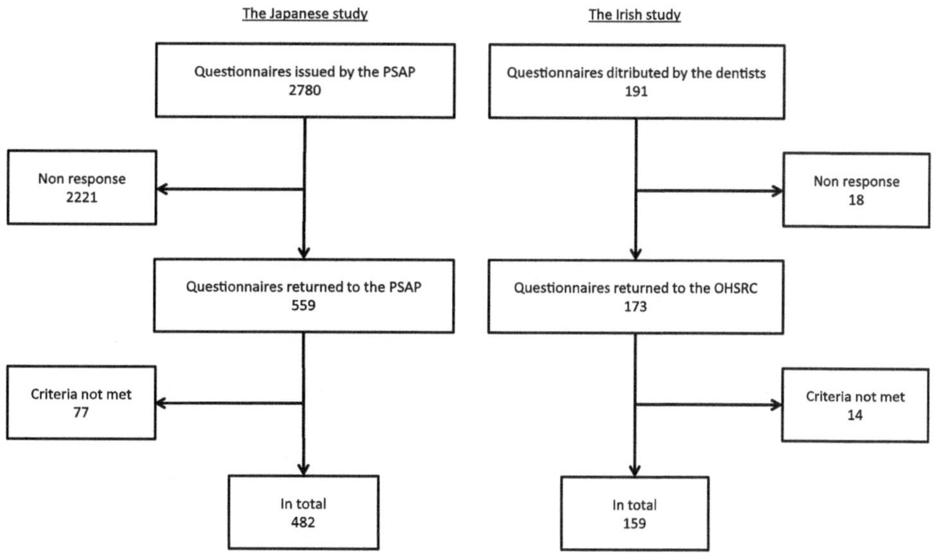

Fig. 1 Flow diagram showing numbers of patients at each stage of the Japanese and Irish studies. PSAP: Promoting Scientific Assessment in Prevention of Tooth Decay and Gum Disease. OHSRC: Oral Health Services Research Centre

as the responses were clearly different between the Japanese and Irish studies. The comparison revealed that the Japanese respondents, who were considered to have a high interest in preventive dentistry, did not always display more knowledge than the Irish respondents, who were considered to be of low socioeconomic status. In particular, the Japanese respondents identified 'Not visiting the dentist for check-up and tooth cleaning' and 'Not using fluoride' less frequently than the Irish respondents as caries risk factors/indicators. A clear reason for the great difference in the identification of dental visits for check-up and tooth cleaning as a caries risk indicator between the two studies is unknown. We checked if the Japanese respondents thought that visiting for check-ups and tooth cleaning might induce more teeth to be drilled but found that only approximately 10% of respondents agreed with the statement 'The more I visit the dentist for check-ups, the more teeth are drilled'.

A possible factor affecting the low identification of this risk factor in Japan is that the introduction of dental visits for check-up and tooth cleaning has been extremely slow in Japan, compared to the Western countries. A national survey reported that visits for dental check-up were only 1.6% of total dental visits in 2014 [23]. Another national survey reported that the uptake of check-up visits by patients during the past one year was 47.8% in 2012 [24], but probably included a simple check-up performed with other operative treatments. In both surveys, professional cleaning was not included. In the current paper, over 90% of the Japanese respondents attended for check-up and tooth cleaning. Nonetheless, they may not be aware that not receiving a check-up and tooth cleaning increases caries risk and may think that scaling (for preventing gum diseases) is the main procedure when attending for check-up and tooth cleaning.

In RoI, visiting the dentist for check-up and tooth cleaning became the norm earlier than in Japan. The earliest available survey [25] showed that in 1979, 20% of Irish adults were already visiting regularly for a check-up; the utilisation rate has since increased [26]. A topical discussion is not only how to increase utilisation, but also whether the common 'six-month' check-up for everyone is evidence-based or not [27]. In the current paper, approximately 70% of the Irish medical-card respondents received check-up and tooth cleaning. This is rather high compared to the average reported for medical-card holders by a national Irish survey (48.4% among 16–24 year olds, 54.2% among 35–44 year olds, 27.9% among 65+ year olds) [26], most likely because our participants were recruited through general dental practices and the national survey was conducted approximately 15 years ago. In addition, caution is necessary because dental practices and their patients in the current study were convenience samples.

It was expected that the Irish medical-card respondents might identify 'Not using fluoride' more frequently than the Japanese health-conscious respondents, because it has been found that the Japanese people, including dentists, are not aware of the significant role of fluoride for caries prevention [3, 4, 28], while RoI has a long history of water fluoridation [9] with on-going active public debates. The percentages of Japanese respondents identifying this item were approximately two-thirds of the Irish ones. However, it was surprising that only approximately 40% of the Irish

Table 3 Percentage (and 95% CI) of respondents from the Japanese and Irish studies identifying each risk factor/indicator[a]

Risk factor/indicator Age group	Yes response by country (%)				Odds ratio (99%CI)[b] Z, Significance level for terms in final model		
	Japanese study		Irish study		Country * Age interaction	Age	Country
Not brushing your teeth properly[c]					e	e	e
20–39	94.8	(89.1–97.6)	94.3	(87.2–98.1)			
40+	91.6	(87.9–94.3)	91.5	(82.5–96.8)			
All ages	92.5	(89.6–94.7)	93.1	(88.0–96.5)			
Bad eating habit[d]					N.A.	e	N.A.
20–39	65.2	(55.8–73.5)					
40+	60.8	(54.4–66.9)					
All ages	62.0	(56.3–67.4)					
Consuming too much sugary foods and drinks[d]					N.A.	e	N.A.
20–39			86.4	(77.4–92.8)			
40+			83.1	(72.3–91.0)			
All ages			84.9	(78.4–90.1)			
Consuming sugary foods and drinks too often[d]					N.A.	e	N.A.
20–39			77.3	(67.1–85.5)			
40+			84.5	(74.0–92.0)			
All ages			80.5	(73.5–86.4)			
Consuming sugary foods and drinks just before bedtime[d]					N.A.	2 (0.804–4.977)	N.A.
20–39			61.4	(50.4–71.6)		$Z = 1.96$	
40+			76.1	(64.5–85.4)		$P = 0.050$	
All ages			67.9	(60.1–75.1)			
Having naturally 'weak teeth'[c]					$Z = 2.18$	N.R.	N.R.
20–39	47.4	(39.0–56.0)	48.9	(38.1–59.8)	$P = 0.029$		
40+	59.9	(55.2–64.6)	40.8	(29.3–53.2)			
All ages	56.4	(51.7–61.0)	45.3	(37.4–53.4)			
Not visiting the dentist for check-up and cleaning[c]					e	e	2.655 (1.550–4.547)
20–39	50.4	(41.7–59.1)	75.0	(64.6–83.6)			$Z = 4.68$
40+	57.3	(51.6–62.9)	78.9	(67.6–87.7)			$P < 0.001$
All ages	55.4	(50.5–60.2)	76.7	(69.4–83.1)			
Not using fluoride[c]							
20–39	32.6	(22.2–45.1)	37.5	(27.4–48.5)	e	e	1.714 (1.049–2.802)
40+	26.5	(21.0–32.9)	43.7	(31.9–56.0)			$Z = 2.82$
All ages	28.2	(22.9–34.2)	40.3	(32.6–48.3)			$P = 0.005$
Having particular bacteria in the mouth that contribute to the development of dental decay[c]					e	e	e
20–39	60.0	(48.8–70.3)	46.6	(35.9–57.5)			
40+	46.4	(39.2–53.8)	49.3	(37.2–61.4)			
All ages	50.2	(43.0–57.4)	47.8	(39.8–55.9)			
Having a reduced amount of saliva (spit) in the mouth[c]					e	e	1.714 (0.159–0.433)
20–39	68.1	(57.8–77.0)	30.7	(21.3–41.4)			$Z = -6.88$
40+	62.8	(55.7–69.4)	33.8	(23.0–46.0)			$P < 0.001$
All ages	64.3	(58.4–69.8)	32.1	(24.9–39.9)			
Having saliva (spit) that does not have the right composition to protect against decay[c]					$Z = -2.42$	N.R.	N.R.

Table 3 Percentage (and 95% CI) of respondents from the Japanese and Irish studies identifying each risk factor/indicator[a] *(Continued)*

20–39	32.6	(24.5–41.9)	22.7	(14.5–32.9)	*P* = 0.016		
40+	24.5	(19.0–30.9)	35.2	(24.2–47.5)			
All ages	26.8	(21.7–32.6)	28.3	(21.5–36.0)			
% of subjects choosing 7 factors/indicators excluding diet item(s)[c]					e	e	e
20–39	11.9	(6.7–20.0)	9.1	(4.0–17.1)			
40+	9.8	(6.9–13.8)	12.7	(6.0–22.7)			
All ages	10.4	(7.6–14.0)	10.7	(6.4–16.6)			

The table includes percentage (and 95% CI) of respondents choosing seven factors/indicators excluding diet item(s) according to age groups
N.A not applicable; *N.R* not relevant when interaction term was significant, *e* eliminated from model due to non-significance
[a]The items were from the Irish study except "Bad eating habit"
[b]Odds ratio, reported for significant main effects in model and not for significant interactions
[c]Step1: full model fitted: Intercept + Age + Country + Country * Age; followed by backward elimination process
[d]Full model fitted: Intercept + Age

medical-card patients identified 'Not using fluoride' as a caries risk factor. It may be because the Irish population were medical-card patients, or/and because some of them interpret fluoride not as a 'risk factor' but as a 'beneficial factor'.

Cultural beliefs and attitudes have an influence on oral health and oral health disparities [29]. One vast difference between the Japanese and Irish culture is their native major religion – Shintoism vs. Christianity. The Japanese culture of cleanliness is partially rooted in their indigenous religion of Shintoism which equates cleanliness with purity [30]; this may account for their different hygiene behaviours compared with Christian countries like RoI. The deep-rooted Japanese belief in pursuing personal hygiene in daily life by themselves may be a reason for their delaying the introduction of dental check-ups and tooth cleaning by dental professionals and the use of fluoridated products.

Another noteworthy point is that among the Irish medical-card patients the percentages of those identifying 'Having a reduced amount of saliva (spit) in the mouth' were comparatively low in both age groups. This knowledge deficiency may present an obstacle to preventing dental caries, including root caries, when they are aged and xerostomia become common. It is not known whether this response was influenced by their lower socio-economic status or by some other country-specific factor; a further study is necessary to confirm the reason.

Common tendencies in both studies were tooth brushing being most frequently identified and saliva buffering capacity being least frequently identified as caries risk factors. In spite of the differing cultural backgrounds and socioeconomic characteristics between the groups, this study reveals a persistent belief in tooth brushing as a means to reduce caries risk, despite the fact that the caries-reducing effect of tooth brushing and other self-administrated oral hygiene interventions per se (without fluoride) is doubtful [31]. In addition, this study shows that saliva's defensive role against caries is not well known.

Although the three breakdown questions on diet (too much sugary diet, too often sugary diet, sugary diet before bedtime) were asked only in the Irish study, the results give insight into public knowledge regarding substrate (diet) factors for caries prevention among this population. The respondents least frequently identified 'Consuming sugary foods and drinks just before bedtime' as a factor increasing caries risk. Considering this result with the low percentages identifying saliva as a risk factor, it would appear that the respondents have little awareness of the full mechanism behind caries development. They may also believe that brushing teeth after consuming sugary foods and drinks before bedtime is

Table 4 Average (and 95% CI) and standard deviation of the number of identified caries risk factor/indicator

Age group	Japanese study			Irish study			Z, Significance level for terms in final model[a]		
	Average	(95% CI)	sd	Average	(95% CI)	sd	Country* Age interaction	Age	Country
20–39	3.87	(3.44–4.31)	1.76	3.58	(3.20–3.96)	1.79	e	e	e
40+	3.71	(3.54–3.88)	1.62	3.76	(3.30–4.22)	1.95			
All ages	3.75	(3.56–3.95)	1.66	3.66	(3.37–3.95)	1.86			

The results were calculated excluding diet item(s) by age group
e: eliminated from model due to non-significance
[a]Full model: Intercept + Age + Country + Country *Age

Table 5 Percentage of Japanese respondents agreeing with the statement by age group ($n = 469$)

Statement	Age group 20–39	40+	All ages
The more I visit the dentist for check-ups, the more teeth, I think, are drilled.			
Strongly/Somewhat agree	12.6	9.9	10.7
Neither agree nor disagree	41.5	45.5	44.3
Strongly/Somewhat disagree	45.9	44.6	45.0

sufficient to prevent tooth decay. Efforts to reduce intake of sugary foods and drinks before bedtime may also have the potential to impact general health under the common risk factor approach [32, 33].

The limitations of the current paper relate to differences in the methodology between the surveys and include: sample representativeness, differences in questionnaire content and remuneration of participants in the Irish study and not the Japanese. In particular, the PSAP was the only source of recruitment in the Japanese study and one dentist recruited more than half of the patients in the Irish study. Therefore, generalisation of the findings is restricted. However, this study illustrates the value of inter-cultural comparison in exploring knowledge and attitudes to risk factors and oral health. The study provides useful new insights worthy of further exploration.

Conclusions

For the risk factors/indicators 'Not visiting the dentist for check-up and cleaning' and 'Not using fluoride', a lower proportion of respondents identified these factors in the Japan study than in the Irish study, indicating that country differences had a stronger influence on patients' knowledge than socio-economic differences. 'Having a reduced amount of saliva (spit) in the mouth' was less known as a caries risk factor among the Irish group. Understanding the influence of a population's social/cultural profile on knowledge deficiency of caries risk is important, particularly when designing programmes to enhance patients' knowledge. Furthermore, persistent belief in tooth brushing for caries prevention and lack of knowledge about saliva buffering capacity were similar tendencies in both study groups despite their different cultural and socioeconomic backgrounds. This implies that there is a general need to inform patients of the defensive role of saliva in both groups from both countries.

Abbreviations

CI: Confidence interval; DTBS: Dental Treatment Benefit Scheme; DTSS: Dental Treatment Services Scheme; GDP: Gross Domestic Product; GP: General Practitioner; IADR: International Association for Dental Research; OHSRC: Oral Health Services Research Centre; OR: Odds ratio; PRSI: Pay-related social insurance; PSAP: Promoting Scientific Assessment in Prevention of Tooth Decay and Gum Disease; PSU: Primary sampling unit; RoI: Republic of Ireland

Acknowledgements

The authors express their thanks to Ms Margaret Cole, Professor Emeritus Denis O'Mullane, Dr Takashi Kumagai, the eight participant Irish dentists, the administrative staff of the PSAP and the staff of the OHSRC.

Funding

The Japanese study was supported by the PSAP. The Irish study was supported by the International Association for Dental Research (IADR) Unilever Social Entrepreneur Approach to Change Oral Health Behaviour Research Award. These two funding bodies did not play any role in the design of the study and collection, analysis, and interpretation of data and in writing the manuscript.

Authors' contributions

For both the Japanese and Irish studies, MN contributed to conception of the studies and acquisition of data. MN and VK contributed to design of both studies, and drafted and finalised the manuscript. HW contributed to design of the Japanese study. MH and FA contributed to design of the Irish study. All authors contributed to analysis and interpretation of data and revising the manuscript critically for important intellectual content. All authors have approved the final version and agreed to be accountable for all aspects of the work.

Competing interests

MN is the chairperson of the board of the PSAP.

Consent for publication

Not applicable.

Ethics approval and consent to participate

The Japanese study was approved by the ethics committee of the Japanese Society for Oral Health (No. 24-4). For the Irish study, ethical approval was given by the Clinical Research Ethics Committee of the Cork Teaching Hospitals (ECM 4 (r) 12/08/14). All patients were informed about the survey and provided written informed consent.

Author details

[1]Oral Health Services Research Centre, University College Cork, Wilton, Cork, Ireland. [2]The School of Dentistry, University of Leeds, Leeds, UK. [3]Faculty of Dentistry, National University of Singapore, Singapore, Republic of Singapore.

References

1. Reich E, Lussi A, Newbrun E. Caries-risk assessment. Int Dent J. 1999;49:15–26.
2. Nishi M, Kumagai T, Whelton H. Access to personalised caries prevention (PCP) programmes was determined by their dentists: a cross-sectional study of current and potential PCP adopters in Japan and their knowledge of caries risk. J Dent Health. 2016;66:399–407.
3. Tsurumoto A, Wright FA, Kitamura T, Fukushima M, Campain AC, Morgan MV. Cross-cultural comparison of attitudes and opinions on fluorides and fluoridation between Australia and Japan. Community Dent Oral Epidemiol. 1998;26:182–93.
4. Hirose M, Murata Y, Fukuda A, Murai Y, Ohoka R, Yahata S, Mizugai H, Igarashi S. Attitudes of elementary and junior high-school students' parents about prevention of dental caries in Shinshinotsu village, Ishikari County, Hokkaido. Jpn J Dent Health. 2011;61:301–9 (In Japanese).

5. ten Cate JM. Contemporary perspective on the use of fluoride products in caries prevention. Br Dent J. 2013;214:161–7.
6. Hashizume LN, Lima YB, Kawaguchi Y, Cury JA. Fluoride availability and stability of Japanese dentifrices. J Oral Sci. 2003;45:193–9.
7. Gunji A, Tamura Y, Hirao K, Machida H, Akita W, Kobayashi N, Fujii A. Recent knowledge of fluoride application for the prevention of caries: focusing on fluoride mouth rinsing. Oral Ther Pharmacol. 2010;29:1–8 (In Japanese).
8. The World Bank: World Bank Open Data. http://data.worldbank.org. Accessed 12 Jan 2017.
9. Clarkson J, McLoughlin J, O'Hickey S. Water fluoridation in Ireland—a success story. J Dent Res. 2003;82:334–7.
10. Prus SG. Comparing social determinants of self-rated health across the United States and Canada. Soc Sci Med. 2011;73:50–9.
11. Flodgren G, Parmelli E, Doumit G, Gattellari M, O'Brien MA, Grimshaw J, Eccles MP. Local opinion leaders: effects on professional practice and health care outcomes. Cochrane Database Syst Rev. 2011;8:CD000125.
12. Promoting Scientific Assessment in Prevention of Tooth Decay and Gum Disease: Hahaha Talk. http://www.honto-no-yobou.jp. Accessed 12 Jan 2017 (In Japanese).
13. The Citizens Information Board: Medical cards. http://www.citizensinformation.ie/en/health/medical_cards_and_gp_visit_cards/medical_card.html. Accessed 12 Jan 2017.
14. Health Service Executive. Primary care reimbursement service. In: Annual report and financial statements 2014. HSE. 2015. https://www.hse.ie/eng/services/publications/corporate/annualreport14.pdf. Accessed 12 Jan 2017.
15. Baelum V, Sheiham A, Burt B. Caries control for populations. In: Fejerskov O, Kidd E, editors. Dental caries: the disease and its clinical management. 2nd ed. Oxford: Wiley-Blackwell; 2008. p. 505–26.
16. Elderton RJ. Preventive (evidence-based) approach to quality general dental care. Med Princ Pract. 2003;12 Suppl 1:12–21.
17. The R Core Team: A language and environment for statistical computing. https://www.r-project.org. Accessed 12 Jan 2017.
18. Vieira AR, Modesto A, Marazita ML. Caries: review of human genetics research. Caries Res. 2014;48:491–506.
19. Benedetti G, Campus G, Strohmenger L, Lingström P. Tobacco and dental caries: a systematic review. Acta Odontol Scand. 2013;71:363–71.
20. Hafez HS, Shaarawy SM, Al-Sakiti AA, Mostafa YA. Dental crowding as a caries risk factor: a systematic review. Am J Orthod Dentofacial Orthop. 2012;142:443–50.
21. Krol DM. Dental caries, oral health, and pediatricians. Curr Probl Pediatr Adolesc Health Care. 2003;33:253–70.
22. Hamamoto DT, Rhodus NL. Methamphetamine abuse and dentistry. Oral Dis. 2009;15:27–37.
23. Ministry of Health Labour and Welfare: Patient survey. http://www.mhlw.go.jp/toukei/list/10-20.html. Accessed 12 Jan 2017 (In Japanese).
24. Ministry of Health Labour and Welfare. Status of dental check-up. In: The National Health and Nutrition Survey Japan, 2012. MHLW. 2014. http://www.mhlw.go.jp/bunya/kenkou/eiyou/dl/h24-houkoku.pdf. Accessed 12 Jan 2017 (In Japanese).
25. Clarkson JJ, O'Mullane DM. Edentulousness in the United Kingdom and Ireland. Community Dent Oral Epidemiol. 1983;11:317–20.
26. Guiney H, Woods N, Whelton H, O'Mullane D. Non-biological factors associated with tooth retention in Irish adults. Community Dent Health. 2011;28:53–9.
27. Riley P, Worthington HV, Clarkson JE, Beirne PV. Recall intervals for oral health in primary care patients. Cochrane Database Syst Rev. 2013;12:CD004346.
28. Kakudate N, Sumida F, Matsumoto Y, Yokoyama Y, Riley JL, Gilbert GH, Gordan VV. Dentists' decisions to conduct caries risk assessment in a Dental Practice-Based Research Network. Community Dent Oral Epidemiol. 2015;43:128–34.
29. Patrick DL, Lee RS, Nucci M, Grembowski D, Jolles CZ, Milgrom P. Reducing oral health disparities: a focus on social and cultural determinants. BMC Oral Health. 2006;6 Suppl 1:S4.
30. Horiuchi S. Major causes of the rapid longevity extension in postwar Japan. Jpn J Popul. 2011;9:162–71.
31. Selwitz RH, Ismail AI, Pitts NB. Dental caries. Lancet. 2007;369:51–9.
32. Kinsey AW, Ormsbee MJ. The health impact of nighttime eating: old and new perspectives. Nutrients. 2015;7:2648–62.
33. Watt RG, Sheiham A. Integrating the common risk factor approach into a social determinants framework. Community Dent Oral Epidemiol. 2012;40:289–96.

Effect of removable functional appliances on mandibular length in patients with class II with retrognathism

Adriana Santamaría-Villegas[1], Rubén Manrique-Hernandez[2], Emery Alvarez-Varela[2] and Claudia Restrepo-Serna[1*]

Abstract

Background: Orthopedic functional devices, are used to improve mandibular length in skeletal class II patients. However, the orthopedic functional device with the best effect to increasing the mandibular length, has not been identified before. Thus, the aim of the present investigation was to evaluate Randomized Controlled Trials (RCT), to determine the best functional appliance improving mandibular length in subjects with retrognathism.

Methods: A systematic review and meta-analysis was performed, including studies published and indexed in databases between 1966 and 2016. RCTs evaluating functional appliances' effects on mandibular length (Condilion-Gnation (Co-Gn) and Condilion-Pogonion (Co-Po)), were included. Reports' structure was evaluated according to 2010 CONSORT guide. The outcome measure was distance between Co-Gn and/or Co-Po after treatment. Data were analyzed with Cochran Q Test and random effects model.

Results: Five studies were included in the meta-analysis. The overall difference in mandibular length was 1.53 mm (Confidence Interval (CI) 95% 1.15–1.92) in comparison to non-treated group. The Sander Bite Jumping reported the greatest increase in mandibular length (3.40 mm; CI 95% 1.69–5.11), followed by Twin Block, Bionator, Harvold Activator and Frankel devices.

Conclusions: All removable functional appliances, aiming to increase mandibular length, are useful. Sander Bite Jumping was observed to be the most effective device to improve the mandibular length.

Keywords: Malocclusion, Angle class II, Retrognathia, Meta-analysis, Orthodontics appliances, Functional

Background

The main reason for using functional removable appliances is to establish muscular balance, eliminate oral dysfunction, and allow a proper length of both the maxilla and the mandible [1]. Several studies have been performed in order to evaluate with different methods, the morphogenic mandibular changes, associated with the use of functional appliances to propulse forward the mandible. Frankel [2, 3], Bionator [4], Bass appliance [5], Herbst [6], Sander Bite Jumping [7], among others; could be found in the literature for this purpose. Individually, many studies have found changes in mandibular length and position, both in the sagittal and vertical plane [2–7]. However, when studies are grouped and analyzed together in systematic reviews and meta-analysis, controversies appear. Some reviews have found no statistically or clinically significant differences between groups treated with functional appliances and controls [8], while other authors have observed those differences to be statistically significant [9]. Additionally, studies have found other results for the treatment with functional appliances, such as secondary statistically significant mandibular elongation [10] and changes in the facial profile, due to incisal inclination [11].

* Correspondence: crestrepo@ces.edu.co
[1]CES-LPH Research Group, Universidad CES, Calle 10A. No. 22-04, Medellín, Colombia
Full list of author information is available at the end of the article

Notwithstanding these results, differentiation of the effects of each type of functional device has not been assessed before. Only the SR published by Cozza et al. [8], evaluated the effect of different appliances on mandibular length. However, they included the Herbst appliance, even when its functional effects are different, due to its fixed mechanism of action. The combination of removable and fixed appliances in the systematic review, hampers a true interpretation of the results.

Due to the above explained premises, the purpose of this study was to evaluate the available scientific evidence in exclusively Randomized Controlled Trials (RCT), regarding the efficacy of each functional appliance found in the literature in improving mandibular length in subjects with class II malocclusion due to retrognathism.

Methods

This SR was conducted in accordance with the guidelines of Transparent Reporting of Systematic Reviews and Meta-analyses (PRISMA-statement) (http://prisma-statement.org/) [12]. The protocol detailing the review method was developed "a priori" following initial discussion between members of the research team.

Ethics and consent statement

Not applicable.

Focused question

In patients with class II skeletal malocclusion, due to retrognathism; which of the different orthopedic functional devices, has the best effect aiming to improve the mandibular length?

Search strategy and literature selection

On 12 January 2016, a systematic search of the medical literature was performed to identify all peer reviewed papers in the English and Spanish literature dealing with the efficacy of the functional appliances in improving mandibular length according to the search strategy described below. Inclusion in the review was based on the type of study, viz., RCTs describing the efficacy of functional appliances in improving mandibular length in children by the adoption of cephalometric measurements. Only those studies assessing the efficacy of removable functional appliances in participants between 6 and 18 years of age were included. In the case of investigations including samples of subjects aged under 6 or over 18, the studies were included in the review only if the children's data could be extracted from the total sample. Studies performed on selected populations that combined fixed orthodontics or appliances with removable functional appliances, were excluded. All search steps and quality assessments were performed by a single author and then carefully checked by all the other authors to minimize bias during the review process. In case of disagreement, decision was reached by consensus of the majority of authors.

As a first step, a search in the National Library of Medicine's PubMed Database, Cochrane, EMBASE and Lilacs databases was performed using the combination of the keyword terms (MeSH when applicable); malocclusion, angle class II, retrognathia, adolescent, child, orthodontic appliances and functional appliances were used to identify a list of potential papers to be included in the review. The search limits were set to papers in English or Spanish language, studies in humans, randomized clinical trial and dates of publication between years 1960 and 2016. From the list of citations, papers were screened on the basis of their title, and those ones clearly not pertinent to this review's aim were excluded. The remaining citations were selected for abstract reading, and those which were of potential interest for this review, based on their abstract contents, were retrieved in full text. Then, the retrieved papers were read to decide on their inclusion/exclusion in the review. As further steps to expand the search, the Scopus and Google Scholar databases and four journal Publishers' website search engines (Elsevier; Wiley-Blackwell; Quintessence Publishing; and Springer) were screened for additional papers of interest. Also, a search within the reference lists of the selected articles, a handmade search within relevant English and Spanish language peer reviewed journals in the pediatric dentistry and orthodontics fields, as well as within Universidad CES electronic library catalogues were performed.

This systematic review was registered in the international Prospective Register of Systematic Review (PROSPERO), registration number CRD42012002858. www.crd.york.ac.uk/prospero/ [Internet]. [cited 2012 sep 4].

Quality assessment

Prior to evaluate the quality of each study, its structure of report was reviewed based on the 2010 CONSORT guidelines for RCT studies [13]. In this review, all items were assessed with respect to the effects of different functional appliances on the length of the mandible, according to the measurements Co-Gn and/or Co-Po. The methodological quality of the included studies was assessed according to the Cochrane systematic review guidelines and recommendations [14–16], and verified with the PRISMA checklist (Transparent Reporting of Systematic Review and Meta-Analyses) [12]. The cut-off criteria for selection of studies are contained in Table 1.

Appraisal of external validity was made according to the following checklist: (i) Sampling of subjects and assessment of sampling bias (i.e., failure to ensure that all

Table 1 Inclusion and exclusion criteria

Inclusion Criteria	Exclusion Criteria
Control group with untreated class II subjects. Treatment group: Patients with Class II malocclusion by retrognathism treated with any of the following appliances: Bionator, Twin Block, Activator, Sander Bite Jumping or Frankel.	Studies which evaluated mandibular length with point Ar.
Minimum 6 months in treatment.	Studies evaluating outcomes with MRI.
Articles in English or Spanish.	Studies which utilized the Herbst appliance. Insufficient data for analysis
Studies in humans	Treatment combined with extractions.
Studies in growing patients (aged between 6 and 18 years old).	Treatment combined with fixed appliances.
Studies evaluated with cephalometric radiographs that included mandibular length measurements using Co-Gn, Co-Po.	Surgical treatment
Randomized clinical trials (RCT) studies	

members of the reference population have a known chance to be recruited in the study sample), (ii) description of mechanism for patient selection, (iii) Exclusion rate and withdrawals of patients for analysis. Appraisal of internal validity provides an assessment of: (i) adequate statistical analysis, (ii) description of control for confusing variables, (iii) blindness for the evaluation of results and (iv) the use of p values or confidence intervals to accompany the effect of the estimation measure. Each criterion was given a value of 1 when accomplished and 0 when failed. The quality of the studies was classified according to the sum of the scores in each criterion. Studies were rated as low (score less than 4), medium (scores between 4 and 5) and high (scores greater than 5).

Data recorded from the selected studies

For each of the included studies, the following data/information were recorded: size and demographic features of the sample [age range (years), gender distribution (% of females)]; type of functional appliance used; duration of treatment (months), and cephalometric points used to measure mandibular length (Co-Gn or Co-Po).

Statistical analysis

Statistical analysis was performed in order to estimate the pooled effect of the different functional appliances on the length of the mandible (Co-Gn or Co-Po), expressed as differences between treatment and control groups, regarding the mean mandibular length, calculated in millimeters.

The heterogeneity analysis between studies was performed with the Q Cochran Test [17, 18] using a critical value of $p < 0.05$, with the objective of determining the model of analysis by fixed or random effects.

Given that in all included studies, mandibular length was measured using the distance in millimeters between Co-Gn and Co–Po, the pooled effect combined was calculated as a weighted mean difference [18].

Due to the high quality of the study reported by Obrien et al. in 2003 [19], and that they reported the mean of length in the treatment and control group with the respective confidence interval; the standard deviation (SD) of the present meta-analysis, was calculated using the standard error of the mean sample of that study.

Availability of data and materials

As this investigation is a Systematic Review and Meta-analysis, the data supporting the findings are available in the databases PubMed, Cochrane, EMBASE and Lilacs. The full-text of the articles were obtained in "Fundadores" library and the available electronic resources of Universidad CES.

Results

Literature search

The Medline, Cochrane, Embase and Lilacs databases search allowed identifying 50 publications, of which ten were excluded on the basis of title screening. Another 33 citations were excluded after abstract reading based on different reasons (i.e. measurements in the investigation didn't include Co-Gn or Co-Po ($n = 13$); include only facial measurements ($n = 5$), control group was lacking ($n = 5$), measurements were based on superimposition of images ($n = 1$), measurements were based on changes on the implant placement ($n = 2$), studies evaluating psychosocial features ($n = 2$), control trials not randomized ($n = 1$), use of fixed appliances ($n = 1$), combination of extra-oral devices and functional appliances ($n = 2$) and results based on cranial base results ($n = 1$)). Seven papers were selected for full-text retrieval.

Full-text reading allowed excluding two more papers, because they did not fullfill the inclusion criteria due to one main reason, viz., there was no random allocation of the control group. Sample was selected by convenience [20, 21]. Search expansion strategy retrieve no more citations. Hence, a total of five publications were found to be relevant to this meta-analysis assessment's aim [7, 19,

22–24]. See Fig. 1 for a flowchart of the literature selection procedure.

Methods of the included studies

An analysis of the methodological quality of the studies with the established criteria by the authors, indicated that two studies had a medium score [23, 24] and the other three [7, 19, 22] were classified as high quality.

The most frequent observed flaw, was that all studies lack of criteria for blindness for evaluation of results. Overall, studies presented acceptable samples sizes for identifying significant differences and sample selection criteria were reported in most of the studies. The four studies that reported the most adequate sample size calculation and inclusion and exclusion criteria, obtained the highest methodological score [7, 19, 22, 24]. One study reported withdrawals between 1% and 16% [22]. The article reported them adequately.

All studies presented suitable report of methods and statistical used to detect and analyze the effect of the intervention. Most of them used the error analysis method for radiographic measurements. Some studies reported the results with confidence intervals (CI) while others reported p values (Tables 2 and 3).

Treatment modalities

Regarding treatment modalities, Harvold Activator was used in one study [22], Twin Block in two studies [19, 22], type II Bionator was evaluated in two studies [23, 24], Frankel in one study [22] and Sander Bite Jumping in one study [7]. These data explain the fact that there are more comparisons than studies in the meta-analysis graphs.

Under the fixed effects model, the effect of functional appliances revealed a statistically significant increase in mandibular length measured as the distance between points Co-Gna or Co-Po (Fig. 2), with a difference in average mandibular length of 1.53 mm (CI 95% 1.15–1.92) with respect to non-treated control groups.

With respect to the efficacy of functional appliances, the Sander Bite Jumping reported the greatest increase in total mandibular length (3.40 mm; CI 95% 1.69–5.11), in comparison with other appliances which included, Twin Block (1.80 mm; CI 95% 0.87–2.73), Bionator (1.41 mm; CI 95% 0.94–1.89), Harvold Activator

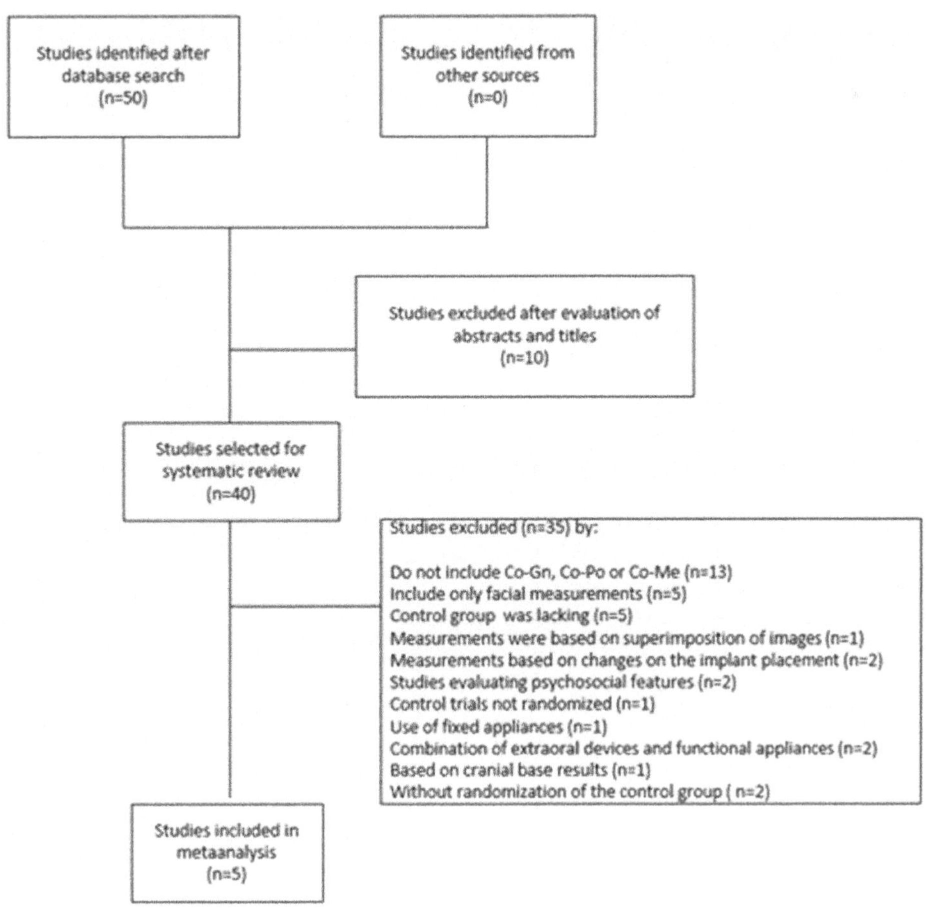

Fig. 1 PRISMA Flowdiagram

Table 2 Included studies

Appliance: sample/ age (years)	Year of publication	Type of study	Measurement method	Type of Appliance	Duration of treatment	Cephalometric points for mandibular changes	Timing of treatment	Maturation analysis and method	Results conclusions of author
Tulloch [23]									
Bionator: 53 /9.4	1997	RCT	CXR[a]	Bionator	15 months	Mandibular length Co-Gn/Co-Pg+ (mm)	1 year before of peak	Carpal	Functional appliances produce mandibular changes with great variation
Control: 61/9.4					15 months				
Martina [7]									
Sander Bite Jumping: 23/10.9	2013	RCT	CXR[a]	Sander Bite Jumping	18 months	Mandibular length (Pg/ OLp+ Co/OLp)	NA[b]	Cervical vertebrae	Treated individuals had a significant increase in mandibular length and molar relationship improvement
Control: 23/10.5					12 months	Mandibular length (Pg/ OLp + Co/OLp)			
Illing [24]									
Twin block: 16/ 11.5	1998	RCT	CXR[a]	Twin Block	9 months	NA[b]	NA[b]	NA[b]	Both appliances demonstrated significant skeletal changes.
Bionator: 18/11.8				Bionator	9 months	Co-Gna(mm)			
Control: 20 /11.2					9 months	NA[b]			
Nelson [22]									
Harvold Activator: 12 /13	1993	RCT	CXR[a]	Classic activator	18 months	Co-Pog (mm)	NA[b]	NA[b]	No evidence supporting that functional appliances alter mandibular
Frankel: 13/13				Frankel	18 months	Co-Pog (mm)			
Control: 17 /13					18 months				
O Brien [19]									
Twin block: 73/9.7	2003	RCT	CXR[a]	Twin block	15 months	Mandibular length (Pg/ OLp + Co/OLp)	Pre-peak	NA[b]	The Twin-block appliance resulted in substantial reduction in the overjets of children with Class II malocclusion.
Control: 74/9.8					15 months	(Pg/OLp + Co/OLp)			

+Measurement not clear in the text
[a]Cephalographic X-ray
[b]Information not available

Table 3 Quality of studies

RCT Studies	Explanation of calculation of sample size	Description of mechanism for patient selection	Explanation of the causes for withdrawal of patients	Statistical analysis adequate to the type of data	Description of the control for confusing factors	Blindness for the evaluation of results	Use of p values or confidence intervals	Evaluation of quality
Nelson 1993 [22]	yes	yes	Yes	yes	yes	no	Yes	High
Tulloch 1997 [23]	yes	yes	No	yes	yes	no	yes	Medium
Illing 1998 [24]	no	yes	Yes	yes	yes	no	yes	medium
O Brien 2003 [19]	yes	yes	Yes	yes	yes	no	yes	high
Martina 2013 [7]	yes	yes	Yes	yes	yes	no	yes	high

RCT Randomized clinical trial

(1.32 mm; CI 95% −0.42–3.06) and Frankel (0.69 mm; CI 95% −0.84–2.22) (Fig. 3), although there were overlapping of the confidence intervals of the effects of Sander Bite Jumping, Twin Block and Bionator.

Discussion

The use of removable functional orthopedic appliances in growing individuals with skeletal Class II, has demonstrated to be effective for the treatment of Class II malocclusion [2, 3, 6, 7, 25]. However, the evidence presents lack of consistency regarding the results shown both in studies [2, 3, 6, 7, 25] and systematic reviews [10, 11]. Additionally, a reliable differentiation of the effects produced by each type of functional appliance, has not been assessed before. Based on these premises, this systematic review evaluated the available scientific evidence in exclusively RCT, aiming to determine the efficacy of each type of functional appliance in improving mandibular length in subjects with class II malocclusion due to retrognathism. The five included investigations were analyzed in order to accomplish the objective.

All the studies included in this systematic review, are RCT. RCTs are the most rigorous way of determining whether a cause-effect relation exists between treatment and outcome and for assessing the cost effectiveness of a treatment, in this case different removable functional appliances. Other study designs, including non-randomized controlled trials, can detect only associations between an intervention and an outcome, but are not able to determine if the association was caused by a third factor linked to both intervention and/or outcome [26]. When these types of studies are included in systematic reviews, aiming to test the effect of a specific treatment (viz., the effects of orthopedic devices in increasing mandibular length), a true interpretation of the results is not possible.

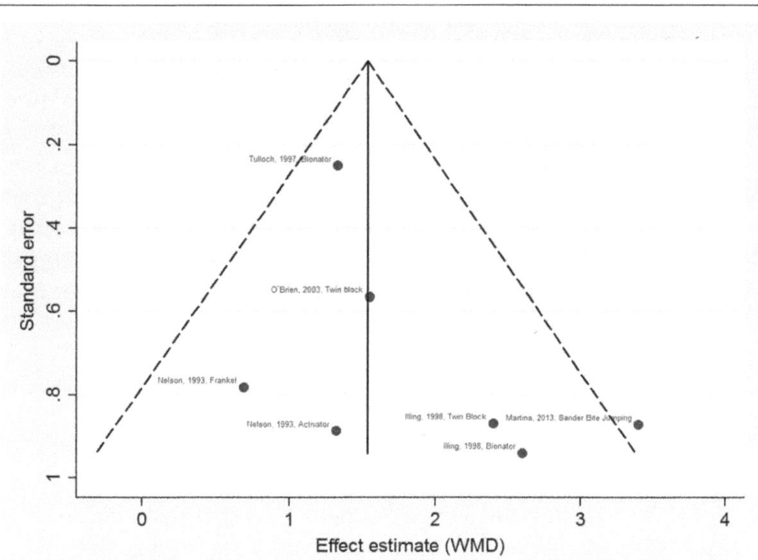

Fig. 2 Funnel diagram of included studies. The funnel plot does not show the existence of publication bias among the included studies

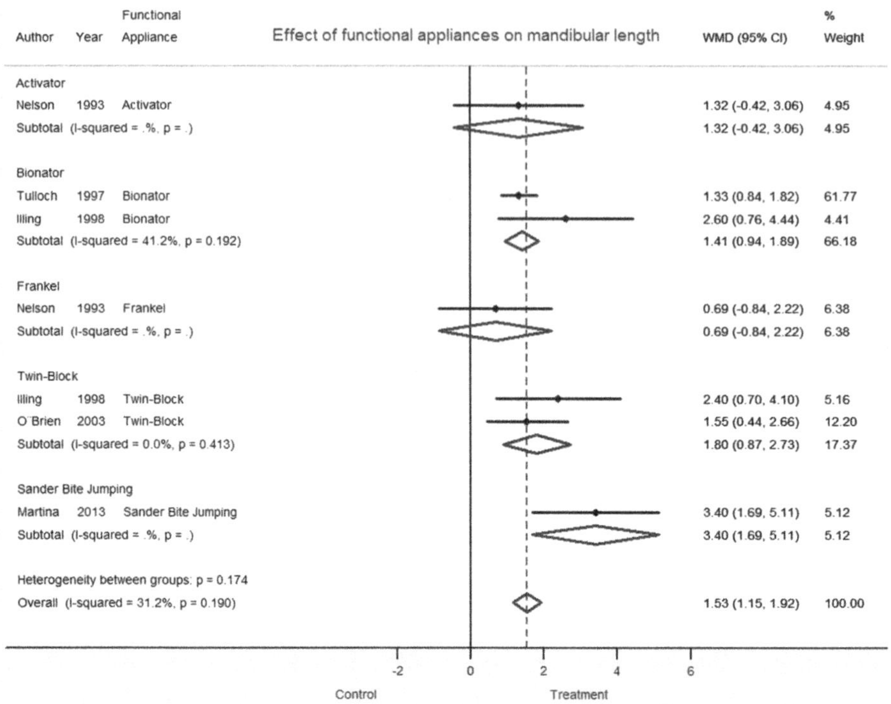

Fig. 3 Effect of functional appliances on mandibular length depending on type of appliance. *WMD* weighted mean difference, *CI* confidence interval 95%

Efforts were made in this investigation to increase the confidence of the results. Treatments which included teeth extractions, were excluded from the sample of this meta-analysis. The reason was that extraction of teeth, compensate the facial and skeletal profile [27]. Thus, is a confounding variable that could have interfered in our purpose of evaluating the effect of removable functional appliances in the increase-to-increase mandibular length.

The most common method to analyze mandibular length in the clinic, is the lateral cephalogram [11]. Actually, linear measurements of mandibular length have been observed to have high reproducibility between different times of measurement [28]. However, the main limitation to compare the measurements of mandibular length among the different studies, is that there is not consistency of measurement. Due to the above reasons, only the RCTs that used measurements in millimeters between Co-Gn and/or Co- Po were included, reducing the potential risk of measurement bias. As a strength of selecting specific points to evaluate the mandibular length, the combined estimate of the effect through weighting, was possible to be calculated. A previous systematic review used this method in order to assess the mandibular length after the use of orthopedic appliances, without determing the effect of each type of appliance [11].

The increase in mandibular length was greatest with the Sander Bite Jumping, followed by Twin Block, Bionator, and Harvold Activator, while the appliance that presented the least variation, was the Frankel. Assuming equal variances, the obtained error was so small to influence the combined estimation of the effect. These results contrast with those reported by Cozza et al. in 2006 [8], who found that the appliance giving the greatest variations was the Herbst followed by the Twin Block. The functional mechanism of action of the Herbst appliance is different from the mechanism of action of the removable functional appliances. Herbst is a fixed appliance, which promotes redirecting of maxillary growth, mesial movement of mandibular teeth and distal movement of maxillary teeth [29]. The different mechanism of action used by Herbst and the removable functional appliances, impedes a true comparison between them.

Clinical success cannot be measured only by mandibular length. Other factors should be considered, such as facial outcomes, solution of parafunctional oral habits and functional changes. This is a limitation not only of this review, but of almost all studies that evaluate treatment for mandibular propulsion. Two more limitations rised; first the studies by Nelson et al. [22], Tulloch et al. [23] and Martina et al. [7], describe the technique of taking the lateral cephalic x-ray in intercuspal position. The remaining studies (O'Brien et al. [19] and Illing et al. [24]), are not clear regarding the mouth position when taking the lateral cephalograms. However, in this systematic review and meta-analysis, we aimed to measure mandibular length, which is not affected by the position of the mandible in the cephalogram. Despite the technique to take the lateral cephalogram with mouth opening or intercuspal position, the measurement of mandibular length is stable.

Second, the age interval of the participants included in this investigation, is wide (6–18 years of age) and allows the result to be affected by the growth of the subjects. However, differentiating the effect of the evaluated removable functional appliances, on improving the mandibular length in children treated during the prepubertal stage and children treated in the pubertal spurt, increase the potential risk of reporting the influence of natural growth of the patients, as effect of the removable functional devices on improving mandibular length.

According to the results of the present investigation, orthopedic functional appliances are effective, independent of the type of appliance. The combined estimation of the effect evaluated by the fixed effect model, revealed a statistically significant increase in mandibular length of treated individuals. Mandibular growth was always greater in treated individuals regardless of the type of appliance used, indicating that functional appliances have a favorable effect on the correction of mandibular retrognathism. The Sander Bite Jumping was observed to be the most effective appliance aiming to improve the mandibular length, followed by the Twin Block. It is important to highlight that the results of the effect of the Sander Bite Jumping was based on only one article, whilst for the other devices, more evidence was presented. The clinical significance of the results has to be elucidated in future studies to weight the pertinence of the treatment with removable functional appliances.

Conclusions

The findings of this meta-analysis, showed a slight increase in mandibular length (Co-Gn and/or Co-Po), after treatment either with Harvold Activator, Twin Block, type II Bionator, Frankel and Sanders Bite Jumping. The Sanders Bite Jumping reported the greatest results. The clinical relevance of this results have to be explored in further studies.

Abbreviations

CI: Confidence interval; Co-Gn: Condilion-Gnation; Co-Po: Condilion-Pogonion; EBD: Evidence based dentistry; EBD: Evidence based dentistry; MA: Meta-analysis; PRISMA: Transparent Reporting of Systematic Reviews and Meta-analyses; PROSPERO: Prospective Register of Systematic Review; RCT: Randomized controlled trial; SR: Systematic review; WMD: Weighted mean difference

Acknowledgement

This study was self-funded by the authors and Universidad CES for all stages of the study. The manuscript was completely drafted and written by the authors, without including any external personnel.

Funding

All funding for this investigation was provided by Universidad CES. Medellín, Colombia.

Authors' contributions

AS conceived the study, screened the list of titles and abstracts resulting from the search, created an overview of the papers selected for full text reading, performed the full text reading, made a selection of the papers that fulfilled the eligibility criteria, collected the data, worked on the interpretation of the data, assisted in the analysis of the data, drafted and designed the manuscript. EA conceived the study, created the search, assisted in the selection strategy of the papers, supervised the data extraction, helped in the drafting of the manuscript. RM Participated in the design and drafting of the study, performed the statistical analysis, revised the manuscript critically for important intellectual content, realized final approval of the manuscript to be published. CR independently screened the list of titles and abstracts resulting from the search, participated in the design, designed and made the drafting of the manuscript, and coordinated the progress. All authors read and approved the final manuscript.

Competing interests

All authors declare that they have no competing interests.

Consent for publication

Not applicable.

Ethics approval and consent to participate

Not applicable.

Author details

[1]CES-LPH Research Group, Universidad CES, Calle 10A. No. 22-04, Medellín, Colombia. [2]Universidad CES, Calle 10A. No. 22-04, Medellín, Colombia.

References

1. Woźniak K, Piątkowska D, Szyszka-Sommerfeld L, Buczkowska-Radlińska J. Impact of functional appliances on muscle activity: a surface electromyography study in children. Med Sci Monit Int Med J Exp Clin Res. 2015;21:246–53.
2. Cevidanes LHS, Franco AA, Gerig G, et al. Assessment of mandibular growth and response to orthopedic treatment with 3-dimensional magnetic resonance images. Am J Orthod Dentofacial Orthop. 2005;128:16–26.
3. Cevidanes LHS, Franco AA, Gerig G, et al. Comparison of relative mandibular growth vectors with high-resolution 3-dimensional imaging. Am J Orthod Dentofacial Orthop. 2005;128:27–34.
4. Araujo AM, Buschang PH, Melo ACM. Adaptive condylar growth and mandibular remodelling changes with bionator therapy–an implant study. Eur J Orthod. 2004;26:515–22.
5. Malmgren O, Omblus J, Hägg U, Pancherz H. Treatment with an orthopedic appliance system in relation to treatment intensity and growth periods. A study of initial effects. Am J Orthod Dentofacial Orthop. 1987;91:143–51.
6. Hägg U, Pancherz H. Dentofacial orthopaedics in relation to chronological age, growth period and skeletal development. An analysis of 72 male patients with Class II division 1 malocclusion treated with the Herbst appliance. Eur J Orthod. 1988;10:169–76.
7. Martina R, Cioffi I, Galeotti A, et al. Efficacy of the Sander bite-jumping appliance in growing patients with mandibular retrusion: a randomized controlled trial. Orthod Craniofac Res. 2013;16:116–26.
8. Cozza P, Baccetti T, Franchi L, De Toffol L, McNamara JA. Mandibular changes produced by functional appliances in Class II malocclusion: a

systematic review. Am J Orthod Dentofacial Orthop. 2006. doi:10.1016/j.ajodo.2005.11.010.
9. Marsico E, Gatto E, Burrascano M, Matarese G, Cordasco G. Effectiveness of orthodontic treatment with functional appliances on mandibular growth in the short term. Am J Orthod Dentofacial Orthop. 2011;139:24–36.
10. Zymperdikas VF, Koretsi V, Papageorgiou SN, Papadopoulos MA. Treatment effects of fixed functional appliances in patients with Class II malocclusion: a systematic review and meta-analysis. Eur J Orthod. 2016;38(2):113–26. doi:10.1093/ejo/cjv034.
11. D'Antò V, Bucci R, Franchi L, Rongo R, Michelotti A, Martina R. Class II functional orthopaedic treatment: a systematic review of systematic reviews. J Oral Rehabil. 2015;42:624–42.
12. Moher D, Liberati A, Tetzlaff J, Altman DG. Preferred reporting items for systematic reviews and meta-analyses: the PRISMA statement. BMJ. 2009. doi:10.1136/bmj.b2535.
13. Schulz KF, Altman DG, Moher D. CONSORT 2010 Statement: updated guidelines for reporting parallel group randomized trials. BMC Med. 2010;8:18.
14. Wright RW, Brand RA, Dunn W, Spindler KP. How to write a systematic review. Clin Orthop. 2007;455:23–9.
15. Siwek J, Gourlay ML, Slawson DC, Shaughnessy AF. How to write an evidence-based clinical review article. Am Fam Physician. 2002;65:251–8.
16. Henderson LK, Craig JC, Willis NS, Tovey D, Webster AC. How to write a Cochrane systematic review. Nephrol Carlton Vic. 2010;15:617–24.
17. Higgins JPT, Thompson SG, Deeks JJ, Altman DG. Measuring inconsistency in meta-analyses. BMJ. 2003;327:557–60.
18. Petitti DB. Meta-analysis, decision analysis, and cost-effectiveness analysis: methods for quantitative synthesis in medicine. 2nd ed. New York: Oxford University Press; 2000.
19. O'Brien K, Wright J, Conboy F, et al. Effectiveness of early orthodontic treatment with the Twin-block appliance: a multicenter, randomized, controlled trial. Part 1: dental and skeletal effects. Am J Orthod Dentofacial Orthop. 2003;124:234–43.
20. Dalci O, Altug AT, Memikoglu UT. Treatment effects of a twin-force bite corrector versus an activator in comparison with an untreated Class II sample: a preliminary report. Aust Orthod J. 2014;30:45–53.
21. Baysal A, Uysal T. Soft tissue effects of Twin Block and Herbst appliances in patients with Class II division 1 mandibular retrognathy. Eur J Orthod. 2013;35:71–81.
22. Nelson C, Harkness M, Herbison P. Mandibular changes during functional appliance treatment. Am J Orthod Dentofacial Orthop. 1993;104:153–61.
23. Tulloch JF, Phillips C, Koch G. The effect of early intervention on skeletal pattern in Class II malocclusion: a randomized clinical trial. Am J Orthod Dentofac Orthop. 1997;111:391–400.
24. Illing HM, Morris DO, Lee RT. A prospective evaluation of Bass, Bionator and Twin Block appliances. Part I–The hard tissues. Eur J Orthod. 1998;20:501–16.
25. Saikoski LZ, Cançado RH, Valarelli FP, de Freitas KM. Dentoskeletal effects of Class II malocclusion treatment with the Twin Block appliance in a Brazilian sample: a prospective study. Dental Press J Orthod. 2014;19:36–45.
26. Schulz KF, Chalmers I, Haynes RJ, Altman DG. Empirical evidence of bias. Dimensions of methodological quality associated with estimates of treatment effects in controlled trials. JAMA. 1995;273:408–12.
27. Booij JW, Goeke J, Bronkhorst EM, Katsaros C, Ruf S. Class II treatment by extraction of maxillary first molars or Herbst appliance: dentoskeletal and soft tissue effects in comparison. J Orofac Orthop. 2013;74:52–63.
28. Haas DW, Martinez DF, Eckert GJ, Diers NR. Measurements of mandibular length: a comparison of articulare vs condylion. Angle Orthod. 2001;71:210–5.
29. Pancherz H. The mechanism of Class II correction in Herbst appliance treatment. A cephalometric investigation. Am J Orthod. 1982;82:104–13.

20

In vitro effects of hyaluronic acid on human periodontal ligament cells

Masako Fujioka-Kobayashi[1,2], Heinz-Dieter Müller[3], Andrea Mueller[4], Adrian Lussi[3], Anton Sculean[5], Patrick R. Schmidlin[4] and Richard J. Miron[3,6,7,8*]

Abstract

Background: Hyaluronic acid (HA) has been reported to have a positive effect on periodontal wound healing following nonsurgical and surgical therapy. However, to date, a few basic *in vitro* studies have been reported to investigating the potential of HA on human periodontal ligament (PDL) cell regeneration. Therefore, the aim of this study was to investigate the effect of HA on PDL cell compatibility, proliferation, and differentiation in vitro.

Methods: Either non-cross-linked (HA_ncl) or cross-linked (HA_cl) HA was investigated. Human PDL cells were seeded in 7 conditions as follows (1) Control tissue culture plastic (TCP) (2) dilution of HA_ncl (1:100), (3) dilution of HA_ncl (1:10), 4) HA_ncl directly coated onto TCP, (5) dilution of HA_cl (1:100), 6) dilution of HA_cl (1:10) and (7) HA_cl directly coated onto TCP. Samples were then investigated for cell viability using a live/dead assay, an inflammatory reaction using real-time PCR and ELISA for MMP2, IL-1 and cell proliferation via an MTS assay. Furthermore, the osteogenic potential of PDL cells was assessed by alkaline phosphatase(ALP) activity, collagen1(COL1) and osteocalcin(OCN) immunostaining, alizarin red staining, and real-time PCR for genes encoding Runx2, COL1, ALP, and OCN.

Results: Both HA_ncl and HA_cl showed high PDL cell viability (greater than 90%) irrespective of the culturing conditions. Furthermore, no significant difference in both mRNA and protein levels of proinflammatory cytokines, including MMP2 and IL-1 expression was observed. Both diluted HA_ncl and HA_cl significantly increased cell numbers compared to the controlled TCP samples at 3 and 5 days. HA_ncl and HA_cl in standard cell growth media significantly decreased ALP staining, COL1 immunostaining and down-regulated early osteogenic differentiation, including Runx2, COL1, and OCN mRNA levels when compared to control samples. When osteogenic differentiation medium (ODM) was added, interestingly, the expression of early osteogenic markers increased by demonstrating higher levels of COL1 and ALP expression; especially in HA 1:10 diluted condition. Late stage osteogenic markers remained inhibited.

Conclusions: Both non-cross-linked and cross-linked HA maintained high PDL cell viability, increased proliferation, and early osteogenic differentiation. However, HA was consistently associated with a significant decrease in late osteogenic differentiation of primary human PDL cells. Future in vitro and animal research is necessary to further characterize the effect of HA on periodontal regeneration.

Keywords: Hyaluronic acid, Hyaluronan, Periodontal regeneration, Soft tissue regeneration, Connective tissue regeneration

* Correspondence: rmiron@nova.edu
[3]Department of Preventive, Restorative and Pediatric Dentistry, School of Dental Medicine, University of Bern, Bern, Switzerland
[6]Department of Periodontology, College of Dental Medicine, Nova Southeastern University, Fort Lauderdale, FL, USA
Full list of author information is available at the end of the article

Background

Hyaluronic acid (HA; also termed hyaluronan or hyaluronate) is an anionic, nonsulfated glycosaminoglycan and considered an optimal biomaterial for tissue engineering, given its broad expression in a connective tissue as well as the significant role it plays during organogenesis, cell migration and development in general [1–4]. Non-cross-linked HA (HA_ncl) is biodegradable, biocompatible, bioresorbable and also well known to improve tissue lubrication in cartilage, guides cell growth and differentiation, and speeds the healing and repair of chronic wounds [5]. Cross-linked HA (HA_cl) has also been utilized for tissue engineering as a scaffold to further improve the overall mechanical performance of the scaffolding material and rigidity supporting the growth of various cells [6–9]. HA has been widely used for patients with knee osteoarthritis due to its ability to provide cartilage tissue integrity [10, 11]. Furthermore, in the oral maxillofacial area, HA injections have been used as a treatment option to manage symptoms of temporomandibular joint disorders [12, 13]. More recently, HA has also been utilized for applications for aesthetic purposes in the oral facial regions primarily to reduce or to eliminate facial creases, interdental papilla loss, and various other abnormalities [8, 14, 15].

Due to the growing use of HA in dentistry, HA has also been hypothesized to have influences on periodontal regeneration [16]. The management of periodontal defects is mainly a result of the cooperative treatment of three unique tissues which comprises the periodontium, the periodontal ligament and the cementum and alveolar bone. [6]. HA is an essential component of the periodontal ligament matrix and has been shown to play various important roles in cell adhesion, migration and differentiation mediated by various HA binding proteins and cell-surface receptors such as CD44 [17]. This CD44 antigen is expressed in periodontal tissues and HA-CD44 interaction has been associated with periodontal ligament (PDL) cell proliferation and mineralization activities [18].

Furthermore, other advantages of HA include its anti-inflammatory activity promoting soft and hard tissue healing response, which may be of significant interest during periodontal regeneration [19]. Based on these assumptions, exogenous HA has already been tested in patients with chronic periodontitis in several clinical studies reporting the beneficial effects of HA on reducing bleeding of probing scores and probing depths [2, 20–23]. However, to date, the in vitro effect of HA on periodontal ligament activity has not been clearly investigated.

Therefore, the aim of the present study was to investigate the effects of HA_ncl and HA_cl on PDL cells by stimulating cells under 3 different conditions of either diluted samples with HA (co-existing at 2 concentrations of 1:10 and 1:100 dilutions) or directly by precoating HA onto tissue culture plastic. The PDL cells cultured with either HA_ncl or HA_cl were assessed for cell viability at 24 h, inflammatory cytokines expression at 1 day, cell proliferation at 1, 3 and 5 days and osteogenic differentiation marker expression at 7 days and 14 days.

Methods

Reagents and cell culture

HA was kindly provided by Regedent (Zürich, Switzerland) utilizing 2 compositions of HA including non-cross-linked native HA (hyaDENT, BioScience GmbH, Dümmer, Germany) as well as a cross-linked HA (hyaDENT BG, BioScience GmbH). HyaDENT (HA_ncl) contains a formulation of 14.0 mg/mL of sodium hyaluronate (synthesized by bacterial fermentation in *Streptococcus* [24], non-cross-linked), and hyaDENT BG (HA_cl) contains 2.0 mg/mL of sodium hyaluronate and 16.0 mg/mL of sodium hyaluronate cross-linked with butanediol diglycidyl ether (BDDE). The seven groups were tested as follows; (1) control tissue culture plastic (TCP) (2) dilution of HA_ncl (1:100), (3) dilution of HA_ncl (1:10), (4) HA_ncl directly coated onto TCP, (5) dilution of HA_cl (1:100), (6) dilution of HA_cl (1:10) and (7) HA_cl directly coated onto TCP based on our previous report [25]. In short, HA was diluted in standard cell culture growth medium consisting of DMEM (Gibco), 10% fetal Bovine serum (FBS; Gibco) and 1% antibiotics (Gibco). The 100 μl of HA were directly pre-coated in per 24-culture well and then the amount of HA was adjusted the same between 1:10 dilution and coating conditions per well in the end post cell seeding.

The primary human PDL cells were obtained from the middle third portion of each tooth extracted from three healthy patients, with no signs of periodontal disease extracted for orthodontic as previously described [26, 27]. Using discarded tissue for research purposes was approved by the Ethical commission of the Canton Bern without an IRB. All patients gave their consent. Briefly, PDL tissues isolated from the center of the root surface with a surgical scalpel were minced, transferred to TCP with media changes every 2 or 3 days. The PDL cells were detached from TCP using 0.25% EDTA-Trypsin (Gibco, Life Technologies, Carlsbad, CA, USA) prior to reaching confluency. Cells used for experimental seeding were from passages 4–6. Cells were cultured in a humidified atmosphere at 37 °C in the cell growth medium. For in vitro experiments, cells were seeded with HA contained within cell culture media at a density of 10,000 cells in 24 well culture plates for cell proliferation experiments and 50,000 cells per well in 24 well dishes for real-time PCR, ELISA, ALP assay, immunostaining and alizarin red experiments. For experiments lasting longer than 5 days, the medium was replaced twice weekly.

Cell viability

Primary human PDL cells were seeded in at a density of 12,500 cells / cm^2 with (1) control TCP (2) dilution of HA_ncl (1:100), (3) dilution of HA_ncl (1:10), (4) HA_ncl directly coated, (5) dilution of HA_cl (1:100), (6) dilution of HA_cl (1:10) and (7) HA_cl directly coated, on chamber slides (Sigma, St. Louis, MO, USA). At 1 day post cell seeding, cells were evaluated using a live-dead staining assay according to the manufacturer's protocol (Enzo Life Sciences AG; Lausen, Switzerland) as previously described [28]. Fluorescent images were quantified with a fluorescent microscope (OLYMPUS BX51, Tokyo, Japan).

Proliferation assay

PDL cells were seeded in 24-well plates at a density of 10,000 cells per well in a 24 well culture plate with the same conditions, (1) control TCP (2) dilution of HA_ncl (1:100), (3) dilution of HA_ncl (1:10), (4) HA_ncl directly coated onto TCP, (5) dilution of HA_cl (1:100), (6) dilution of HA_cl (1:10) and (7) HA_cl directly coated onto TCP. Cells were quantified using a fluorescent MTS assay (Promega, Madison, WI, USA) at 1, 3 and 5 days for cell proliferation as previously described [29]. At desired time points, cells were washed with phosphate-buffered saline (PBS, pH = 7.4) and quantified using a ELx808 Absorbance Reader (BIO-TEK, Winooski, VT, USA).

Real-time PCR analysis

PDL cells were first cultured for 1 day with HA in order to investigate its inflammatory marker expressions, including matrix metalloproteinase-2 (MMP2) and interleukin-1 (IL-1). Moreover, in order to investigate the effects of HA on the osteogenic differentiation, the cells were stimulated for 7 days within each concentration of HA with and without osteogenic differentiation medium (ODM), which consisted of DMEM supplemented with 10% FBS, 1% antibiotics, 50 μg/mL ascorbic acid (Sigma) and 10 mM β-glycerophosphate (Sigma) to promote osteogenic differentiation as previously described [30]. The RNA expressions of runt-related transcription factor 2 (Runx2), collagen1a2 (COL1a2), alkaline phosphatase (ALP), osteocalcin (OCN) in either condition were measured. The total RNA was harvested using High Pure RNA Isolation Kit (Roche, Basel, Switzerland). Primer and probe sequences were fabricated with primer sequences according to Table 1. A Nanodrop 2000c (Thermo, Wilmington, DE, USA) was used to quantify the total RNA levels. Real-time RT-PCR was performed using FastStart Universal SYBR Green Master mix (Roche) and quantified on an Applied Biosystems 7500 Real-Time PCR machine. The amplification profile was 40 cycles at 95 °C for 15 s (annealing), followed by 60 °C for 60 s (elongation). The ΔΔCt method was used to calculate gene expression levels normalized to the expression of glyceraldehyde 3-phosphate dehydrogenase (GAPDH).

Table 1 PCR primers for genes encoding MMP2, IL-1, Runx2, ALP, COL1a2, OCN and GAPDH

Gene	Primer Sequence
hMMP2 F	ccccaaaacggacaaaga
hMMP2 R	cttcagcacaaacaggttgc
hIL-1 F	ggttgagtttaagccaatcca
hIL-1 R	ggtgatgacctaggcttgatg
hRunx2 F	tcttagaacaaattctgcccttt
hRunx2 R	tgctttggtcttgaaatcaca
hCOL1a2 F	cccagccaagaactggtatagg
hCOL1a2 R	ggctgccagcattgatagtttc
hALP F	gacctcctcggaagacactc
hALP R	tgaagggcttcttgtctgtg
hOCN F	agcaaaggtgcagcctttgt
hOCN R	gcgcctgggtctcttcact
hGAPDH F	agccacatcgctcagacac
hGAPDH R	gcccaatacgaccaaatcc

Inflammatory cytokine quantification with ELISA

The supernatant culture media were collected at 1 and 3 days post cell seeding. MMP2 (DY902, range = 0.625–20.00 ng/mL) and IL-1β/IL-F2 (DY201, range = 3.91–250 pg/mL) were quantified using an ELISA assays (R&D Systems, Minneapolis, MN, USA) according to manufacturer's protocol as previously described [31, 32]. Briefly, 100 μL of assay diluents and 100 μL of sample were incubated for 2 h at room temperature in antibody-precoated 96-well plates. Wells were washed 3 times with washing buffer, incubated for 2 h with peroxidase-conjugated antibody solution, washed again, followed by the addition of 100 μL of substrate solution for 20 min and 50 μL of stopping solution for 20 min. Absorbance was measured at 450 nm and 570 nm on an ELx808 Absorbance Reader and subtract at 570 nm from the readings at 450 nm.

ALP activity assay

PDL cells were stimulated within each concentration of HA with and without ODM. At 7 days, cells were quantified for alkaline phosphatase expression utilizing a cell imaging system. Alkaline phosphatase activity was monitored using a Leukocyte alkaline phosphatase kit (procedure No. 86, Sigma) as previously described [33]. PDL cells were fixed by immersion in a citrate-acetone-formaldehyde fixative solution for 5 min. The alkaline-dye mixture was prepared by mixing 1 mL Sodium

Nitrite Solution and 1 mL of a fast red violet alkaline solution dissolved in 45 mL of distilled water and 1 mL of Naphtol AS-Bl alkaline solution. Surfaces were then placed in an alkaline dye mixture solution for 15 min protected from light followed by rinsing in deionized water. All images were captured on a Wild Heerbrugg M400 ZOOM Makroskop (WILD HEERBRUGG, Heerbrugg, Switzerland) at the same magnification and light intensity and imported into Image J software (NIH, Bethesda, MD, USA). Image segmentation (Thresholding) was used to generate percent stained values for each field of view.

Immunofluorescent staining

At 14 days post PDL cell seeding, the cells were fixed with 4% formaldehyde for 10 min, followed by permeabilized within PBS containing 0.2% Triton X-100 and blocked in PBS containing 1% bovine serum albumin (BSA, Sigma) for 1 h. Subsequently, cells incubated overnight at 4 °C either with a polyclonal rabbit to collagen type I antibody (sc-28657, Santa Cruz, CA, USA) or a polyclonal rabbit to osteocalcin antibody (sc-30044, Santa Cruz) at a dilution of 1:75 in PBS containing 1% BSA. After washing with PBS, cells were incubated for 1 h at 37 °C with TR-conjugated-goat-anti-rabbit antibodies (sc-2780, Santa Cruz) (1:100) diluted in PBS containing 1% BSA. Prior to viewing, samples were mounted with Vectashield containing DAPI nuclear staining (Vector, Burlingame, CA, USA). Images were captured from each surface with an OLYMPUS BX51 fluorescence microscope. The optical density (OD) of the fluorescent staining was quantified from 3 independent experiments using Image J software.

Mineralization assay

Alizarin red staining was performed to determine the presence of extracellular matrix mineralization. PDL cells were stimulated for 14 days within each concentration of HA in ODM. After 14 days, cells were fixed in 96% ethanol for 15 min and stained with 0.2% alizarin red solution (Alizarin Red S, Sigma) in water (pH 6.4) at room temperature for 1 h as previously described [30]. All images were captured and the percentage of staining was evaluated in the same manner as the ALP assay.

Statistical analysis

All experiments were performed in triplicate with three independent experiments for each condition. Mean and standard error (SE) were analyzed for statistical significance using a one-way analysis of variance with Tukey post hoc test (*, p values < 0.05 was considered significant) by GraphPad Prism 6.0 software (GraphPad Software, Inc., La Jolla, CA, USA).

Results

Cell viability and proliferation in response to HA

To investigate the biocompatibility of HA towards human PDL cells, the alive / dead assay was utilized. It was determined that both HA_ncl or HA_cl maintained a high level of cell viability (over 90%) in the presence of HA at various concentrations (Fig. 1). Moreover, the mRNA expression of inflammatory cytokine genes encoding MMP2 and IL-1 of PDL cells treated with either HA_ncl or HA_cl demonstrated little differences at 1 day post seeding when compared to control samples (Fig. 2a, c). Inflammatory cytokine release of MMP and IL-1 from PDL cells treated with either HA_ncl or HA_cl was investigated at 1 day and 3 days post cell seeding (Fig. 2b, d). There was no significant difference

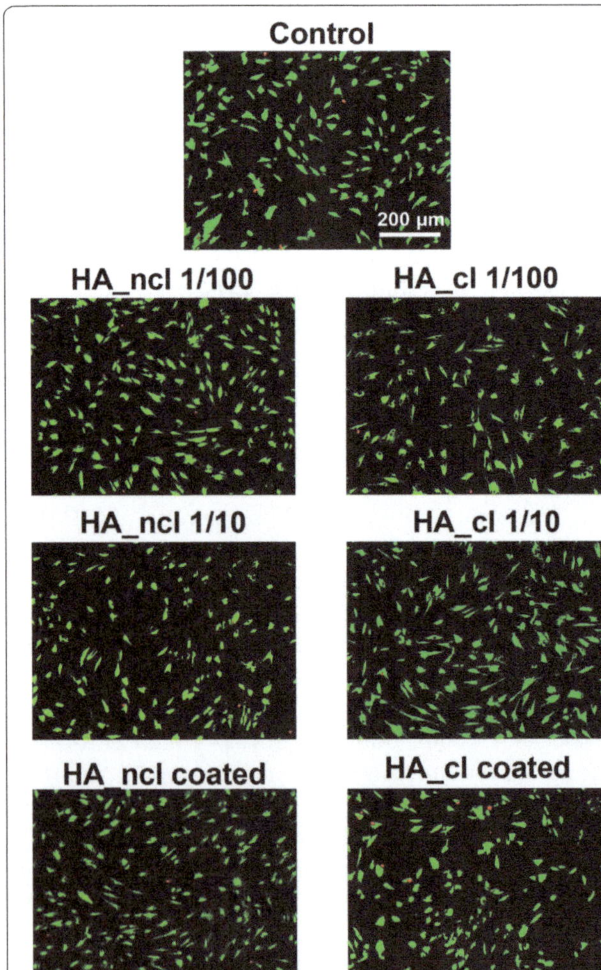

Fig. 1 Cell viability staining of primary human primary PDL cells exposed to control (TCP), non-cross-linked HA (HA_ncl) and cross-linked HA (HA_cl) surfaces. For cell viability, Live-Dead staining was done with viable cell appearing in green and dead cells in red. The results from these experiments demonstrated that both HA_ncl and HA_cl are highly biocompatible at dilutions of 1:100 and 1:10 as well as pre-coated onto cell culture plastic

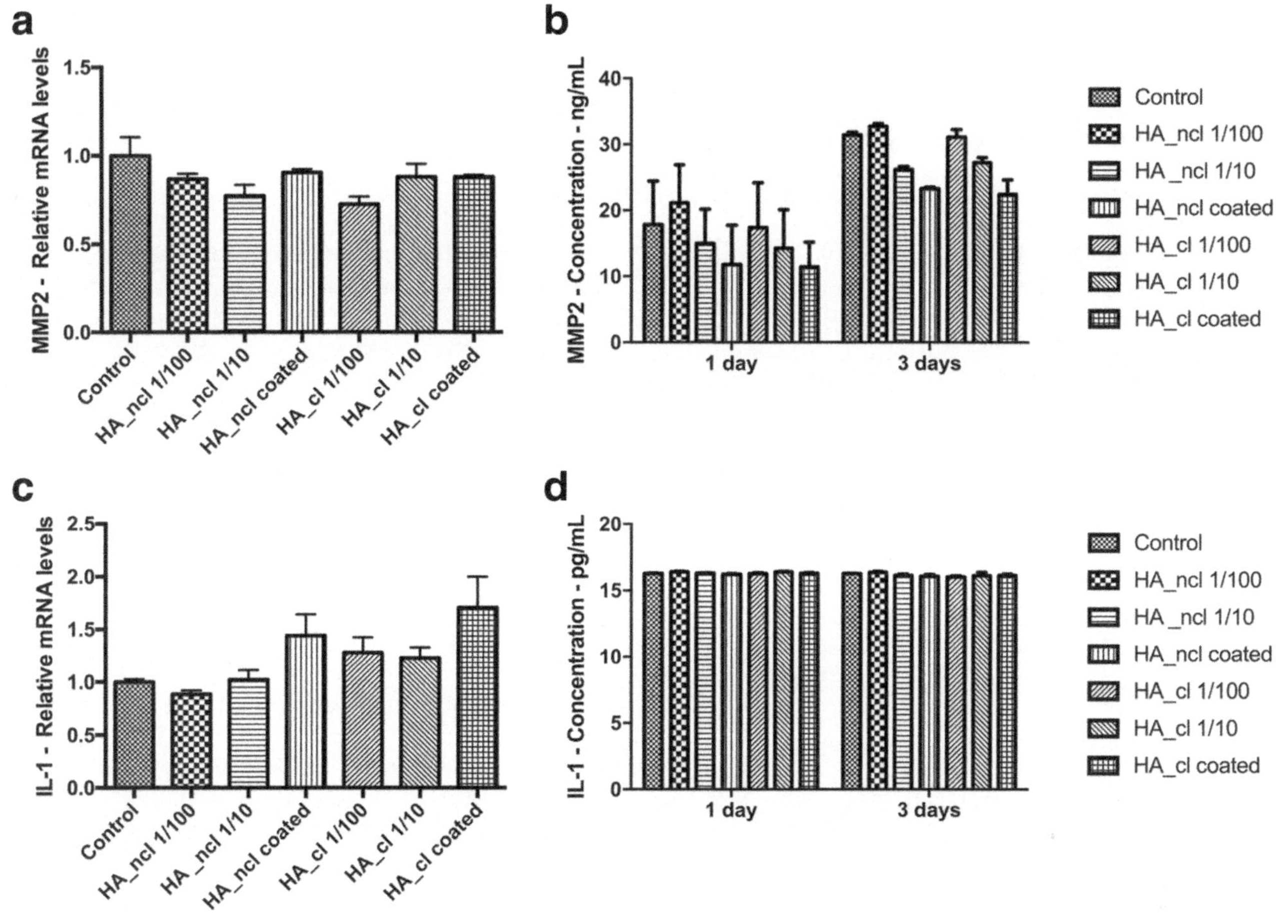

Fig. 2 Real-time PCR of PDL cells seeded with HA_ncl and HA_cl for genes encoding (**a**) matrix metalloproteinase-2 (MMP2), (**c**) Interleukin-1 (IL-1), at 1 days post seeding. Protein release at 1 and 3 days of (**b**) MMP2, (**d**) IL-1, (** denotes significantly higher than all other modalities among HA treated groups, $p < 0.05$)

between MMP2 and IL-1 release among both HA_ncl and HA_cl treated groups as well as mRNA expression (Fig. 2b, d). Thereafter, PDL cell proliferation was investigated in response to HA_ncl and HA_cl at 1, 3 and 5 days post seeding (Fig. 3). It was found that while cell numbers were indifferent at 1 day post seeding (Fig. 3a), a significant increase was observed at 3 and 5 days in either diluted condition for both HA_ncl and HA_cl (Fig. 3b, c).

Cell differentiation in response to HA

Thereafter, the primary human PDL cells were investigated for their ability to differentiate when cultured with HA_ncl and HA_cl (Figs. 4, 5, 6 and 7). The mRNA expression of osteogenic markers was compared by real-time PCR for genes encoding Runx2, COL1a2, ALP and OCN at 7 days (Fig. 4). All HA_ncl and HA_cl treatments significantly downregulated Runx2, COL1a2, ALP and OCN mRNA levels when compared with control samples (Fig. 4a, c, e, g), in normal growth medium. When ODM supplement was added to culture media, it was found that no significant difference was observed in the Runx2 mRNA expression (Fig. 4b), whereas both HA_ncl and HA_cl in 1:10 diluted condition demonstrated a 3-fold significant increase in COL1a2 mRNA levels (Fig. 4d) and a 20-fold increase in ALP levels. Nevertheless, the OCN mRNA expression was still significantly downregulated in either 1:10 diluted or coated conditions for both HA_ncl and HA_cl despite culture with ODM at 7 days post cell seeding (Fig. 4h).

Moreover, it was generally found that HA_ncl significantly decreased ALP staining. HA_cl treatment demonstrated no significant changes in the ALP staining at 7 days likely as a result of the cross-linking HA (Fig. 5a). Interestingly, when ODM was added to cell culture media to promote osteogenic differentiation, HA_ncl at a dilution of 1:10 significantly increased up to 5-fold ALP staining when compared to all other treatment modalities (Fig. 5b, depicted by **). In addition, both HA_ncl and HA_cl coated samples demonstrated a significant increase in ALP staining under ODM supplement

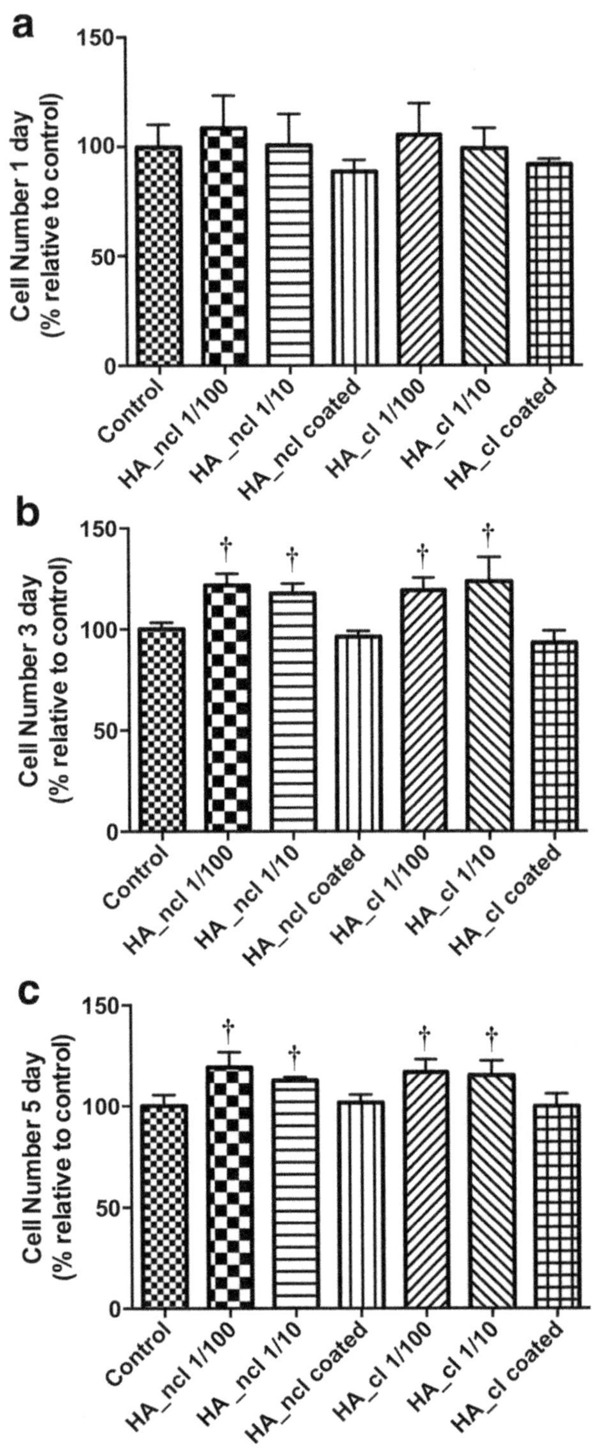

Fig. 3 Proliferation assay of PDL cells seeded with HA_ncl and HA_cl at (**a**) 1, (**b**) 3 and (**c**) 5 days post seeding. It was found that both HA and HA_cl at dilutions of 1:100 and 1:10 significantly increased cell numbers at 3 days and 5 days post seeding when compared to control samples († denotes significantly higher than control, $p < 0.05$)

when compared to control TCP at 7 days (Fig. 5b). Thereafter, it was demonstrated that both HA_ncl and HA-cl significantly decreased COL1 immunofluorescent staining at 14 days post seeding (Fig. 6a, c) as well as mRNA expression via real-time PCR at 7 days (Fig. 4c).

Cells were further investigated by OCN immunostaining and alizarin red staining when induced by HA_ncl and HA_cl treatment (Figs. 6b, d, and 7). All HA_ncl and HA_cl treatment significantly decreased OCN protein expression and alizarin red staining when compared to control samples as well as OCN mRNA expression (Fig. 4g, h).

Discussion

In the present study, the effect of high molecular weight (HMW) HA_ncl and HA_cl were evaluated on in vitro periodontal ligament cell behavior. It was first found that both HA_ncl and HA_cl did not elucidate PDL cell apoptosis even at high concentrations (Fig. 1). Both compositions of HA were shown to be biocompatible on PDL cells without any noticeable differences between their in vitro conditions (diluted in culture media versus pre-coated onto TCP).

We then sought to investigate the inflammatory response of HA on PDL cells. It has previously been shown that low molecular weight (LMW, 100–500 kDa) HA, but not the native HMW HA molecules (~4,000 kDa), stimulated inflammatory cells [34]. Nakatani et al. reported that the expression of MMP-1 in cultured human PDL cells was enhanced by the treatment with HA-oligo through p38MAPK signaling pathway, suggesting that the degradation of the periodontal tissues under pathologic conditions may involve MMP-1 induction by HA-oligo [35]. On the other hand, the majority of products used in connection with periodontal therapy contain HMW HA [8]. The mechanism of anti-inflammatory effects of HMW HA has been widely investigated previously due to the pronounced impact and desire for treatment modalities in the field of osteoarthritis and periodontitis. HA has been shown to modulate inflammation in articular chondrocytes and synoviocytes, due to the specific inhibition of MMPs [19, 36] and down-regulation of TNF-α, IL-8, and inducible nitric oxide synthase [37]. In the present study, HMW HA and HA_cl did not affect the mRNA expressions of inflammatory cytokines, including MMP-2 and IL-1 at 1 day post seeding in healthy PDL cells (Fig. 2). The present study was assessed only in utilizing healthy human PDL cells, whereas in the presence of inflammation, HMW HA within these tissues is reportedly broken down to LMW HA by reactive oxygen species or by bacterial hyaluronidase [8, 38–40]. Therefore, these combined results suggest that although HA demonstrated the little influence on the inflammation in the current study utilizing healthy PDL cells, a more pronounced effect could be observed in diseased tissues due to gingival tissue inflammation in periodontitis.

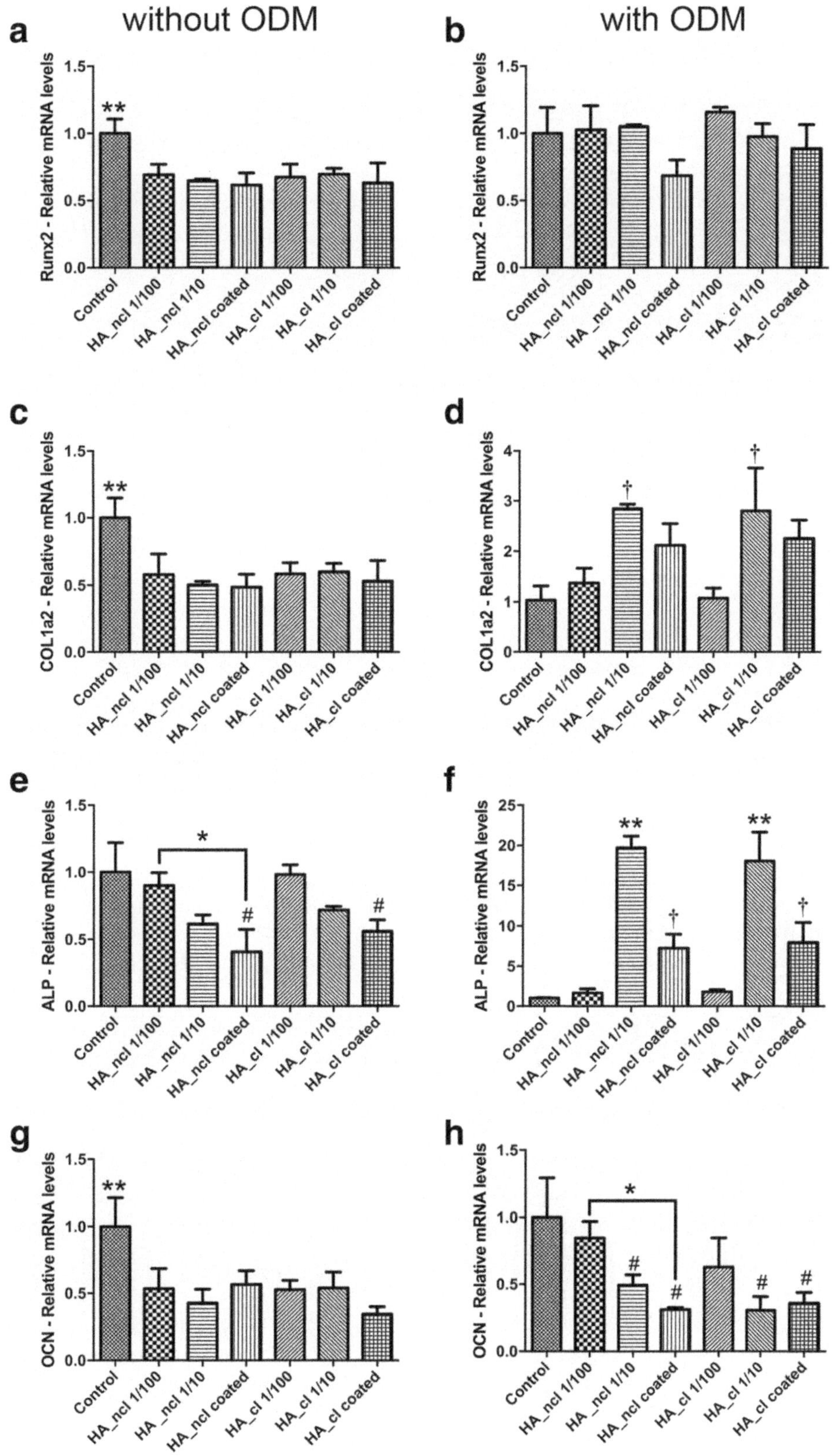

Fig. 4 (See legend on next page.)

(See figure on previous page.)
Fig. 4 Real-time PCR of PDL cells seeded with HA_ncl and HA_cl treatment for genes encoding (**a**, **b**) Runx2, (**c**, **d**) Collagen 1 alpha 2 (COL1a2), (**e**, **f**) alkaline phosphatase (ALP) and (**g**, **h**) osteocalcin (OCN) at 7 days post seeding. Cells were treated (**a**, **c**, **e**, **g**) in regular growth medium or (**b**, **d**, **f**, **h**) with ODM. (* denotes significant difference, $p < 0.05$; # denotes significantly lower than control, $p < 0.05$; † denotes significantly higher than control, $p < 0.05$; ** denotes significantly higher than all other treatment modalities, $p < 0.05$)

Thereafter, the effects of HA demonstrated an increase in PDL cell proliferation (Fig. 3). During the granulation phase of periodontal tissue repair, HA has been shown to be a key protein highly expressed in various tissues responsible for promoting cell proliferation, migration, and granulation tissue organization [19]. In non-mineralized tissues, HA is transiently elevated during the formation of tissue repair and helps with the re-establishment of the epithelium [38]. In our study, both 1:100 and 1:10 dilution of HA_ncl, as well as HA_cl, promoted cell proliferation at 3 and 5 days post PDL cell seeding (Fig. 3). It was previously shown by Takeda et al. in the same manner that HMW HA enhanced cell adhesion and proliferation of human periodontal ligament cells [9]. In our study, both diluted HA compositions and pre-coated HA promoted PDL cell proliferation, which suggests a positive effect for periodontal tissue regeneration.

The effect of HMW HA on cell differentiation has however had controversial findings. To date, most studies reported that cell differentiation was increased by low-MW HA [16, 41–43]. Huang et al. [41] reported an osteogenic cell behavior of HMW HA in a concentration-dependent manner on rat mesenchymal stem cells. Moreover, it was demonstrated that sulfated HMW HA could enhance the osteogenic differentiation of human mesenchymal stem cells [44]. On the other hand, studies have also shown that cell differentiation was not affected by HMW HA [16, 45–48]. For example, Kaneko et al. demonstrated that HA inhibited BMP-induced osteoblastic differentiation through the CD44 receptor in osteoblasts [45]. Noteworthy, in a pure bone defect model, it was demonstrated that HA-gelatin hydrogels loaded into biphasic calcium phosphate (BCP) ceramics in rabbit femurs promoted the new bone formation and collagen mineralization [46]. HA gel has further been shown to accelerate the healing process in the tooth sockets of rats, stimulating the expression of osteogenic proteins such as bone morphogenetic protein (BMP)-2 and osteopontin (OPN) in vivo [47]. On the other hand, Atilgan et al. reported that the demineralized bone matrix (DBM) + tricalcium phosphate + HA combination showed more new bone formation without HA [48]. Therefore, there remains great interest to determine what may be causing the reported variability in the literature.

In the present study, the expression of osteogenic markers stimulated by HA_ncl and HA_cl was investigated with and without ODM. Both HA_ncl and HA_cl down-regulated Runx2, COL1a2 and OCN mRNA levels, suggesting that HA treatment of PDL cells inhibits osteogenesis in a regular cell culture medium (Fig. 4). Moreover, it was observed that HA significantly decreased ALP activity at 7 days, COL1 and OCN

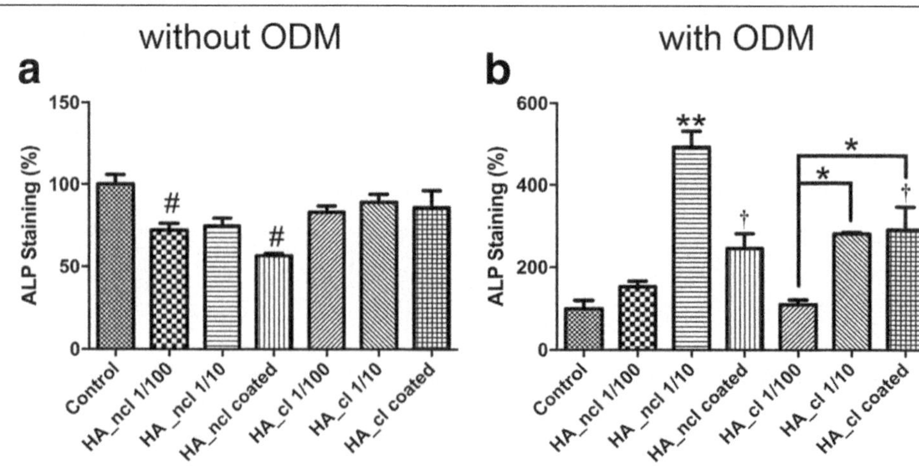

Fig. 5 Alkaline phosphatase staining of PDL cells treated by HA_ncl and HA_cl (**a**) in growth medium or (**b**) within ODM at 7 days post seeding. Both HA_ncl and HA_cl significantly decreased ALP staining without ODM while with ODM both HA_ncl and HA_cl significantly increased ALP staining when compared to control samples (* denotes significant difference, $p < 0.05$; # denotes significantly lower than control, $p < 0.05$; † denotes significantly higher than control, $p < 0.05$; ** denotes significantly higher than all other treatment modalities, $p < 0.05$)

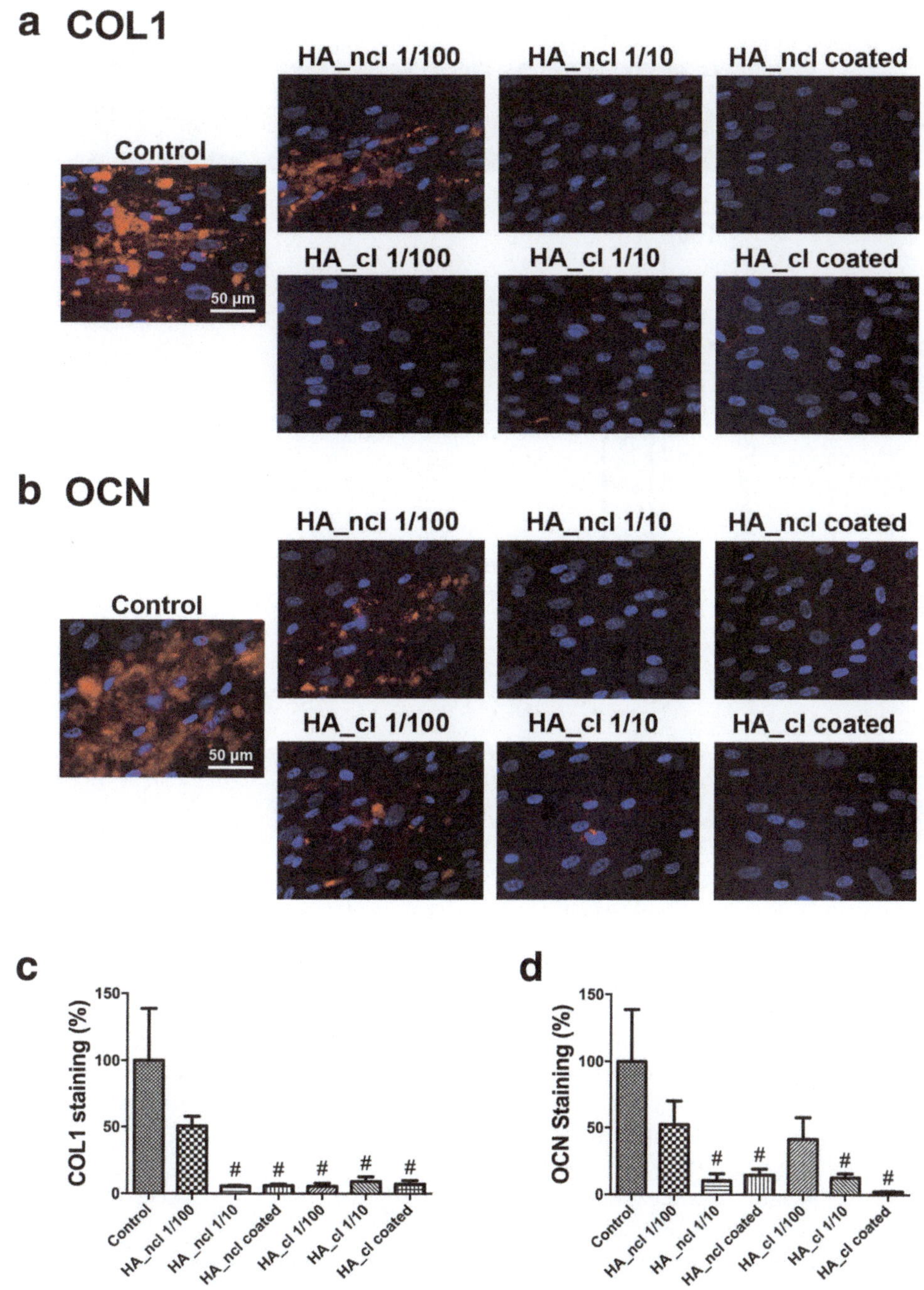

Fig. 6 Immunofluorescent COL1 staining and OCN staining at 14 days post cell seeding with HA_ncl and HA_cl. (**a**) The merged images of immunofluorescent detection of COL1 (red) and DAPI (blue). (**b**) The merged images of immunofluorescent detection of OCN (red) and DAPI (blue). (**c**, **d**) Quantified data of (**c**) COL1 and (**d**) OCN immunostaining at 14 days (# denotes significantly lower than control, $p < 0.05$)

immunofluorescent staining at 14 days when compared to control samples (Figs. 5a, 6). Interestingly, however, when ODM was added to promote osteoblast differentiation, it was found that both HA_ncl or HA_cl in 1:10 diluted condition demonstrated a 3-fold and 20-fold increase in COL1a2 and ALP mRNA levels respectively in ODM (Fig. 4d, f). Moreover, HA_ncl at a dilution of 1:10 demonstrated a 5-fold significant increase in ALP staining compared to control samples in the presence of ODM (Fig. 5b). Therefore, it may be concluded that if granted the right culture conditions, the HA may be used to promote early osteogenic differentiation. Interestingly, however, was the finding that irrespective of the addition of ODM, both HA compositions consistently down-regulated late osteoblast differentiation as assessed by OCN mRNA expression as well as alizarin red staining (Fig. 7).

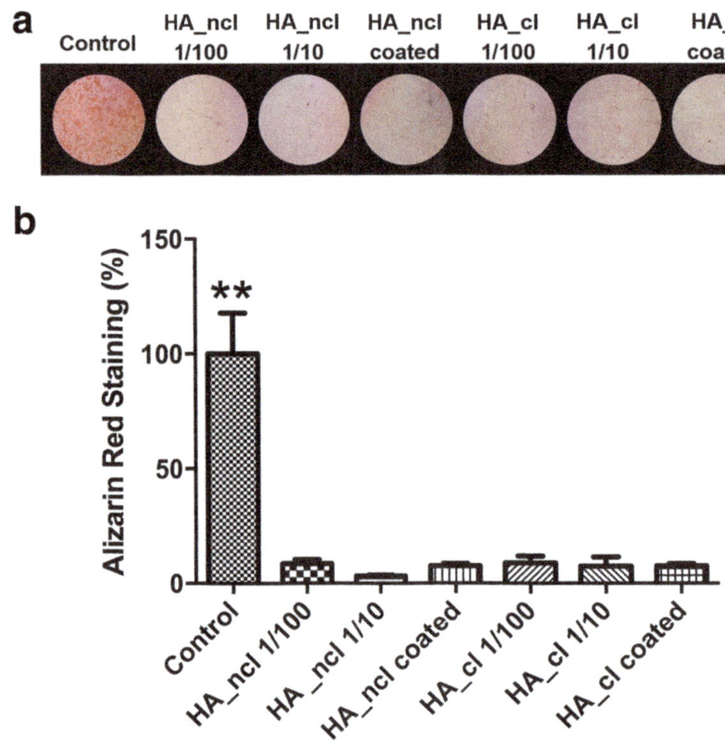

Fig. 7 Alizarin red staining denoting mineralization at 14 days post seeding. (**a**) Alizarin red staining images and (**b**) quantified data of alizarin red staining from colour thresholding software for PDL cells treated with HA_ncl or HA_cl (** denotes significantly higher than all other treatment modalities, $p < 0.05$). It was found that both HA_ncl and HA_cl treatment significantly decreased alizarin red staining

For periodontal regeneration, HMW HA has previously been investigated in a dog intrabony defect model and neither significant periodontal tissue nor bone tissue regeneration was observed [9]. Interestingly, in another canine model, Kim et al. reported that HA improved wound healing and bone formation of hemisection performed extraction sockets with communication of the periodontal lesion [49]. The effect of HMW-HA on periodontal regeneration remains somewhat controversial, however, its contradiction might be explained due to the variety of HA molecular weight, modification methods, concentration, existence of inflammation and also cell types. It may be that HA requires an osteoconductive matrix during periodontal regeneration to improve the osteogenic phase of PDL regeneration, however, this hypothesis certainly requires further investigation.

Conclusion

Both HA_ncl and HA_cl were shown to be extremely biocompatible and at both concentrations were associated with a significant increase in PDL cell numbers. The early osteogenic differentiation markers such as Runx2, COL1 and ALP were significantly downregulated in standard cell growth media. Interestingly, with the addition of ODM, the expression of early osteogenic markers was shown to significantly increase COL1 and ALP levels, especially at higher concentration (1:10) utilizing both HA_ncl and HA_cl diluted condition. Nevertheless, the late stage osteogenic marker such as OCN as well as calcium formation was inhibited regardless of the ODM addition. Future in vitro models including in inflammatory conditions, as well as animal research, are necessary to further characterize the optimal uses as well as delivery systems of HA for improved clinical use.

Abbreviations

ALP: Alkaline phosphatase; BCP: Biphasic calcium phosphate; BDDE: Butanediol diglycidyl ether; BSA: Bovine serum albumin; COL: Collagen; DBM: Demineralized bone matrix; DMEM: Dulbecco's modified eagle medium; EDTA: Ethylenediaminetetraacetic acid; FBS: Fetal Bovine serum; GAPDH: Glyceraldehyde 3-phosphate dehydrogenase; HA: Hyaluronic acid; HA_cl: Cross-linked HA; HA_ncl: Non-cross-linked hyaluronic acid; HMW: High molecular weight; IL-1: Interleukin-1; LMW: Low molecular weight; MMP2: Matrix metalloproteinase-2; MTS: 3-(4,5-dimethylthiazol-2-yl)-5-(3-carboxymethoxyphenyl)-2-(4-sulfophenyl)-2H-tetrazolium; OCN: Osteocalcin; OCN: Osteocalcin; OD: Optical density; ODM: Osteogenic differentiation medium; OPN: Osteopontin; PBS: Phosphate buffered saline; PDL: Periodontal ligament; RT-PCR: Reverse transcription polymerase chain reaction; Runx2: Runt-related transcription factor 2; SE: Standard error; TCP: Tissue culture plastic.

Acknowledgement

The authors thank Catherine Solioz for her careful technical assistance in helping with the experiments.

Funding

The authors received funding from Regedent who provided the HA materials utilized in the present manuscript.

Authors' contributions

MFK, HDM, AM, AL, AS, PRS and RJM have made substantial contributions to conception and design, MFK, HDM, AM and PRS have made the acquisition of data, and MFK, HDM, AL, AS, and RJM have performed analysis and interpretation of data. MFK, AS and RJM have been involved in drafting the manuscript or revising it critically for important intellectual content. MFK, HDM, AM, AL, AS, PRS and RJM have given final approval of the version to be published.

Competing interests

Patrick Schmiddlin has received a research grant from Regedent, Switzerland. Both non-cross-linked and cross-linked HA utilized in the present study were also provided by Regedent. All other authors declare that they have no competing interests to disclose.

Consent for publication

Not applicable.

Ethics approval and consent to participate

Not applicable. The primary human PDL cells within the present manuscript did not require an ethical approval as the tissues were to be discarded and was performed in accordance with the Declaration of Helsinki and approved by the Ethics Committee of the Canton of Bern, University of Bern, Switzerland. All patients gave their consent.

Author details

[1]Department of Cranio-Maxillofacial Surgery, Bern University Hospital, Inselspital, Bern, Switzerland. [2]Department of Oral Surgery, Institute of Biomedical Sciences, Tokushima University, Tokushima, Japan. [3]Department of Preventive, Restorative and Pediatric Dentistry, School of Dental Medicine, University of Bern, Bern, Switzerland. [4]Clinic of Preventive Dentistry, Periodontology and Cariology, Center of Dental Medicine, University of Zurich, Zürich, Switzerland. [5]Department of Periodontology, School of Dental Medicine, University of Bern, Bern, Switzerland. [6]Department of Periodontology, College of Dental Medicine, Nova Southeastern University, Fort Lauderdale, FL, USA. [7]Cell Therapy Institute, Center for Collaborative Research, Nova Southeastern University, Fort Lauderdale, FL, USA. [8]Department of Periodontics and Oral Medicine, University of Michigan School of Dentistry, Ann Arbor, MI, USA.

References

1. Toole BP. Hyaluronan in morphogenesis. Semin Cell Dev Biol. 2001;12(2):79–87.
2. Bertolami CN, Messadi DV. The role of proteoglycans in hard and soft tissue repair. Crit Rev Oral Biol Med. 1994;5(3–4):311–37.
3. Pilloni A, Rimondini L, De Luca M, Bernard GW. Effect of hyaluronan on calcification-nodule formation from human periodontal ligament cell culture. J Appl Biomater Biomech. 2003;1(1):84–90.
4. Chen WY, Abatangelo G. Functions of hyaluronan in wound repair. Wound Repair Regen. 1999;7(2):79–89.
5. Donegan GC, Hunt JA, Rhodes N. Investigating the importance of flow when utilizing hyaluronan scaffolds for tissue engineering. J Tissue Eng Regen Med. 2010;4(2):83–95.
6. Bartold PM, Xiao Y, Lyngstaadas SP, Paine ML, Snead ML. Principles and applications of cell delivery systems for periodontal regeneration. Periodontol. 2006;41:123–35.
7. Choi SC, Yoo MA, Lee SY, Lee HJ, Son DH, Jung J, Noh I, Kim CW. Modulation of biomechanical properties of hyaluronic acid hydrogels by crosslinking agents. J Biomed Mater Res A. 2015;103(9):3072–80.
8. Collins MN, Birkinshaw C. Hyaluronic acid based scaffolds for tissue engineering—A review. Carbohydr Polym. 2013;92(2):1262–79.
9. Takeda K, Sakai N, Shiba H, Nagahara T, Fujita T, Kajiya M, Iwata T, Matsuda S, Kawahara K, Kawaguchi H, et al. Characteristics of high-molecular-weight hyaluronic acid as a brain-derived neurotrophic factor scaffold in periodontal tissue regeneration. Tissue Eng A. 2011;17(7–8):955–67.
10. Ishijima M, Nakamura T, Shimizu K, Hayashi K, Kikuchi H, Soen S, Omori G, Yamashita T, Uchio Y, Chiba J, et al. Intra-articular hyaluronic acid injection versus oral non-steroidal anti-inflammatory drug for the treatment of knee osteoarthritis: a multi-center, randomized, open-label, non-inferiority trial. Arthritis Res Ther. 2014;16(1):R18.
11. Brzusek D, Petron D. Treating knee osteoarthritis with intra-articular hyaluronans. Curr Med Res Opin. 2008;24(12):3307–22.
12. Manfredini D, Piccotti F, Guarda-Nardini L. Hyaluronic acid in the treatment of TMJ disorders: a systematic review of the literature. Cranio. 2010;28(3):166–76.
13. Guarda-Nardini L, Cadorin C, Frizziero A, Ferronato G, Manfredini D. Comparison of 2 hyaluronic acid drugs for the treatment of temporomandibular joint osteoarthritis. J Oral Maxillofac Surg. 2012;70(11):2522–30.
14. Cohen JL, Dayan SH, Brandt FS, Nelson DB, Axford-Gatley RA, Theisen MJ, Narins RS. Systematic review of clinical trials of small- and large-gel-particle hyaluronic acid injectable fillers for aesthetic soft tissue augmentation. Dermatol Surg. 2013;39(2):205–31.
15. Becker W, Gabitov I, Stepanov M, Kois J, Smidt A, Becker BE. Minimally invasive treatment for papillae deficiencies in the esthetic zone: a pilot study. Clin Implant Dent Relat Res. 2010;12(1):1–8.
16. Zhao N, Wang X, Qin L, Zhai M, Yuan J, Chen J, Li D: Effect of hyaluronic acid in bone formation and its applications in dentistry. J Biomed Mater Res A. 2016;104(6):1560-9. doi:10.1002/jbm.a.35681. Epub 2016 Apr 9.
17. Oksala O, Salo T, Tammi R, Hakkinen L, Jalkanen M, Inki P, Larjava H. Expression of proteoglycans and hyaluronan during wound healing. J Histochem Cytochem. 1995;43(2):125–35.
18. Yeh Y, Yang Y, Yuan K. Importance of CD44 in the proliferation and mineralization of periodontal ligament cells. J Periodontal Res. 2014;49(6):827–35.
19. Dahiya P, Kamal R. Hyaluronic Acid: a boon in periodontal therapy. N Am J Med Sci. 2013;5(5):309–15.
20. Johannsen A, Tellefsen M, Wikesjo U, Johannsen G. Local delivery of hyaluronan as an adjunct to scaling and root planing in the treatment of chronic periodontitis. J Periodontol. 2009;80(9):1493–7.
21. Bertl K, Bruckmann C, Isberg PE, Klinge B, Gotfredsen K, Stavropoulos A. Hyaluronan in non-surgical and surgical periodontal therapy: a systematic review. J Clin Periodontol. 2015;42(3):236–46.
22. Briguglio F, Briguglio E, Briguglio R, Cafiero C, Isola G. Treatment of infrabony periodontal defects using a resorbable biopolymer of hyaluronic acid: a randomized clinical trial. Quintessence Int. 2013;44(3):231–40.
23. Fawzy El-Sayed KM, Dahaba MA, Aboul-Ela S, Darhous MS. Local application of hyaluronan gel in conjunction with periodontal surgery: a randomized controlled trial. Clin Oral Investig. 2012;16(4):1229–36.
24. Saranraj P. Hyaluronic Acid Production and its Applications A Review. Int J Pharm Biol Arch. 2013;4(5):853-59.
25. Mueller A, Fujioka-Kobayashi M, Mueller HD, Lussi A, Sculean A, Schmidlin PR, Miron RJ: Effect of hyaluronic acid on morphological changes to dentin surfaces and subsequent effect on periodontal ligament cell survival, attachment, and spreading. Clin Oral Investig. 2016. [Epub ahead of print].
26. Miron RJ, Bosshardt DD, Hedbom E, Zhang Y, Haenni B, Buser D, Sculean A. Adsorption of enamel matrix proteins to a bovine-derived bone grafting material and its regulation of cell adhesion, proliferation, and differentiation. J Periodontol. 2012;83(7):936–47.
27. Miron RJ, Caluseru OM, Guillemette V, Zhang Y, Gemperli AC, Chandad F, Sculean A. Influence of enamel matrix derivative on cells at different maturation stages of differentiation. PLoS One. 2013;8(8):e71008.
28. Sawada K, Caballe-Serrano J, Bosshardt DD, Schaller B, Miron RJ, Buser D, Gruber R: Antiseptic solutions modulate the paracrine-like activity of bone chips: differential impact of chlorhexidine and sodium hypochlorite. J Clin Periodontol. 2015;42(9):883-91. doi:10.1111/jcpe.12447. Epub 2015 Sep 28.
29. Miron RJ, Saulacic N, Buser D, Iizuka T, Sculean A. Osteoblast proliferation and differentiation on a barrier membrane in combination with BMP2 and TGFbeta1. Clin Oral Investig. 2013;17(3):981–8.
30. Miron RJ, Hedbom E, Saulacic N, Zhang Y, Sculean A, Bosshardt DD, Buser D. Osteogenic potential of autogenous bone grafts harvested with four different surgical techniques. J Dent Res. 2011;90(12):1428–33.
31. Kobayashi E, Flückiger L, Fujioka-Kobayashi M, Sawada K, Sculean A, Schaller B, Miron RJ: Comparative release of growth factors from PRP, PRF, and advanced-PRF. Clin Oral Investig. 2016;20(9):2353-60. Epub 2016 Jan 25.
32. Sawada K, Fujioka-Kobayashi M, Kobayashi E, Schaller B, Miron RJ. Effects of Antiseptic Solutions Commonly Used in Dentistry on Bone Viability, Bone Morphology, and Release of Growth Factors. J Oral Maxillofac Surg. 2016;74(2):247–54.

33. Miron RJ, Oates CJ, Molenberg A, Dard M, Hamilton DW. The effect of enamel matrix proteins on the spreading, proliferation and differentiation of osteoblasts cultured on titanium surfaces. Biomaterials. 2010;31(3):449–60.
34. Eberlein M, Scheibner KA, Black KE, Collins SL, Chan-Li Y, Powell JD, Horton MR. Anti-oxidant inhibition of hyaluronan fragment-induced inflammatory gene expression. J Inflamm (Lond). 2008;5:20.
35. Nakatani Y, Tanimoto K, Tanaka N, Tanne Y, Kamiya T, Kunimatsu R, Tanaka E, Tanne K. Effects of hyaluronan oligosaccharide on the expression of MMP-1 in periodontal ligament cells. Arch Oral Biol. 2009;54(8):757–63.
36. Prasadam I, Mao X, Shi W, Crawford R, Xiao Y. Combination of MEK-ERK inhibitor and hyaluronic acid has a synergistic effect on anti-hypertrophic and pro-chondrogenic activities in osteoarthritis treatment. J Mol Med (Berl). 2013;91(3):369–80.
37. Wang CT, Lin YT, Chiang BL, Lin YH, Hou SM. High molecular weight hyaluronic acid down-regulates the gene expression of osteoarthritis-associated cytokines and enzymes in fibroblast-like synoviocytes from patients with early osteoarthritis. Osteoarthritis Cartilage. 2006;14(12):1237–47.
38. Bartold PM, Page RC. The effect of chronic inflammation on gingival connective tissue proteoglycans and hyaluronic acid. J Oral Pathol. 1986;15(7):367–74.
39. Yamalik N, Kilinc K, Caglayan F, Eratalay K, Caglayan G. Molecular size distribution analysis of human gingival proteoglycans and glycosaminoglycans in specific periodontal diseases. J Clin Periodontol. 1998;25(2):145–52.
40. Scott D, Siboo R, Chan EC, Siboo R. An extracellular enzyme with hyaluronidase and chondroitinase activities from some oral anaerobic spirochaetes. Microbiology. 1996;142(Pt 9):2567–76.
41. Huang L, Cheng YY, Koo PL, Lee KM, Qin L, Cheng JC, Kumta SM. The effect of hyaluronan on osteoblast proliferation and differentiation in rat calvarial-derived cell cultures. J Biomed Mater Res A. 2003;66(4):880–4.
42. Gu H, Huang L, Wong YP, Burd A. HA modulation of epidermal morphogenesis in an organotypic keratinocyte-fibroblast co-culture model. Exp Dermatol. 2010;19(8):e336–339.
43. Zou L, Zou X, Chen L, Li H, Mygind T, Kassem M, Bunger C. Effect of hyaluronan on osteogenic differentiation of porcine bone marrow stromal cells in vitro. J Orthop Res. 2008;26(5):713–20.
44. Hempel U, Moller S, Noack C, Hintze V, Scharnweber D, Schnabelrauch M, Dieter P. Sulfated hyaluronan/collagen I matrices enhance the osteogenic differentiation of human mesenchymal stromal cells in vitro even in the absence of dexamethasone. Acta Biomater. 2012;8(11):4064–72.
45. Kaneko K, Higuchi C, Kunugiza Y, Yoshida K, Sakai T, Yoshikawa H, Nakata K. Hyaluronan inhibits BMP-induced osteoblast differentiation. FEBS Lett. 2015;589(4):447–54.
46. Nguyen TB, Lee BT. A combination of biphasic calcium phosphate scaffold with hyaluronic acid-gelatin hydrogel as a new tool for bone regeneration. Tissue Eng A. 2014;20(13–14):1993–2004.
47. Mendes RM, Silva GA, Lima MF, Calliari MV, Almeida AP, Alves JB, Ferreira AJ. Sodium hyaluronate accelerates the healing process in tooth sockets of rats. Arch Oral Biol. 2008;53(12):1155–62.
48. Atilgan HI, Demirel K, Kankaya Y, Oktay M, Sahiner C, Korkmaz M, Koca G, Kocer U, Kankaya D. Scintigraphic and histopathologic evaluation of combined bone grafts. J Craniofac Surg. 2013;24(6):1902–7.
49. Kim JJ, Song HY, Ben Amara H, Kyung-Rim K, Koo KT: Hyaluronic Acid Improves Bone Formation in Extraction Sockets With Chronic Pathology: A Pilot Study in Dogs. J Periodontol. 2016;87(7):790-5. doi:10.1902/jop.2016.150707. Epub 2016 Mar 18.

21

Clinical registry of dental outcomes in head and neck cancer patients (OraRad): rationale, methods, and recruitment considerations

Rajesh V. Lalla[1*], Leslie Long-Simpson[2], James S. Hodges[2], Nathaniel Treister[3,4], Thomas Sollecito[5], Brian Schmidt[6], Lauren L. Patton[7], Michael T. Brennan[8] for the OraRad Study Group

Abstract

Background: Most head and neck (H&N) cancer patients receive high-dose external beam radiation therapy (RT), often in combination with surgery and/or chemotherapy. Unfortunately, high-dose RT has significant adverse effects on the oral and maxillofacial tissues, some of which persist for the life of the patient. However, dental management of these patients is based largely on individual and expert opinion, as few studies have followed patients prospectively to determine factors that predict adverse oral sequelae. In addition, many previous studies were conducted before widespread adoption of intensity-modulated radiation therapy (IMRT) and concurrent chemotherapy. The objective of this multi-center study is to systematically evaluate the oral health of subjects for 2 years after commencement of RT, with the goal of identifying risk factors that predict adverse oral outcomes post-RT.

Methods: This is a prospective multi-center longitudinal cohort study of H&N cancer patients who receive high-dose RT with curative intent. Planned enrollment is 756 subjects at 6 primary clinical sites (and their affiliated sites) in the USA. A baseline visit is conducted prior to the beginning of RT. Follow-up visits are conducted at 6, 12, 18 and 24 months from the start of RT. The primary outcome measure is the 2-year rate of tooth loss in patients who have received at least one session of external beam RT for H&N cancer. Secondary outcome measures include the incidence of exposed intraoral bone; incidence of post-extraction complications; change in Decayed Missing and Filled Surfaces (DMFS); change in periodontal measures; change in stimulated whole salivary flow rates; change in mouth opening; topical fluoride utilization; chronic oral mucositis incidence; changes in RT-specific quality of life measures; and change in oral pain scores.

Discussion: This study will contribute to a better understanding of the dental complications experienced by these patients. It will also enable identification of risk factors associated with adverse outcomes such as tooth loss and osteoradionecrosis. These findings will support the development of evidence-based guidelines and inform the planning of future interventional studies, with the goal of advancing improvements in patient care and outcomes.

Trial registration: ClinicalTrials.gov Identifier NCT02057510, registered 5 February 2014.

Keywords: Head and neck cancer, Radiation therapy, Protocol, Tooth loss, Exposed bone, Osteoradionecrosis, Salivary flow, Periodontal disease, Caries, Recruitment

* Correspondence: Lalla@uchc.edu
[1]Section of Oral Medicine, MC1605, University of Connecticut Health, 263, Farmington Avenue, Farmington, CT 06030-1605, USA
Full list of author information is available at the end of the article

Background

Most head and neck (H&N) cancer patients receive high-dose external beam radiation therapy (RT), often in combination with surgery and/or chemotherapy [1]. Unfortunately, high-dose RT has significant adverse effects on the oral and maxillofacial tissues, some of which persist for the life of the patient [2]. The salivary glands are often included in the fields of radiation, which frequently leads to irreversible hyposalivation [3], resulting in increased rates of dental caries and tooth loss post-radiation [4]. Radiation-induced soft tissue fibrosis can lead to restricted mouth opening (trismus), which reduces the ability to maintain oral hygiene [5]. Furthermore, radiation impairs bone homeostasis and ability to heal, leading to a life-long risk of jaw osteoradionecrosis (ORN), which is often precipitated by dental extractions [6]. Consequently, these patients are caught in a vicious circle, being at higher risk of needing dental extractions, but with extractions to be avoided post-RT due to the risk for ORN.

To attempt to reduce the frequency of such complications, pre-RT dental evaluation and management is considered a best practice and standard of care in the USA and many other countries. However, pre-RT dental management practices vary widely among centers, due to a lack of reliable data on dental morbidity in these patients and on outcomes of dental management strategies. Although some studies indicate that these patients have significant dental morbidity post-RT, definitive data to document the extent, severity and risk factors for these complications do not exist. Consequently, pre-RT dental management is largely based on expert opinion [7]. For example, an international survey of dentists/oral surgeons experienced in providing pre-RT care found that approximately 50% would extract a mandibular tooth in the radiation field with a small periapical lesion and pain on percussion, while 50% would treat the tooth endodontically [8]. Clinicians mentioned that the lack of adequate data reduced their confidence in their treatment decisions. Such disparate decision-making can result in sub-optimal dental and medical outcomes for these complex patients.

The objective of this prospective observational cohort study is to collect data on dental outcomes in patients who have received RT to the H&N region. Systematic collection of this data in a large multi-center cohort will lead to a better understanding of the dental complications experienced by these patients. In addition, it will enable the identification of risk factors associated with negative outcomes such as tooth loss and ORN. These findings will support the development of evidence-based guidelines and should lead to improvements in patient care and outcomes. The purpose of this manuscript is to describe the study protocol (version 4, 29 October 2015) for this important ongoing study and provide insight based on our experience related to subject recruitment and complexity of study procedures.

Methods

Study design

This is a prospective multi-center longitudinal cohort study of H&N cancer patients who receive high-dose RT.

Outcome measures

The primary outcome measure is the 2-year rate of tooth loss in patients who have received at least one session of external beam RT with curative intent for H&N cancer.

"Tooth loss" is defined as a dental extraction that has been performed or recommended. Teeth that are lost without the involvement of a healthcare professional are also included in this definition. Since dental extractions are often avoided in this population because of the increased risk of ORN, tooth loss also includes teeth having a dental procedure to avoid extraction of a tooth that would have been extracted if the individual had not received RT. The following categories constitute teeth that would otherwise be recommended for extraction: non–restorable because of fracture or extent of caries; amputated crown with root remaining; uncontrolled or persistent periodontal or odontogenic infection. Such teeth are classified as "hopeless teeth" for the purposes of this study.

Secondary outcome measures include the following additional oral health outcomes associated with RT in H&N cancer patients and potential risk factors for negative outcomes:

- Incidence of exposed intraoral bone, suggestive of ORN. This will be defined as exposed maxillary or mandibular bone with an avascular appearance in a quadrant that has received RT;
- Incidence of post-extraction complications;
- Change in Decayed, Missing, and Filled Surfaces (DMFS);
- Change in periodontal measures;
- Change in stimulated whole salivary flow rates;
- Change in mouth opening in mm;
- Use of fluoride to prevent new caries;
- Incidence of chronic oral mucositis;
- Change in RT-specific quality of life measures; and
- Change in pain scores as measured with the UCSF Oral Cancer Pain Scale.

Study organization and funding

Subjects are enrolled at six primary clinical study sites, which are (in alphabetical order): Brigham and Women's Hospital, Carolinas Medical Center, New York University, University of Connecticut Health, University of North

Carolina, and University of Pennsylvania. Personnel at each site include the site Principal Investigator (PI), study coordinator(s), and clinical examiner(s). Some of the primary clinical sites have also established local affiliated sites. The Data Coordinating Center (DCC) for the study is located at the University of Minnesota (Division of Biostatistics) and includes the site PI/study statistician, study manager, and database administrator. The study is funded by the US National Institute for Dental and Craniofacial Research (NIDCR) through a cooperative agreement (U01) mechanism. NIDCR staff are closely involved in the development and oversight of the study.

Safety of human subjects and data integrity

Approval from the Institutional Review Board (IRB) at each clinical study site was obtained before beginning enrollment at that site. Any changes are also communicated to IRB and other stakeholders as appropriate. In addition, each site was individually activated by the NIDCR after passing all relevant requirements for human subjects safety and personnel training. All subjects participate in an informed consent process conducted by the study coordinator, including the signing of a written informed consent document. An independent Data and Safety Monitoring Board (DSMB) has been constituted by the NIDCR to ensure subject safety. It has 3 members, all of whom are free from competing interests. It meets annually and additional meetings can be called as needed. The DSMB reviews any adverse events as well as other study data. No safety concerns have been identified to date.

Study data is entered into a secure database, hosted at the DCC, using web-based data-entry screens created for this study. DCC staff monitor study data to identify missing data or forms and communicate with the clinical sites to resolve these issues. Formal monitoring of study records is conducted by an independent contract research organization. Study Monitors visit each clinical site annually for formal study monitoring.

Training and calibration

All study personnel receive training on the activities they conduct in the study. This includes training on carrying out clinical assessments as well as training on completing study forms, data entry, and all non-clinical procedures. In addition, annual in-person calibration on healthy volunteers is conducted for all clinical examiners for DMFS and periodontal measurements. Clinical examiners must meet minimum standards for intra- and inter-rater consistency annually for these measurements. Specifically, examiners must achieve at least 95% intra-examiner reproducibility within ± 2 mm for both clinical attachment loss and pocket depth; at least 75% inter-examiner agreement for pocket depth within ± 1 mm; and at least 60% inter-examiner agreement for clinical attachment loss within ± 1 mm. Examiners also receive hands-on training on measuring furcation involvement and tooth mobility.

Subject selection criteria

Inclusion criteria

To be eligible to participate in this study, a subject must meet all of the following criteria:

- Diagnosed with H&N squamous cell carcinoma (SCC) or a salivary gland cancer (SGC), and intends to receive external beam RT with curative intent (tumor eradication), with or without concomitant chemotherapy;
  OR
  Diagnosed with a non-SCC, non-SGC malignancy of the H&N region, and intends to receive RT, with or without concomitant chemotherapy. The subject must be expected to receive at least 4500 cGy to at least 1 of 26 specified sites in the H&N region;
- Aged 18 years and older;
- Willing and able to provide signed and dated consent form;
- At least 1 natural tooth remaining or expected to remain in the mouth after completion of the pre-RT dental extractions, if any;
- Willing to comply with all study procedures; and
- Willing to participate for the duration of the study.

After the completion of the baseline study visit, it must be verified that the subject has received at least one session of RT, to confirm eligibility for continued follow-up in the study.

Exclusion criteria

A potential subject who meets any of the following criteria will be excluded from participation in this study:

- Receiving palliative RT;
- History of prior curative RT to the H&N region to eradicate a malignancy;
- Incarcerated at time of screening; or
- Anything that would place the subject at increased risk or preclude the subject's full compliance with or completion of the study.

Study assessments

Figure 1 depicts the sequence of events in a subject's participation. A baseline visit is conducted before the beginning of RT but after completing any recommended pre-RT extractions and other invasive oral procedures. Follow-up visits are conducted at 6, 12, 18, and 24 months

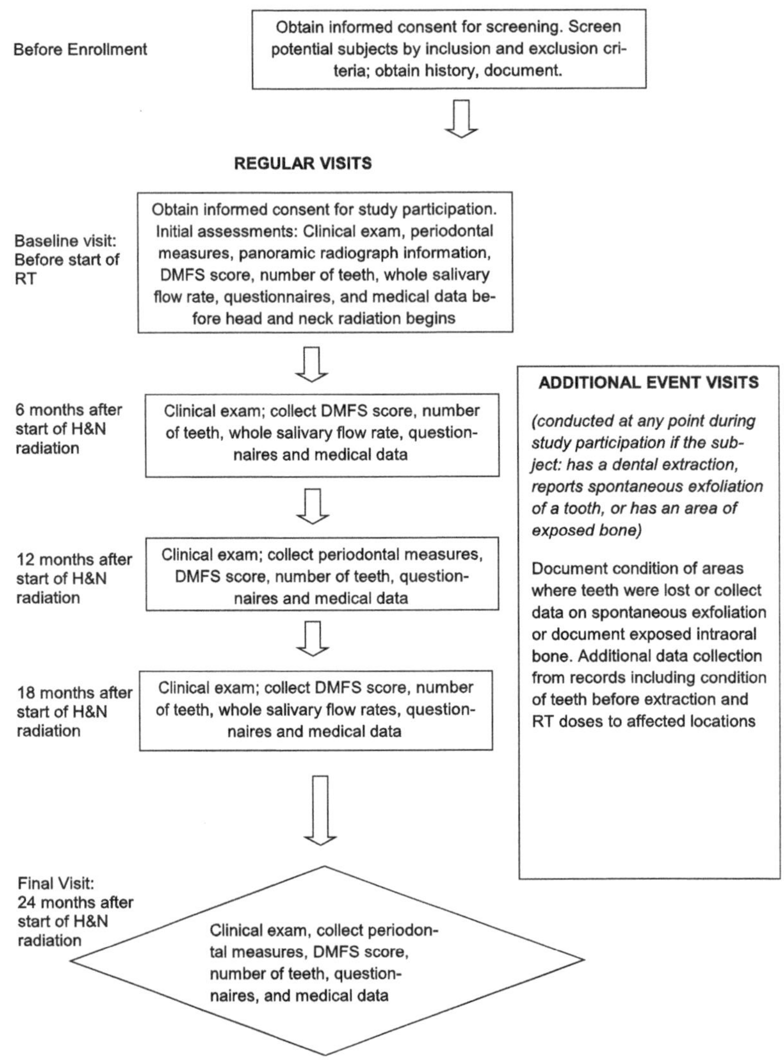

Fig. 1 Sequence of a subject's participation

(+/- 30 days) from the start of RT. Table 1 summarizes the procedures conducted at each study visit.

Details of study assessments, including instruments/scales used, are as follows:

- A panoramic radiograph taken within 180 days before the baseline study visit is evaluated to assess the presence of intrabony devices, periapical lesions and impacted teeth.
- Periodontal measures are collected at baseline, 12, and 24 month visits. Probing depths and the distance from the cemento-enamel junction to the gingival margin are measured using a UNC 15 probe at six sites on each tooth. The clinical attachment level is calculated by the DCC using these two recorded measurements. The presence of bleeding upon probing is documented at the six periodontal probing sites. These assessments are obtained on all teeth other than third molars. Additionally, at the baseline visit, a plaque score is recorded for the Ramfjord teeth, furcation involvement is measured using a Naber's probe, and tooth mobility is assessed [9]. The invasive periodontal measures are not performed on patients needing antibiotic prophylaxis prior to invasive dental procedures.
- Decayed, missing, filled surfaces (DMFS) are recorded at baseline, 6, 12, 18, and 24 month visits. The dentition is examined for active decay, missing teeth because of extraction and/or spontaneous exfoliation, and teeth that have restorations. A No. 23 explorer or a No. 2A explorer is used to detect decay. Five tooth surfaces on the posterior teeth and four tooth surfaces on the anterior teeth are scored for DMFS. The DMFS is also used to reconcile newly missing teeth between study visits.

Table 1 Study Procedures at each time-point (per SPIRIT guidelines)

Procedures		Screening	Baseline Visit (0 – 42 days before RT begins)	Baseline records review after RT	Follow-up Visit 1 (182 ± 30 days after RT begins)	Follow-up Visit 2 (364 ± 30 days after RT begins)	Follow-up Visit 3 (546 ± 30 days after RT begins)	Follow-up Visit 4 (728 ± 30 days after RT begins)	Early Withdrawal Visit	Unscheduled Visit
Consent for screening, assess eligibility, record basic demographic data		X								
Obtain signed study consent form, confirm eligibility			X							
Review medical and dental records	Diagnosis and treatment plan	X	X							
	Medication use		X		X	X	X	X	X	
	Pre-RT dental care delivered			X						
	Data on extractions and complications		X		X	X	X	X	X	
	Total amount of radiation received			X						
Oral/Dental Assessment	DMFS		X		X	X	X	X	X	
	Number of teeth, removable prostheses		X		X	X	X	X	X	
	Presence of intrabony devices		X							
	Periodontal measures[a]		X			X		X	X[c]	
	WHO oral mucositis scale		X		X	X	X	X	X	
	Mouth opening measurement		X		X	X	X	X	X	
	Panoramic radiograph[b]		X							
	Tooth loss, ORN, dental infection/complication		X		X	X	X	X	X	
Measure salivary flow rate			X		X		X		X[c]	
Obtain participant-reported data	Demographics, tobacco and alcohol use		X							
	Fluoride use and oral hygiene practices		X		X	X	X	X	X	
	Oral cancer pain assessment		X		X	X	X	X	X	
	Oral health-related quality of life (RT-specific)		X		X	X	X	X	X	
Post-extraction/exfoliation/exposed bone assessment (if applicable)			X		X	X	X	X	X	X

[a]Periodontal measures at baseline include clinical attachment loss, bleeding on probing, pocket depth, gingival recession, plaque index, tooth mobility and furcation involvement; at follow-up visits, plaque index, tooth mobility and furcation involvement are not recorded
[b]Findings from clinical radiograph are recorded; radiograph is taken for study only if a current (<180 days) radiograph from routine clinical care is not available
[c]Measured at early withdrawal visit only if it would have been done at next scheduled visit

- Salivary flow rate is collected at baseline, 6, and 18 month visits. Participants are provided with unflavored paraffin (gum base) and two 50 ml test tubes. They are instructed to chew the gum base for 2 min, meanwhile expectorating saliva into one of two test tubes. This is done as practice to standardize the technique and stabilize the flow rate. The same chewing/expectorating method is used for 5 min for the final flow rate assessment, timed using a digital timer. The saliva collected in 5 min is weighed and recorded.
- Additional assessments completed at all visits include clinical examination of the subject's oral cavity for "hopeless teeth" (using criteria described above), grading of oral mucositis using the World Health Organization (WHO) mucositis scale [10], inspection of both the mandible and maxilla for exposed intraoral bone, and measurement of maximal mouth opening using a Therabite® Range of Motion Scale in millimeters.
- Patient-reported questionnaires are administered at all study visits. These questionnaires collect information on the participant's daily oral hygiene habits, oral pain using the UCSF Oral Cancer Pain Scale [11], and quality of life related to their oral health using items from the EORTC QLQ-H&N35 scale [12].
- Additional "Event visits" are conducted if a subject has any of the following "events": has a dental extraction, reports spontaneous exfoliation of a tooth, or has an area of exposed intraoral bone. Any signs and symptoms the subject may present with at the visit are recorded, including those related to infection and wound healing. Additional data, related to the event, is collected from the medical and dental records, including radiation doses to affected locations and the condition of the teeth before extraction.

Statistical considerations

Sample size and power considerations

Total planned enrollment is 756 subjects across all clinical sites. The primary outcome used to determine sample size is the rate of tooth loss after the end of RT. Although ORN is an important outcome in these patients, the relative infrequency of ORN [13] makes it unfeasible to conduct a study with ORN as a primary outcome measure. Tooth loss is an ideal outcome measure because it is more common than ORN, it is easily measured, and ORN in this population often results from post-RT dental extractions.

Previous studies found that 20 of 168 patients either had or were recommended to have a dental extraction after median follow-up of 7.6 months after end of H&N RT [14], and that 10 of 50 patients (20%) reported having had an extraction or a procedure to avoid an extraction at a median follow-up of 728 days after the end of RT, with median time of 442 days from the end of RT to the procedure (Unpublished data, University of Connecticut). We also estimated that up to 30% of enrolled participants would withdraw from study participation, be lost to follow-up, or become deceased during 2 years of follow-up. Based on the foregoing, we assumed 20% of subjects would have an extraction or a procedure to avoid an extraction by 2 years after RT, so that 756 enrolled subjects would yield 529 participants with 2-year follow-up data on tooth loss and an expected 95% confidence interval (around 20%) of 16.7%–23.7%, which we deemed adequately narrow. If the actual rate of tooth loss is lower than 20%, a 95% confidence interval will be narrower; if the actual rate of tooth loss is higher than 20%, a 95% confidence interval will be wider. Under these assumptions, 88–125 subjects will have a tooth-loss event. Based on common rules of thumb, this suffices to consider 8–12 predictors (risk factors) for tooth loss [15].

Planned analyses

The study's primary objective is descriptive so the analyses are mainly descriptive. The primary objective can be interpreted in two ways: What fraction of subjects had a tooth-loss event in the two years after RT? And how many teeth were lost per year? Analyses of the former will use time-to-event (survival) methods, where the event is the first tooth loss. This type of analysis accounts for partial follow-up. The 2-year fraction with tooth-loss events will be estimated using the survivor function and associated confidence interval. To estimate the rate of teeth lost per year, each subject's outcome is the number of teeth they lost, analyzed using a negative binomial model with log link and offset log follow-up time (in years) and no predictors. This model's intercept, raised to the power e (the base of the natural logarithm), estimates the rate of teeth lost per year. (The negative binomial model allows analysis of a count outcome with a flexible error variance. Obviously this model is inappropriate if many participants lose large numbers of teeth but this seems unlikely.) Secondary analyses will cull potential risk factors for tooth loss events and for increased rate of tooth loss by considering them as predictors in the regression analyses described above. Other secondary analyses will consider the secondary outcomes, many of which are measured at multiple follow-up visits, so their analyses will be longitudinal, accounting for the presumed correlation of a subject's multiple measurements.

One complication of these analyses is how a subject's initial number of teeth affects tooth loss. We will examine this question in preliminary analyses that include in the regression a flexible function of the initial number of teeth (e.g., a 4°-of-freedom spline). A further complication arises from subjects who have incomplete follow-up due to death. We account for this by defining the outcome being estimated as "rate [or chance] of tooth loss assuming survival to 2 years", which can be estimated by various methods that accommodate participants with incomplete follow-up, e.g., inhomogeneous Poisson processes or logistic regression including a flexible function of follow-up time as an adjuster.

Discussion

The results of this ongoing study are expected to be valuable for several reasons. First, this study will definitively document the oral and dental morbidity resulting from high-dose RT to the H&N region. This includes the impact on salivary flow, mouth opening, caries, periodontal disease, tooth loss, and development of ORN. A better understanding of these downstream effects of RT will inform the pre-RT dental evaluation and reinforce its importance to all stakeholders including patients, medical and dental providers, and third-party payers. Second, this study should allow the identification of risk factors for adverse oral and dental outcomes. As mentioned previously, the pre-RT dental management of these patients varies widely and is largely based on expert opinion. Identification of specific risk factors will allow for evidence-based decision making and better clinical outcomes. Thus, our findings have the potential to lead to significant changes in clinical practice. Third, this study provides a unique opportunity to compare pre-RT dental management practices across a number of different sites. An assessment of important factors, such as number of pre-RT dental extractions, duration between extractions and start of RT, and subsequent development of ORN, in this large cohort can be highly informative.

There are some limitations of this study design. Two years is a relatively short follow-up period as tooth loss may occur after this time. While a longer follow-up period would be desirable, funding constraints did not allow for this and it can also be challenging to follow such medically complex patients for longer periods. Important assessments such as periodontal measurements and salivary flow are not conducted at each follow-up visit. These are completed at alternating follow-up visits to reduce the length of the follow-up visits and burden on the subject. Although the study Manual of Procedures recommends that each subject should be examined by the same clinical examiner at all visits, in practice this has been difficult to achieve due to scheduling issues and staff turnover. However, all clinical examiners are calibrated to strict standards for inter- and intra-rater consistency.

Recruitment presents a challenge in most clinical studies and especially in the oncology population. It has been estimated that only about 3% of patients with cancer participate in a clinical trial and even at some tertiary academic centers, the rate may be below 10% [16]. A barrier to recruitment for the present study is that in order for the baseline visit to be conducted prior to the start of RT, patients may need to be approached soon after their cancer treatment plan has been determined. At this time, patients are often emotionally fragile and overwhelmed with details from various providers on planned surgery, chemotherapy, and RT. In the context of a life-threatening diagnosis, patients can be bewildered about being approached for participation in an observational dental study that does not offer any direct impact on their cancer prognosis. Indeed, as of December 2015, the most common reason (60%) for an approached patient not being formally screened is that they are "not interested/too busy". Careful and patient explanation of the dental and oral complications of RT, and possible benefits of study participation, can be helpful, particularly if reinforced by the radiation oncologist. It is highly desirable to have a team-based approach, where all parties recognize and reinforce the importance of the study and benefits of participation, to the subject and to society. Potential benefits to the subject include the regular and detailed monitoring of their oral and dental status at no charge, which can facilitate the earlier diagnosis and management of potential oral complications. Appropriate monetary compensation is also provided to subjects for their time and effort in attending study visits. However, the study does not directly provide or support clinical care, which may have a negative effect on some patients' interest in study participation.

An important aspect of recruitment is access to the patient population. It is standard practice in the USA for these patients to be referred to a dentist for a pre-RT dental assessment [1]. This dental assessment may occur at the cancer treatment site itself or at a community dental practice. Our experience at the different clinical sites has shown that recruitment is enhanced when the study team works closely with the clinical dental providers receiving the clinical referral and/or the oncology team managing the medical care of these patients. However, the pre-RT clinical dental evaluation can also be a reason patients decline study participation. Specifically, when the pre-RT dental evaluation by regular clinical providers includes periodontal probing, patients have sometimes been unwilling to then undergo the additional detailed periodontal examinations conducted at the baseline study visit by the calibrated study examiner.

The number of eligible patients also varies across sites, with sites located in large urban centers or tertiary care centers usually having a larger patient population.

Indeed, such higher profile referral centers have been the strongest enrolling sites. However, a proportion of patients at such magnet referral centers travel from a distance for their cancer care but may receive follow-up closer to home. This can lead to sub-optimal compliance with the subsequent follow-up visits after treatment. Thus, appropriate selection of patients is important. The main barrier to recruitment at smaller centers is access to an adequate number of eligible patients. The smaller sites, however, also tend to have better attendance at follow-up visits. Strategies we have adopted at sites with lower enrollment include the establishment of a satellite study location at a nearby healthcare facility, where enrollment activities and/or study visits can take place. While this has had a modest positive impact on enrollment, it does create new challenges in terms of obtaining medical records from the satellite site.

An additional factor affecting recruitment is adequate staffing, given the ongoing demands related to scheduling and conducting follow-up visits as well as data management. To better optimize use of the study staff's time, the amount of medications data being collected at follow-up visits was significantly reduced after about 250 subjects had been enrolled. An analysis of the medications data collected to that point revealed that, beyond the 6 month visit, very few subjects were using the medications being collected. Therefore, collection of detailed medications data from medical records after that point was determined as not being critical to achieve the main study objectives.

Notwithstanding all of the above-mentioned recruitment considerations, over 450 subjects have been enrolled to the study so far. Thus, this landmark study is expected to meet its planned enrollment target and result in significant advances in the care of patients receiving RT to the H&N region.

Acknowledgements
The authors gratefully acknowledge the significant contributions of Dr. Jane C. Atkinson of the NIDCR to the development of the study protocol, Ms. Mary Cutting of the NIDCR for editing the study protocol, and the contributions of Ms. Helen Voelker of the Data Coordinating Center in establishing the study database.

Funding
This study is supported by the National Institute for Dental and Craniofacial Research (NIDCR) through grant U01DE022939 with Principal Investigators Dr. Michael T. Brennan and Dr. Rajesh V. Lalla. The NIDCR did not have any role in the decision to submit this manuscript for publication.

Authors' contributions
RVL prepared the first draft of this manuscript and the study protocol, made revisions to this manuscript and the study protocol for important intellectual content, incorporated comments from other authors into this manuscript, and finalized the manuscript. LLS made revisions to this manuscript and the study protocol for important intellectual content. JSH made revisions to this manuscript and the study protocol for important intellectual content. NT made revisions to this manuscript and the study protocol for important intellectual content. TS made revisions to this manuscript and the study protocol for important intellectual content. BS made revisions to this manuscript and the study protocol for important intellectual content. LLP made revisions to this manuscript and the study protocol for important intellectual content. MTB prepared the first draft of the study protocol, and made revisions to this manuscript and the study protocol for important intellectual content. All authors have read and approved the final manuscript.

Competing interests
The authors declare that they have no competing interests.

Consent for publication
Not applicable. This manuscript does not contain any individual person's data in any form.

Ethics approval and consent to participate
The study received ethical approval from the following institutional review boards (IRBs): Carolinas HealthCare System IRB, University of Connecticut Health IRB, University of Pennsylvania IRB, Dana-Farber Cancer Institute IRB, New York University IRB, University of North Carolina IRB, and University of Minnesota IRB. All subjects participate in an informed consent process including the signing of a written informed consent document.

Author details
[1]Section of Oral Medicine, MC1605, University of Connecticut Health, 263, Farmington Avenue, Farmington, CT 06030-1605, USA. [2]Division of Biostatistics, School of Public Health, University of Minnesota, 2221 University Ave SE Suite 200, Minneapolis, MN 55414, USA. [3]Division of Oral Medicine and Dentistry, Brigham and Women's Hospital, 1620 Tremont Street, 3rd Floor, Boston, MA 02120, USA. [4]Department of Oral Medicine, Infection and Immunity, Harvard School of Dental Medicine, 188 Longwood Avenue, Boston MA 02115, USA. [5]Department of Oral Medicine, University of Pennsylvania School of Dental Medicine, 240 South 40th Street, Philadelphia, PA 19104, USA. [6]Department of Oral & Maxillofacial Surgery and Bluestone Center for Clinical Research, New York University College of Dentistry, 421 First Avenue, New York, NY 10010, USA. [7]Department of Dental Ecology, School of Dentistry, University of North Carolina, Chapel Hill, NC CB 7450, USA. [8]Department of Oral Medicine, Carolinas Medical Center, 1000 Blythe Blvd, Charlotte, NC 28203, USA.

References
1. Pfister DG, Spencer S, Brizel DM, et al. Head and neck cancers, version 1. 2015. J Natl Compr Canc Netw. 2015;13(7):847–55. quiz 856.
2. Lalla RV, Brennan MT, Schubert MM. Oral Complications of Cancer Therapy. In: Yagiela J, editor. Pharmacology and Therapeutics for Dentistry. St. Louis, MO: Lippincott Williams & Wilkins; 2010.
3. Jensen SB, Pedersen AM, Vissink A, et al. A systematic review of salivary gland hypofunction and xerostomia induced by cancer therapies: prevalence, severity and impact on quality of life. Support Care Cancer. 2010;18(8):1039–60.
4. Hong CH, Napenas JJ, Hodgson BD, et al. A systematic review of dental disease in patients undergoing cancer therapy. Support Care Cancer. 2010; 18(8):1007–21.
5. Buglione M, Cavagnini R, Di Rosario F, et al. Oral toxicity management in head and neck cancer patients treated with chemotherapy and radiation: Xerostomia and trismus (Part 2). Literature review and consensus statement. Crit Rev Oncol Hematol. 2016;102:47–54.
6. Buglione M, Cavagnini R, Di Rosario F, et al. Oral toxicity management in head and neck cancer patients treated with chemotherapy and radiation: Dental pathologies and osteoradionecrosis (Part 1) literature review and consensus statement. Crit Rev Oncol Hematol. 2016;97:131–42.
7. Brennan MT, Woo SB, Lockhart PB. Dental treatment planning and management in the patient who has cancer. Dent Clin North Am. 2008; 52(1):19–37. vii.

8. Bruins HH, Jolly DE, Koole R. Preradiation dental extraction decisions in patients with head and neck cancer. Oral Surg Oral Med Oral Pathol Oral Radiol Endod. 1999;88(4):406–12.
9. Ramfjord SP. Indices for prevalence and incidence of periodontal disease. J Periodontol. 1959;30:51–9.
10. World Health Organization. Handbook for reporting results of cancer treatment. Geneva: World Health Organization; 1979.
11. Connelly ST, Schmidt BL. Evaluation of pain in patients with oral squamous cell carcinoma. J Pain. 2004;5(9):505–10.
12. European Organisation for Research and Treatment of Cancer. EORTC QLQ - H&N35. [Internet document] 2009 [cited 2011 9 November]; Available from: http://groups.eortc.be/qol/sites/default/files/img/specimen_for_printing_hn35.pdf.
13. Peterson DE, Doerr W, Hovan A, et al. Osteoradionecrosis in cancer patients: the evidence base for treatment-dependent frequency, current management strategies, and future studies. Support Care Cancer. 2010;18(8): 1089–98.
14. Gomez DR, Estilo CL, Wolden SL, et al. Correlation of osteoradionecrosis and dental events with dosimetric parameters in intensity-modulated radiation therapy for head-and-neck cancer. Int J Radiat Oncol Biol Phys. 2011;81(4): e207–13.
15. MacCallum RC, Widaman KF, Zhang S, Hong S. Sample size in factor analysis. Psychol Methods. 1999;4:84–99.
16. Unger JM, Hershman DL, Albain KS, et al. Patient income level and cancer clinical trial participation. J Clin Oncol. 2013;31(5):536–42.

Do children's previous dental experience and fear affect their perceived oral health-related quality of life (OHRQoL)?

Leena Merdad[1*] and Azza A. El-Housseiny[2,3]

Abstract

Background: Oral health-related quality of life (OHRQoL) has been used to describe the consequences of oral health conditions and treatments in children. A better understanding of OHRQoL and its relationship with dental fear and previous dental experience is necessary to improve children's oral health status. The aim of this study was to investigate the association of dental history and experience with dental fear and the OHRQoL of children aged 11 to 14 years.

Methods: A cross-sectional study was conducted using a multi-stage stratified sample of 1,312 middle school children. Information regarding OHRQoL was collected from the children using the Child Perceptions Questionnaire (CPQ_{11-14}), and information regarding dental fear was collected using the Children's Fear Survey Schedule-Dental Subscale (CFSS-DS). Information on past dental experiences and sociodemographic data were collected from the parents using self-administered questionnaires. Dental examinations were performed to assess caries experience.

Results: The multivariable model indicated that dental fear was the strongest predictor of OHRQoL as the fearful children had on average CPQ_{11-14} scores that were 10 units higher than those of the non-fearful children. Regarding past dental experience, pain as the reason for the most recent dental visit was associated with poor OHRQoL, while receiving a filling during the previous dental visits was significantly associated with better OHRQoL. In addition, a larger number of siblings, a lower family income, a lower paternal education level, health problems and prior hospitalization were significantly associated with poor OHRQoL.

Conclusion: This study identified that dental fear and some factors related to previous dental experience are associated with OHRQoL. In dental practice, children with dental fear should be identified, guided and treated early to avoid deterioration of their OHRQoL.

Keywords: Oral health-related quality of life, CPQ, CPQ_{11-14}, Children, Dental fear, Dental experience, predictors

Background

It is important to assess the influence of oral health on the everyday life of children because oral diseases may not only limit children's current physical, social and psychological well-being but may also affect their future development and academic achievement. Oral health-related quality of life (OHRQoL) is a multidimensional construct that consists of subjective assessments of oral health, emotional and functional well-being and self-esteem [1]. It has commonly been used to describe the outcomes of oral health conditions and treatments in children [1]. The late childhood/pre-adolescence stage is frequently characterized by a potentially high caries rate, a tendency toward poor nutritional habits, dental phobia, eating disorders, pre-occupation with others' views and unique social and psychological needs [2]. A better understanding of OHRQoL and its influencing dental and clinical factors in pre-adolescent children is necessary to provide them with optimum oral health care and treatment and improve their oral health.

Many questionnaires have been developed to assess OHRQoL in children. The Child Perceptions Questionnaire

* Correspondence: Lmerdad@kau.edu.sa
[1]Department of Dental Public Health, Faculty of Dentistry, King Abdulaziz University, P.O. Box 80209 21589 Jeddah, Saudi Arabia
Full list of author information is available at the end of the article

(CPQ) is one of the most commonly used self-report scales [3]. This questionnaire was developed for and validated in children in Canada and showed adequate reliability and validity [4]. The CPQ items cover four health domains: oral symptoms, functional limitations, emotional well-being and social well-being [4]. The CPQ has been translated into many languages and has been adapted and validated for other cultures [3].

Dental fear and previous dental experience play a significant role in dental practice. Dental fear and anxiety are not uncommon among children and adolescents and present a challenge for dentists [5, 6]. Children's dental anxiety has been recognized as a factor associated with behavior management problems [6] and as the most important factor in whether children will require general anesthesia during dental treatment [7]. Previous dental experience has also been reported to be related to children's negative behavior at the dental clinic [8].

The relationship between previous dental experience and ORHQoL has been minimally investigated in the literature. A few studies have investigated the relationship between patterns of dental visits and OHRQoL [9, 10]. A study of Brazilian adults reported that compared with subjects who visit the dentist regularly, those who did not reported poor OHRQoL [9]. Studies on dental fear and OHRQoL are also limited, and the mechanism behind the relationship is unclear. A low to moderate correlation was found between dental anxiety/fear and OHRQoL in subjects aged 16 years and older [11]. A study that investigated dental fear in 11- to 14-year-olds in relation to OHRQoL suggested that dental fear negatively influenced children's OHRQoL. In addition, the study found that the association between the social well-being and emotional well-being domains of the OHRQoL and dental fear was modified by orthodontic treatment [12]. Regarding caries experience, the relationship between caries and OHRQoL remains controversial. Some studies have reported a significant association between caries and poor OHRQoL [13], while others have reported no association [14].

Few studies have investigated the association between previous dental experience and the OHRQoL of preadolescent children and the possible impairment effect of dental fear. Thus, the main aim of this study was to investigate the factors associated with OHRQoL among children aged 11 to 14 years, with a focus on past dental history, experience and fear.

Methods

Study design & sampling

This cross-sectional analytical study was undertaken between September 2013 and May 2014 in the city of Jeddah, Saudi Arabia. Using a linear regression model and conservatively assuming a small effect size (0.02) with 18 predictors that have been reported in the literature to be associated with OHRQoL, a significance level of 0.05 and a power of 0.9, the estimated sample size was 1,273 children. The sample size was increased to 1,500 to account for non-responders.

A multistage stratified random sampling technique was used to select the population from children enrolled in middle schools in the city. According to the Ministry of Education, a total of 109,710 children (59,460 male and 50,250 female) were registered in 431 middle schools. The schools were randomly selected from the city's school list, which was stratified according to gender (male or female), funding source (public or private) and district (North, East, South or West). A total of 16 middle schools were selected. In each school, one class from each grade (7th to 9th grades) was randomly selected for inclusion in the study. Students aged 11 to 14 years old in the selected classrooms were included in the study. The response rate was approximately 87%. Ethical approval was obtained from the Research Ethics Committee, Faculty of Dentistry, King Abdulaziz University. Permission to conduct the study was also obtained from the Ministry of Education and the schools' principals.

Questionnaires

Two questionnaires were used in this study. The first was the child questionnaire, which consisted of two parts. The first part was the Child Perceptions Questionnaire (CPQ_{11-14}), which is used to measure OHRQoL in children aged 11 to 14 years [4]. It is composed of 37 items that cover four health domains: oral symptoms, functional limitations, emotional well-being and social well-being. In this study, the validated Arabic version of the CPQ_{11-14} questionnaire, which has been reported to have good psychometric properties [15], was used. The Arabic version is composed of 36 items; the question about difficulties playing musical instruments was omitted because the participating children rarely studied music [15]. The participants were asked about the frequency of certain events in the last three months. They had 5 response categories to choose from: 0 = Never, 1 = Once or twice, 2 = Sometimes, 3 = Often and 4 = Every day or almost every day. The total score ranges from a minimum of 0 to a maximum of 144, and higher scores indicate worse OHRQoL.

The second part of the child questionnaire was the Children's Fear Survey Schedule-Dental Subscale (CFSS-DS), which is the most commonly, used scale to measure dental fear in children [16]. The CFSS-DS is composed of 15 items related to different types of dental treatment, such as "injections" and "drilling". Each item is rated on a 5-point Likert scale with scores ranging from 1, "not afraid at all", to 5, "very afraid". The total score ranges from a minimum of 15 to a maximum of 75. A higher score reveals higher dental fear [17]. The validated Arabic version of CFSS-DS was used in this study [18].

The second questionnaire used in this study was the parent questionnaire (Additional file 1), which was used to assess the different factors associated with the child's OHRQoL. It included questions about the child's age, gender, birth order, number of siblings, family income, parents' education, and general medical history (including the presence of medical health problems and any prior hospitalization). It also included questions about dental history and dental experiences (including the frequency and patterns of dental visits, the reason for the most recent dental visit and the procedures involved and behavior during previous visits).

A package was sent to the children's parents that included a letter explaining the objectives of the study, the study questionnaires and the consent form. The investigators collected the parent questionnaires from the students, and only those with a signed informed consent were asked to complete the child questionnaire. Instructions on how to complete both the CPQ_{11-14} and CFSS-DS were given to the children by a trained investigator, who read each item aloud in the classroom, explained unclear questions and made sure that the children completed the items independently.

Dental examination

After the children completed the questionnaires, dental examinations were performed to determine the presence of caries. The examination was conducted using a sterile, flat-surfaced mouth mirror and a Community Periodontal Index (CPI) probe (Nordent, Elk Grove Village, IL, USA) under adequate lighting and proper infection control measures. The children were seated on a chair with a backrest in front of the examiner. The index for decayed, missing and filled primary teeth (dmft) and permanent teeth (DMFT) was recorded according to the 1997 WHO criteria [19]. Caries examinations were performed out by two trained and calibrated examiners (Kappa = 0.93).

Variables

The main outcome in this study was the total CPQ_{11-14} score. It was calculated for each child by summing the score for all the items of the CPQ_{11-14}. The predictors measured in this study were the child's age, gender, birth order, and number of siblings; family income; parents' education; history of health problems; history of hospitalization; dental visits, dental visits in the last 3 months; main reasons for the most recent dental visit; main procedure during the previous dental visits; history of poor behavior reported by parents during the previous dental visits, dental fear, measured with the CFSS-DS; and caries in the primary and permanent dentition. Regarding the fear score, for each child, the total score was calculated by adding the fear scores for each of the 15 items on the CFSS-DS. A cutoff score of 32 was used to divide the children into fearful and non-fearful groups [20–22]. The D/d component of the DMFT/dmft was used to identify untreated carious teeth.

Statistical analysis

Categorical data were described as frequencies and percentages, and continuous data were described as means and standard deviations (SD). The associations between the predictors and the total CPQ_{11-14} score were tested using *t*-tests and one-way analysis of variance (ANOVA). Tukey post-hoc tests were used if the one-way ANOVA showed significant differences between the groups. The association between the DMFT and CPQ_{11-14} scores was assessed using Pearson's correlation. A stepwise linear regression with an entry of 0.05 and a removal of 0.1 was used to identify significant predictors of the total CPQ_{11-14} score. The significance level was set at 0.05. STATA version 13 (StataCorp, College Station, Texas, USA) was used to analyze the data.

Results

Descriptive statistics

A total of 1,312 children completed the questionnaire and participated in the study. The sociodemographic and health-related characteristics of the study population are displayed in Table 1. Approximately half of the children were 11 to 12 years old, and the other half were 13 to 14 years old. Females constituted 45% of the sample. The majority reported middle family income (71%). Regarding the educational level of the children's mothers, a large percentage had a secondary education (39%); regarding the children's fathers, 50% had a university education. Approximately 15% of children had health problems, with the majority of those children reporting a history of asthma (36%) or allergies (39%). Twenty-four percent reported a history of hospitalization, with the main causes reported as an operation (45%), followed by an emergency (40%).

Table 1 summarizes the patterns of dental visits, behavior and fear among the study population. Approximately 90% of the children had ever visited a dentist, and 33% had visited the dentist in the last 3 months. The main reason for the most recent dental visit was pain (61%), followed by fillings (36%). The main procedures undergone at the previous dental visits were fillings (44%), examinations (42%) and extractions (35%). Approximately 34% of the parents reported that their child behaved poorly during their previous visits, and according to the CFSS-DS, 20% of the children were fearful. Regarding caries, 77% of the children had untreated caries, and the mean DMFT was 4.0 ± 3.3.

Table 1 Characteristics of the study population

Sociodemographic variables	N	%	Dental history and experience	N	%
Age (years) (*n* = 1,312)			Dental visit ever (*n* = 1,295)		
11–12	653	50	Yes	1,158	89
13–14	659	50	No	137	11
Gender (*n* = 1,312)			Dental visit in the last 3 months (*n* = 1,271)		
Male	719	55	Yes	414	33
Female	593	45	No	857	67
Birth order (*n* = 1,312)			Reason for most recent dental visit (*n* = 1,287)[a]		
First	302	23	Regular check-up	101	8
2-3	510	39	Pain	782	61
4+	500	38	Filling	464	36
Number of siblings (*n* = 1,312)			Esthetic	148	12
0–3	455	35	Other	119	9
4–5	476	36	Procedure at previous dental visit/s (*n* = 1,286)[a]		
6+	381	29	Examination	536	42
Family income (*n* = 1,312)			Local anesthesia	186	15
Low	119	9	Extraction	448	35
Middle	933	71	Filling	565	44
High	260	20	Prophylaxis	189	15
Mother's education (*n* = 1,308)			Other	82	6
Less than secondary	334	26	Behavior during previous dental visit/s (*n* = 1,295)[b]		
Secondary	508	39	Good	744	57
University	466	36	Poor	444	34
Father's education (*n* = 1,289)			I don't know	107	8
Less than secondary	200	16	Fear (CFSS-DS) (*n* = 1,312)		
Secondary	449	35	Fearful (score ≥32)	265	20
University	640	50	Non-fearful	1,047	80
General health variables			Untreated caries (*n* = 1,312)		
Health problems (*n* = 1,269)			Yes	1,012	77
Yes	188	15	No	300	23
No	1,081	85	DMFT (mean (SD))	4.0 (3.2)	
Hospitalization (*n* = 1,283)					
Yes	308	24			
No	975	76			

Abbreviations: *DMFT* Decayed Missing and Filled Permanent Teeth; *CFSS-DS* Children's Fear Survey Schedule-Dental Subscale; *SD* Standard deviation.
[a]Answer categories are not mutually exclusive
[b]Reported by parents

Bivariate analysis

Table 2 shows the association between total CPQ_{11-14}scores and sociodemographic and health-related characteristics. The CPQ_{11-14} scores ranged from 0 to 100. The mean ± standard deviation of CPQ_{11-14} score was 24.6 ± 17.2 while the median and interquartile range (IQR) was 21 (12–34). Regarding sociodemographic characteristics, the CPQ_{11-14} scores were significantly associated with the number of siblings, family income, the mother's education and the father's education (P-value < 0.001). In addition, higher mean scores were significantly associated with the presence of health problems (P-value < 0.001) and prior hospitalization (P-value = 0.001). The CPQ_{11-14} scores were not significantly affected by age, gender or birth order.

Table 3 presents the associations between total CPQ_{11-14} scores and the patterns of dental visits, behavior and fear. The children who reported pain as the main reason for their most recent dental visit reported significantly higher CPQ_{11-14} scores than those who did not (P-value < 0.01). In

Table 2 Total OHRQoL (CPQ_{11-14}) scores by sociodemographic and general health variables

Sociodemographic variables	Mean	SD	Median	IQR	*P*-value[a]
Total score	24.6	17.2	21	12–34	—
Age (years)					
11-13	25.1	17.2	21	12–33	0.328
14-15	24.2	17.2	20	12–35	
Gender					
Male	25.0	17.6	21	12–35	0.357
Female	24.2	16.7	20	12–33	
Birth order					
First	24.5	17.0	20	12–34	0.156
2-3	23.7	17.1	20	11–33	
4+	25.7	17.3	23	12–36	
Number of siblings					
0-3	23.3	16.5	19	12–32	0.002[b]
4-5	23.8	17.0	20	11–32	
6+	27.2	18.0	24	13-37	
Family income					
Low	30.3	19.7	27	15–43	<0.001[c]
Middle	24.6	16.9	21	12–34	
High	22.2	16.6	19	10–31	
Mother's education					
Less than secondary	27.0	18.4	22	13–37	0.007[d]
Secondary	24.3	16.7	21	12–34	
University	23.2	16.6	19	12–31	
Father's education					
Less than secondary	29.3	18.8	28	14–41	<0.001[e]
Secondary	24.0	17.0	20	12–33	
University	23.7	16.5	20	12–33	
General health variables					
Health problems					
Yes	28.3	18.4	26	14–39	<0.001
No	23.7	16.6	20	12–33	
Hospitalization					
Yes	27.2	17.8	23	14–38	0.001
No	23.7	16.8	20	12–33	

Abbreviations: *OHRQoL* Oral health related quality of life; *CPQ_{11-14}* Child Perceptions Questionnaire for 11- to 14-year-olds; *SD* Standard deviation; *IQR* Interquartile range.
[a]Two-sample *t*-test, One-way ANOVA test and Tukey post-hoc test were used
[b]0–3 < 6+; 4–5 < 6+
[c]High < Low; Middle < Low
[d]University < Less than secondary
[e]Secondary < Less than secondary; University < Less than secondary

addition, the children who reported that the main procedure at their previous dental treatment was an extraction or filling had higher scores than those who did not (*P*-value < 0.05). The children whose parents reported that the child behaved poorly at previous dental visit/s had higher scores than those whose parents reported good behavior (*P*-value < 0.001). Fearful children reported higher CPQ_{11-14} scores compared with non-fearful ones (*P*-value < 0.001). CPQ_{11-14} scores had a weak, positive and non-significant correlation with DMFT scores ($\rho = 0.03$, *P*-value = 0.356) and were not significantly associated with untreated caries.

Regression analysis

The significant predictors of OHRQoL determined with linear regression are displayed in Table 4. Number of siblings, family income, parental education, health problems, hospitalization, dental fear, pain as the reason for the most recent dental visit, and filling as the procedure performed during the previous dental visits were significantly associated with OHRQoL. For every unit increase in the number of siblings, there was a 0.5-unit increase in the CPQ_{11-14} score (*P*-value < 0.05). Compared with children with a low family income, children with a high family income had CPQ_{11-14} scores that were 5.2 units lower (*P*-value < 0.01). Compared with children whose fathers had less than a secondary education, children whose fathers had a secondary or university education had CPQ_{11-14} scores that were approximately 4 units lower (*P*-value < 0.01). Regarding general health, those who reported a history of hospitalization or health problems had CPQ_{11-14} scores 3.1 units higher than those who did not (*P*-value < 0.05). Regarding dental history, those who reported pain as the main reason for their most recent dental visit had scores 2.2 units higher than those who did not (*P*-value < 0.05), and those who reported receiving a filling during previous dental visits had scores 2.7 units lower than those who did not (*P*-value < 0.01). Fear was a strong predictor of CPQ_{11-14} scores, and fearful children had scores 9.9 units higher than non-fearful children (*P*-value < 0.001).

Discussion

This school-based cross-sectional study investigated the effects of past dental history, dental experience, dental fear and sociodemographic factors on the OHRQoL of children aged 11 to 14 years. Our findings revealed that dental fear, pain as the reason for the most recent dental visit, a larger number of siblings, lower family income, a lower paternal education level, health problems and prior hospitalization were significantly associated with lower OHRQoL. Having received a filling during the previous dental visits was significantly associated with better OHRQoL.

In our study, dental fear was a strong and significant predictor of poor OHRQoL. Similarly, dental fear in 11- to 14-year-old children has been reported to negatively influence their OHRQoL [12]. This association could be explained by known risk factors that are associated with dental fear, such as irregular dental visits and high

Table 3 Total OHRQoL (CPQ_{11-14}) scores by patterns of dental visits, behavior and fear among the study population

Dental history & experience	Mean	SD	Median	IQR	*P*-value[a]
Dental visit ever					
Yes	24.7	17.2	21	12–34	0.855
No	25.0	17.8	20	12–35	
Dental visit in the last 3 months					
Yes	24.3	16.9	21	12–34	0.674
No	24.7	17.3	20	11–34	
Reason for most recent dental visit					
Regular check-up					
Yes	23.0	16.9	18	10–33	0.307
No	24.8	17.2	21	12–34	
Pain					
Yes	25.7	17.7	22	13–35	0.004
No	22.9	16.2	20	11–33	
Filling					
Yes	25.4	18.0	22	12–36	0.226
No	24.2	16.8	20	12–33	
Esthetic					
Yes	24.1	16.5	20	11–35	0.673
No	24.7	17.3	21	12–34	
Procedure at previous dental visit/s					
Examination					
Yes	24.3	16.2	21	12–34	0.549
No	24.9	17.9	21	12–35	
Local anesthesia					
Yes	25.9	18.2	22	12–36	0.279
No	24.4	17.0	21	12–34	
Extraction					
Yes	26.1	18.3	22	13–36	0.027
No	23.9	16.6	20	12–33	
Filling					
Yes	25.9	18.3	22	12–37	0.016
No	23.6	16.3	20	12–32	
Prophylaxis					
Yes	23.1	16.4	20	11–33	0.181
No	24.9	17.3	21	12–35	
Behavior during previous dental visit/s[b]					
Good	23.5	16.9	20	11–33	<0.001
Poor	26.9	17.9	23	14–37	
Fear (CFSS-DS)					
Fearful (score ≥32)	32.6	18.8	31	18–40	<0.001
Non-fearful	22.6	16.2	19	11–30	
Untreated caries					
Yes	24.8	17.3	21	12–34	0.648
No	24.2	16.8	20	12–35	
DMFT (Pearson's ρ)	0.03				0.356

Abbreviations: *OHRQoL* Oral health related quality of life; CPQ_{11-14} Child Perceptions Questionnaire for 11- to 14-year-olds; *SD* Standard deviation; *IQR* Interquartile range; *CFSS-DS* Children's Fear Survey Schedule-Dental Subscale.

[a]Two-sample *t*-test was used

[b]Reported by parents

Table 4 Linear regression results (coefficients, SEs, 95% CIs and *P*-values) for predictors of OHRQoL (CPQ_{11-14}) scores

Significant Predictors	Coefficient	SE	95% CI	*P*-value
Number of siblings	0.5	0.2	(0.1, 0.9)	0.017
Income				
Low	Ref	—	—	—
Middle	−3.2	1.8	(−6.6, 0.3)	0.075
High	−5.2	2.0	(−9.1, −1.3)	0.009
Father's education				
Less than secondary	Ref	—	—	—
Secondary	−4.3	1.5	(−7.1, −1.4)	0.004
University	−3.9	1.4	(−6.7, −1.0)	0.008
Ever hospitalized	3.1	1.1	(0.9, 5.3)	0.007
Health problem	3.1	1.1	(0.5, 5.7)	0.022
Dental fear (Fearful = 1)	9.9	1.2	(7.6, 12.2)	<0.001
Pain as reason for most recent dental visit	2.2	1.0	(0.3, 4.1)	0.011
Received a filling at previous dental visit/s	−2.7	0.9	(−4.5, −0.8)	0.005

Abbreviations: *OHRQoL* Oral health related quality of life; CPQ_{11-14} Child Perceptions Questionnaire for 11- to 14-year-olds; *SE* Standard error; *CI* Confidence interval

numbers of caries. A previous survey conducted among Swedish adults found that dental anxiety was associated with irregular dental care and low OHRQoL [23]. In addition, fearful children (aged 4–11 years old) and fearful preschoolers were reported to have had more caries experience and more avoidance patterns than those without fear [24, 25]. Therefore, the early recognition and management of childhood dental fear is essential for delivering effective child dental treatment, reducing dental avoidance and behavior management problems and improving children's overall oral health and OHRQoL. However, it must be noted that the relationship between dental fear and OHRQoL is likely to be bi-directional as poor OHRQoL could also cause or exacerbate dental-related fear.

Children who reported pain as the main reason for their most recent dental visit reported significantly higher CPQ scores than those who did not. In a previous study, two-thirds of 11- to 14-year-olds visited the dentist because of pain that had a significant impact on their daily activities [26]. Dental pain has been reported to be significantly associated with poor OHRQoL in 10- to 19-year-olds [27] and 8- to 12-year-olds [28]. Dental pain is highly likely to be an indicator of dental caries [26–28], and sporadic dental treatment prompted by pain usually requires invasive procedures and extractions that are associated with fear [29]. School-based preventive strategies should be encouraged to reduce the prevalence of caries and dental pain and to improve OHRQoL.

Receiving a dental filling during the previous visits was a significant predictor of better OHRQoL. This finding is in line with previous studies that found significant improvement in OHRQoL in 12-year-old children who had undergone dental treatment compared with children who had untreated carious teeth [30] and in preschoolers after complete dental treatment [31]. Such results are expected, as restoration of teeth eliminates pain and restores function.

The pattern of dental visits did not show any significant effect on the OHRQoL. This finding is surprising, particularly because irregular dental visits have been reported to be associated with more numerous caries and untreated caries [32, 33]. Our findings also contradict other studies, in which poor OHRQoL was associated with not having visited the dentist in the previous year [10]. Afonso-Souza et al. [9] suggested that subjects with a high socioeconomic status who have good oral health usually make regular dental visits, unlike subjects with a low socioeconomic status and poor oral health. They added that any protective effect of regular visits on perceived oral health that they found in their results would be small or null because of residual confounders. The effect of the pattern of previous dental visits remains unclear and needs further investigation.

We found several sociodemographic characteristics that were associated with poor OHRQoL; higher mean CPQ_{11-14} scores were significantly associated with a greater number of siblings, lower family income and parents with lower education. A recent longitudinal study found that the socioeconomic factors parental education and income were a consistent predictor of OHRQoL for 10- to 14-year-old children [34]. In addition, a Brazilian study reported that low family income, mothers with less than 9 years of education, and living with two or more siblings were significantly associated with poor OHRQoL [14]. Children of mothers with low education who did not visit the dentist regularly were found to be at risk of not receiving dental care [35].

In the present study, children who had fathers with low education had poor OHRQoL. This finding can be attributed to the fact that in the community in which the participants lived, the father is the earner in the family. In addition, taking children for dental care is the responsibility of the parents, and because oral health knowledge and beliefs are gained through education and reflected in attitudes and behaviors, fathers with low education might not value the need to seek early dental care for prevention and treatment.

Higher mean CPQ_{11-14} scores were significantly associated with previous health problems and a history of hospitalization. Poor self-reported oral health has been associated with poor general health in 12- and 15-year-olds [10]. A systematic review suggested that the deterioration of oral health in hospitalized patients could have an impact on their health and quality of life by increasing the risk of acquired infections [36]. The interaction between general health and oral health is bidirectional and complex. There is a potential for oral pathogens and their toxins to spread to other organs and tissues, while the drugs and techniques used to treat systemic diseases can produce a low salivary flow or xerostomia, which affects mastication, swallowing, taste, speech, halitosis and esthetics [37].

The CPQ_{11-14} scores had a weak, positive and non-significant association with DMFT scores and were not significantly associated with untreated caries. This finding contradicts a study that reported a significant association between caries and CPQ_{11-14} scores in 12-year-old Ugandan children [38]. A higher number of caries was significantly associated with higher CPQ scores for 8- to 10-year-old Australian children, but not 11- to 13-year-olds [13]. Similar to our findings, a UK study reported no association between DMFT in 11- to 14-year-olds and CPQ scores [39]. In addition, no association was found between caries and oral symptoms and the functional limitation domains of the CPQ_{11-14} in Brazilian 12-year-olds [14]. The authors of the Brazilian study attributed their findings to the low caries prevalence because approximately 60% of their sample had zero DMFT. However, in our study, a high percentage of the children (77%) had untreated caries. Our non-significant findings may be explained by the fact that 11- to 14-year-old children usually have newly erupted permanent teeth in which caries extension is limited and superficial and might not cause severe discomfort or functional impairments.

This study has some limitations. The OHRQoL is a complex construct and has a bidirectional relationship with many factors; consequently, the cross-sectional design limits the ability to draw causal inferences because the temporality of the reported relationships cannot be established. Self-reported questionnaires rely on the participants' ability to understand the questions and the answer options provided. To overcome this limitation in a relatively young population, the questionnaire was provided to students who had at least 6 years of formal education in their native language, and a trained investigator was available to clarify any ambiguous item or answer any questions. This study only included 11- to 14-year-old children and excluded other age groups because the CPQ_{11-14} is the only scale that measures OHRQoL that has been validated in the Arabic language. Research is ongoing to validate scales used for other age groups, which will facilitate researchers' investigations of OHRQoL in Arabic populations. Finally, although the study was conducted among a multi-stage stratified sample of school children living in Jeddah, Saudi Arabia, the results might not be generalizable to children living in other regions or other parts of the world.

Conclusions

The present study confirmed the association between dental fear and previous dental experience and OHRQoL. Significant associations were observed between dental fear, pain as the reason for the most recent dental visit, a larger number of siblings, lower family income, lower paternal education levels, health problems and prior hospitalization and poor OHRQoL, while having received a filling during the previous dental visits was significantly associated with better OHRQoL. Patterns of previous dental visits and caries were not associated with OHRQoL. Nonetheless, fear plays an important role in dental practice, and the early recognition of fearful children is necessary to guide their behavior and overcome the effects of fear on their OHRQoL. In addition, oral health education should be directed toward low socioeconomic families to improve their children's oral health and OHRQoL. Further studies are needed to assess the association between these factors and specific domains of OHRQoL. Longitudinal studies are also needed to study the cause and effect of different variables on OHRQoL.

Abbreviations

ANOVA: Analysis of variance; CFSS-DS: Children's Fear Survey Schedule-Dental Subscale; CPI: Community Periodontal Index; CPQ: Child Perceptions Questionnaire; DMFT: Index for decayed, missing and filled permanent teeth; Dmft: Index for decayed, missing and filled primary teeth; OHRQOL: Oral health related quality of life

Acknowledgments

The authors acknowledge that this research was not funded and was written in full by the authors. The authors would like to thank Prof Najat Farsi for her valuable feedback and for reviewing the manuscript, and all the schoolteachers who helped in distributing and collecting the questionnaires.

Authors' contributions
LM analyzed and interpreted the data and contributed to writing the manuscript. AE designed the study, collected the data and contributed to writing the manuscript. Both authors read and approved the final manuscript.

Competing interests
The authors have no competing interests to declare.

Consent for publication
Not applicable.

Ethics approval and consent to participate
Ethical approval was obtained from the Research Ethics Committee, Faculty of Dentistry, King Abdulaziz University. Permission to conduct the study was also obtained from the Ministry of Education and the schools' principals. A signed informed consent was collected from children's parents.

Author details
[1]Department of Dental Public Health, Faculty of Dentistry, King Abdulaziz University, P.O. Box 80209 21589 Jeddah, Saudi Arabia. [2]Department of Pediatric Dentistry, Faculty of Dentistry, King Abdulaziz University, Jeddah, Saudi Arabia. [3]Department of Pediatric Dentistry, Faculty of Dentistry, Alexandria University, Alexandria, Egypt.

References

1. Sischo L, Broder HL. Oral health-related quality of life: what, why, how, and future implications. J Dent Res. 2011;90:1264–70.
2. American Academy of Pediatric Dentistry. Guideline on adolescent oral health care. Reference manual 15/16. Pediatr Dent. 2015;37:151–58.
3. Gilchrist F, Rodd H, Deery C, Marshman Z. Assessment of the quality of measures of child oral health-related quality of life. BMC Oral Health. 2014;14:40.
4. Jokovic A, Locker D, Stephens M, Kenny D, Tompson B, Guyatt G. Validity and reliability of a questionnaire for measuring child oral-health-related quality of life. J Dent Res. 2002;81:459–63.
5. de Carvalho RW, de Carvalho Bezerra Falcao PG, de Luna Campos GJ, de Souza Andrade ES, do Egito Vasconcelos BC, da Silva Pereira MA. Prevalence and predictive factors of dental anxiety in Brazilian adolescents. J Dent Child (Chic). 2013;80:41–6.
6. Wogelius P, Poulsen S, Toft SH. Prevalence of dental anxiety and behavior management problems among six to eight years old Danish children. Acta Odontol Scand. 2003;61:178–83.
7. Savanheimo N, Vehkalahti MM, Pihakari A, Numminen M. Reasons for and parental satisfaction with children's dental care under general anaesthesia. Int J Paediatr Dent. 2005;15:448–54.
8. Baier K, Milgrom P, Russell S, Mancl L, Yoshida T. Children's fear and behavior in private pediatric dentistry practices. Pediatr Dent. 2004;26:316–21.
9. Afonso-Souza G, Nadanovsky P, Chor D, Faerstein E, Werneck GL, Lopes CS. Association between routine visits for dental checkup and self-perceived oral health in an adult population in Rio de Janeiro: the Pro-Saude Study. Community Dent Oral Epidemiol. 2007;35:393–400.
10. Pattussi MP, Olinto MT, Hardy R, Sheiham A. Clinical, social and psychosocial factors associated with self-rated oral health in Brazilian adolescents. Community Dent Oral Epidemiol. 2007;35:377–86.
11. Mehrstedt M, John MT, Tonnies S, Micheelis W. Oral health-related quality of life in patients with dental anxiety. Community Dent Oral Epidemiol. 2007;35:357–63.
12. Luoto A, Lahti S, Nevanpera T, Tolvanen M, Locker D. Oral-health-related quality of life among children with and without dental fear. Int J Paediatr Dent. 2009;19:115–20.
13. Do LG, Spencer A. Oral health-related quality of life of children by dental caries and fluorosis experience. J Public Health Dent. 2007;67:132–9.
14. de Paula JS, Leite IC, de Almeida AB, Ambrosano GM, Mialhe FL. The impact of socioenvironmental characteristics on domains of oral health-related quality of life in Brazilian schoolchildren. BMC Oral Health. 2013;13:10.
15. Brown A, Al-Khayal Z. Validity and reliability of the Arabic translation of the child oral-health-related quality of life questionnaire (CPQ11-14) in Saudi Arabia. Int J Paediatr Dent. 2006;16:405–11.
16. Porritt J, Buchanan H, Hall M, Gilchrist F, Marshman Z. Assessing children's dental anxiety: a systematic review of current measures. Community Dent Oral Epidemiol. 2013;41:130–42.
17. Cuthbert MI, Melamed BG. A screening device: children at risk for dental fears and management problems. ASDC J Dent Child. 1982;49:432–6.
18. El-Housseiny A, Farsi N, Alamoudi N, Bagher S, El Derwi D. Assessment for the children's fear survey schedule-dental subscale. J Clin Pediatr Dent. 2014;39:40–6.
19. World Health Organization. Oral health surveys: basic methods. 4th ed. Geneva, Switzerland: World Health Organization; 1997.
20. Hembrecht EJ, Nieuwenhuizen J, Aartman IH, Krikken J, Veerkamp JS. Pain-related behaviour in children: a randomised study during two sequential dental visits. Eur Arch Paediatr Dent. 2013;14:3–8.
21. Krikken JB, van Wijk AJ, ten Cate JM, Veerkamp JS. Measuring dental fear using the CFSS-DS. Do children and parents agree? Int J Paediatr Dent. 2013;23:94–100.
22. ten Berge M, Veerkamp JS, Hoogstraten J, Prins PJ. Childhood dental fear in the Netherlands: prevalence and normative data. Community Dent Oral Epidemiol. 2002;30:101–7.
23. Carlsson V, Hakeberg M, Wide BU. Associations between dental anxiety, sense of coherence, oral health-related quality of life and health behavior–a national Swedish cross-sectional survey. BMC Oral Health. 2015;15:100.
24. Klingberg G, Berggren U, Carlsson SG, Noren JG. Child dental fear: cause-related factors and clinical effects. Eur J Oral Sci. 1995;103:405–12.
25. Milsom KM, Tickle M, Humphris GM, Blinkhorn AS. The relationship between anxiety and dental treatment experience in 5-year-old children. Br Dent J. 2003;194:503–6.
26. Pau A, Khan SS, Babar MG, Croucher R. Dental pain and care-seeking in 11–14-years-old adolescents in a low-income country. Eur J Oral Sci. 2008;116:451–7.
27. Mashoto KO, Astrom AN, David J, Masalu JR. Dental pain, oral impacts and perceived need for dental treatment in Tanzanian school students: a cross-sectional study. Health Qual Life Outcomes. 2009;7:73.
28. Schuch HS, Correa MB, Torriani DD, Demarco FF, Goettems ML. Perceived dental pain: determinants and impact on brazilian schoolchildren. J Oral Facial Pain Headache. 2015;29:168–76.
29. Karjalainen S, Olak J, Soderling E, Pienihakkinen K, Simell O. Frequent exposure to invasive medical care in early childhood and operative dental treatment associated with dental apprehension of children at 9 years of age. Eur J Paediatr Dent. 2003;4:186–90.
30. Severo Alves L, Dam-Teixeira N, Susin C, Maltz M. Association among quality of life, dental caries treatment and intraoral distribution in 12-year-old South Brazilian schoolchildren. Community Dent Oral Epidemiol. 2013;41:22–9.
31. Abanto J, Paiva SM, Sheiham A, Tsakos G, Mendes FM, Cordeschi T, et al. Changes in preschool children's OHRQoL after treatment of dental caries: responsiveness of the B-ECOHIS. Int J Paediatr Dent. 2015;26:259–65.
32. Coolidge T, Skaret E, Heima M, Johnson EK, Hillstead MB, Farjo N, et al. Thinking about going to the dentist: a Contemplation Ladder to assess dentally-avoidant individuals' readiness to go to a dentist. BMC Oral Health. 2011;11:4.
33. Wigen TI, Skaret E, Wang NJ. Dental avoidance behaviour in parent and child as risk indicators for caries in 5-year-old children. Int J Paediatr Dent. 2009;19:431–7.
34. Gururatana O, Baker SR, Robinson PG. Determinants of children's oral-health-related quality of life over time. Community Dent Oral Epidemiol. 2014;42:206–15.
35. Goettems ML, Ardenghi TM, Demarco FF, Romano AR, Torriani DD. Children's use of dental services: influence of maternal dental anxiety, attendance pattern, and perception of children's quality of life. Community Dent Oral Epidemiol. 2012;40:451–8.
36. Terezakis E, Needleman I, Kumar N, Moles D, Agudo E. The impact of hospitalization on oral health: a systematic review. J Clin Periodontol. 2011; 38:628–36.
37. Johnson NW, Glick M, Mbuguye TN. (A2) Oral health and general health. Adv Dent Res. 2006;19:118–21.
38. Robinson PG, Nalweyiso N, Busingye J, Whitworth J. Subjective impacts of dental caries and fluorosis in rural Ugandan children. Community Dent Health. 2005;22:231–6.
39. Marshman Z, Rodd H, Stern M, Mitchell C, Locker D, Jokovic A, et al. An evaluation of the child perceptions questionnaire in the UK. Community Dent Health. 2005;22:151–5.

23

Odontogenic tumors in Ethiopia: eight years retrospective study

Bruktawit Kebede[1*], Dawit Tare[2], Birke Bogale[3] and Fessahaye Alemseged[4]

Abstract

Background: Odontogenic tumor (OT) comprises a large heterogeneous group of lesions arising from tooth producing tissues or its remnants. Studies on OTs are scarce in Ethiopia. Thus, the present study aimed to assess the pattern of OTs in Ethiopia.

Methods: An 8 years retrospective study was conducted at the Dental and Maxillofacial Department, St. Paul's referral hospital, Addis Ababa, Ethiopia. Data were collected by reviewing the medical records of patients who visited the Department from September 2008 to August 2015. All the collected data were coded, checked, edited and entered to SPSS windows 18. Lastly, descriptive statistics, and logistic regression were performed for data analysis.

Results: A total of 448 patient's socio-demographic, and clinical data were reviewed from the registry book of patients diagnosed with OT. Of these, only 163 patient's records were complete and suitable for the study. 88 (54%) of the study subjects (163) were males, while the remaining 75 (46%) were females. The mean age of patients was 34, ranging between 8 and 80 years. 132 (81.0%) of the OTs were benign, and the rest 31 (19.0%) were malignant type. 126 (77.3%) of OTs occurred in the mandible, and the remaining 37 (22.3%) were located in the maxilla. 135 (82.8%) of the patients had primary surgical treatment. Continuity defect, facial disfigurement and malocclusion were the most frequently encountered complications after surgery. Living in rural areas showed statistically significant association with complication after surgery [Adjusted OR = 2.13, (95% CI: 0.98, 4.6)]. In addition, tumor size had statistically significant association with complication after surgery [Adjusted OR = 4.24, (95% CI: 1.76, 10.21)].

Conclusion: OTs were mainly found in males than their females counterpart. Benign OT was predominant over malignant OTs. Regular checkup and/or visit to dentists could help early case detection, and management of OTs.

Keywords: Complication, Ethiopia, Pattern, Surgical treatment, Odontogenic tumors

Background

Odontogenic tumors (OTs) are rare tumors that are specifically seated in the jaw bones. They constitute a heterogeneous group of lesions due to the different degrees of intertissue interaction and various growth patterns. OTs are derived from epithelial, ectomesenchymal and/or mesenchymal elements of the odontogenic tissues. OTs show variable clinical and histopathological features. Among all, the ability of OTs to transit from one form to another complicates the formal classification of OTs. As a result, World Health Organization (WHO) was obligated to revise its 1971 classification of OTs in 1992 to have consensus all over the world [1, 2]. Nevertheless, this revision could not resolve the controversial classification of OTs. In 2005, WHO published the latest third edition of OTs histological typing that brought non-negligible consensus. Of note, the WHO classification has divided OTs as epithelial, mesenchymal, and mixed based on the tissue they originated [3–6].

Many retrospective studies have been conducted in different continents of the world such as Africa, Asia, Europe, and North and South America to assess the distribution of OTs. These studies reported different distribution rates of OTs that ranged from 1 to 28%. The overall and relative frequency of individual OTs differ from region to region. It is speculated that the differences in the observed frequencies are attributed to variations in geographic or cultural settings [7].

* Correspondence: birukkeb@gmail.com
[1]Oral and Maxillofacial Surgery case team, Department of Dentistry, Jimma University, Jimma, Ethiopia
Full list of author information is available at the end of the article

Importantly, most forms of tumors are age related. In Ethiopia, the average life expectancy at birth in 2014 was 64.1 years [8].

The cause(s) of OTs remain(s) unclear. Nonetheless, the majority of OTs seem to arise *de novo*, without an apparent causative factor [9–11]. It has been reported that OTs have a predilection for the entire facial region specifically, for the mandible and maxilla [12]. The treatment of choice for OT is surgical operation; extirpation and curettage for benign type, and segmental resection for malignant type of OT. If left untreated, it could result in death within four to six months of diagnosis [12]. Despite these consequences, little is known about the magnitude of OT in Ethiopia. Therefore, this study determined pattern of odontogenic tumors in Ethiopian population.

Methods

This study received ethical approval from Jimma University, College of Public Health and Medical Sciences Ethical and Review office. Patient confidentiality was strictly maintained by not mentioning patient's name and any potential identifier on the checklist.

A retrospective cross-sectional study design was conducted to determine the pattern of OTs in Ethiopia at Dental and Maxillofacial Department, St. Paul's referral hospital, Addis Ababa, Ethiopia. The hospital has a catchment population of more than 5 million (https://en.wikipedia.org/wiki/St._Paul%27s_Hospital_Millennium_Medical_College). This Department is one of the largest and pioneer centers for maxillofacial surgery in Ethiopia. The vast majority of the cases investigated at this Department are patients who are referred from all over the country. To this end, we reviewed the medical recordings of patients who were diagnosed as OT from September 2008 to August 2015 at the Department.

Complete medical records of patients with unambiguous histopathological diagnosis of OT were included in this study. Importantly, histopathological examinations were done by senior pathologists for the purpose of patient diagnosis. All the necessary data such as age, gender, present address, duration of OT lesion, location of the OT lesion, size of OT lesion, histopathology findings, type of operation and complication after surgery were collected by well oriented nurses working at the Department. The completeness and quality of all collected data were assessed at the end of each data collection dates by the principal investigator.

Lastly, descriptive statistics and logistic regression analysis were performed using Statistical Package for Social Sciences (SPSS) version 18. Odds ratios were used as measures of association between the independent and outcome variables. A p-value of less than or equal to 0.05 was considered statistically significant.

Results

Recruitments

A total of 448 patient's medical records with the diagnosis of OT were reviewed. Of these, 285 recording were excluded from this study due to various reasons. First, 132 (29.5%) medical records had an incomplete medical recording. Second, 57 (12.7%) records were missed and replaced with new records upon the consecutive follow-up appointments. Third, 96 (21.4%) records revealed inconsistent histopathological investigation reports of biopsy and fine needle aspiration cytology upon repeated examinations. As such, only 163 (36.4%) patients' medical records were complete and found to be suitable for the study (Fig. 1).

Socio-demographic characteristics

From the total of 163 reviewed medical records, 88 (54%) were males, while the remaining 75 (46%) were females. The majority, 82 (50.3%), of patients were within age group of 20–39 years. 96 (58.9%) of the participants were living in rural areas of the country (Table 1).

Pattern of odontogenic tumors

Of the 163 cases, 80.4% were benign tumors, while the remaining 19.6%, were malignant tumors. Ameloblastoma 75 (46%) was the most frequent type of benign OT, followed by odontogenic myxioma (8.6%). On the other hand, primary intraosseous squamous cell carcinoma (IOSCC) was the most common type of malignant OT (Table 2). The majority, 112 (68.7%), of OT cases were presented after 1 year of onset of symptoms. On the other hand, 51 (31.3%) of the cases were presented before 1 year of onset of symptoms (Fig. 2).

Distribution of OT cases by gender

Ameloblastoma was the predominant type of OT diagnosed among the male patients with male to female sex

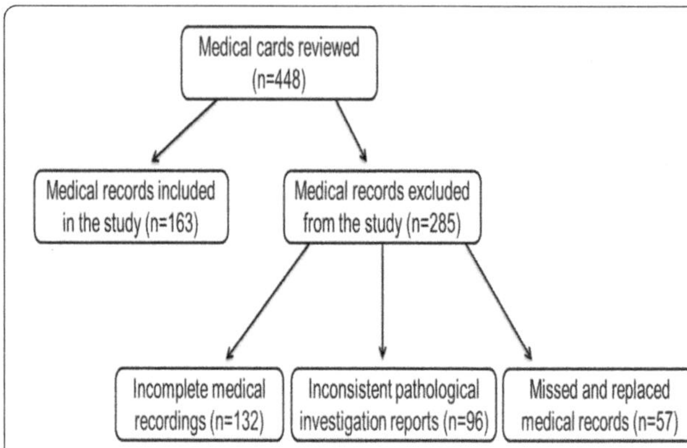

Fig. 1 Flow diagram of recruitments. Medical records of patients who were diagnosed as OT from September 2008 to August 2015 were reviewed

Table 1 Socio-demographic characteristics of patients with the diagnosis of OT at St. Paul's referral hospital, Addis Ababa, Ethiopia

Socio-demographic characteristics	Frequency (%)
Gender	
Male	88 (54)
Female	75 (46)
Age	
0–19	34 (20.8)
20–39	82 (50.3)
> = 40	47 (28.8)
Address	
Urban	67 (41.1)
Rural	96 (58.9)

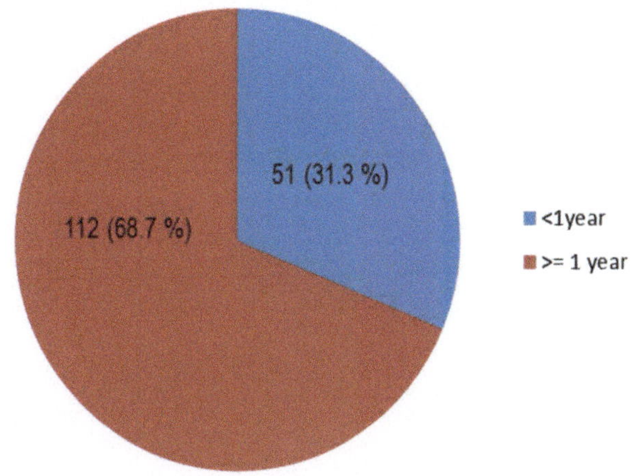

Fig. 2 Presentation of odontogenic tumors. OT cases presented less than or greater than 1 year of onset of symptoms were presented

ratio of 1.27. Similarly, ameloblastoma and primary intra osseous SCC were the two most frequently diagnosed OTs among females. However, odontoma had equal distribution among both genders (Table 3).

Distribution of OT cases by age

The age of patients diagnosed with OT ranged from 8 to 80 years with a mean age of 34 years. 40 (24.5%) ameloblastoma cases were within the age group of 20–39 years. Primary IOSCC was seen predominantly among the age group of greater than or equals to 40 years. Odontogenic myxioma, odontogenic fibroma and odontoma were commonly seen among the age group of 20–39 years which accounted 7 (50%), 6 (75%) and 4 (66.7%), respectively. 5 (50%) of KCOT were diagnosed with the age range of 0–19 years old. Similar number of ameloblastic fibroma was seen in patients age group of 0–19 and 20–39. 11 (73.3%) of other type of OTs were seen in the age group of 20.39 years old (Table 4).

Distribution of OT case by location

OTs were located in different sites of maxillofacial areas. Mandible was the most frequently affected site constituting 126 (77.3%) of OT cases, while the maxilla was affected in 37 (22.7%) of OT cases. Of the different classes of OTs, ameloblastoma, primary IOSCC, odontogenic myxioma, and odontogenic fibroma were the most frequent forms OTs that were diagnosed in the mandible. Similarly, ameloblastoma, primary IOSCC and KCOT were the commonest OT types that affected maxilla (Table 5).

Table 2 Frequency distribution of odontogenic tumors at St. Paul's referral hospital, Addis Ababa, Ethiopia

Types of odontogenic tumor		Frequency (%)	Frequency (%)
Being tumors	Ameloblastoma	75 (46.0)	131 (80.4%)
	Odontogenic myxioma	14 (8.6)	
	Keratocystic OT	10 (6.1)	
	Odontogenic fibroma	10 (6.1)	
	Ameloblatic fibroma	9 (4.3)	
	Odontoma	6 (3.7)	
	Others	9 (5.4)	
Malignant tumors	Primary intra osseous SCC	26 (16.8)	32 (19.6%)

Surgical treatment and its complications

Out of the total 163 patients, 135 (82.8%) received surgical treatment while 28 (17.2%) were referred to other oncology centers. From the 135 patients who received primary treatment at SPRH, 80 (49.1%) of patients had segmental resection whilst 20 (12.3%) had marginal resection. In addition, enucleation and curettage were done for 35 (21.5%) of the treated patients (Table 6).

Facial disfiguration, malocclusion, numbness, recurrence, and continuity defects were the complications observed after surgical treatment in 66 (40.5%), 56 (36.2%), 13 (8.0%), 20 (12.3%) and 80 (49.1%) patients, respectively. Of note,

Table 3 Distribution of odontogenic tumors by sex at St. Paul's referral hospital, Addis Ababa, Ethiopia

Types of OTs	Gender		Total	Male to female ratio
	Male	Female		
Ameloblastoma	42	33	75	1.27
Primary intra osseous SCC	16	10	26	1.6
Odontogenic myxioma	10	4	14	2.5
Keratocystic OT	2	8	10	0.25
Odontogenic fibroma	4	6	10	0.67
Ameloblatic fibroma	6	3	9	2
Odontoma	3	3	6	1
Others	6	9	15	0.67
Total OTs cases	89	74	163	1.2

Table 4 Distribution of odontogenic tumors by age at St. Paul's referral hospital, Addis Ababa, Ethiopia

Odontogenic tumors	Age (years)		
	0-19	20-39	> = 40
Ameloblastoma	17	40	18
Primary intra osseous SCC	0	7	19
Odontogenic myxioma	5	7	2
Keratocystic OT	5	3	2
Odontogenic fibroma	1	6	1
Ameloblatic fibroma	4	4	1
Odontoma	1	4	1
Others	1	11	3
Total OTs cases	34	82	47

out of these 135 patients who had surgical treatment, 47 of them had no any complication after surgery (Table 6).

Bivariate logistic regression analysis was conducted to assess the relationship between complications after surgery and different variables such as gender, age, place of residence, size and time of OT presentation. Importantly, complication after surgery had statistically significant relation with place of residence and tumor size. Living in the rural areas had more likely chance of having complication after surgery than living in the urban areas [Adjusted OR = 2.13, (95% CI: 0.98, 4.6)]. Similarly, as size of tumor increases the chances of having complication after surgery also increases [Adjusted OR = 4.24, (95% CI: 1.76, 10.21)]. However, gender, age, time of OT presentation were not statistically significant ($P > 0.05$) (Table 7).

Discussion

Studies of OT among population are crucial for identification of the population group at risk, possible factors associated to OT development, and to develop more precisely differential diagnosis [13]. OTs studies are very scarce in Ethiopia. Therefore, we aimed at investigating the pattern of OTs in Ethiopia over a period of 8 years. In the current study, there were significant number of medical records that were excluded from the analysis. Of note, most of the complete records were for patients who had surgical treatment. In fact, most patients who had surgical treatment were with benign OT, which might in turn have led to the over representation of benign tumors over malignant ones. Therefore, it is important that the readers keep this in mind and interpret the date carefully.

Classes of OTs can either be benign or malignant. However, when considered globally, there is a considerable racial predilection for specific types of tumor. In this study, about 80.4% of the cases were benign OTs. This finding is slightly lower than reports from Nigeria (96.8%) [14] and (96.6%) [15], India (100%) [16], Turkey (93.2%) [12], and Brazil (94.5%) [13]. Some forms of benign OTs such as KCOT, odontoma do not exhibit clinical symptom. As a result, the chances of detecting them are really low unless otherwise patients had routine dental examination, which is unusual practice in Ethiopia. This might be a reason for low incidence of benign tumors in the current study. On the other hand, about 19.6% of this study cases were found to be malignant. This finding is higher than reports from Nigeria (3.2%) [14] and (3.4%) [15], Turkey (6.8%) [12] and Brazil (5.5%) [13]. The observed differences in the distribution of malignant OTs might be due to the geographical and cultural variation among the different study population. For instance, some of our study participants were using traditional medicines such as leaves, stems, and roots of some plants before coming to the hospital. Nevertheless, these traditional medications are not successful in curing

Table 5 Distribution of odontogenic tumors by site of occurrence at St. Paul's referral hospital, Addis Ababa, Ethiopia

Odontogenic tumors	Maxilla	Mandible	Maxilla: Mandible
Ameloblastoma	8	67	0.18
Primary intra osseous SCC	8	18	0.44
Odontogenic myxioma	3	11	0.27
Keratocystic OT	6	4	1.5
Odontogenic fibroma	3	7	0.43
Ameloblatic fibroma	4	5	0.8
Odontoma	0	6	-
Others	5	10	0.5
Total OTs cases	37	126	0.3

Table 6 Frequency distribution of surgical treatment and its complications of odontogenic tumors at St. Paul's referral hospital, Addis Ababa, Ethiopia

Variables			Frequency (%)
Surgical treatment	Jaw Resection	Segmental	80 (49.1)
		Marginal	20 (12.3)
	Enucleation and curettage		35 (21.5)
	Referral to oncology center		28 (17.2)
Surgical Complication	Yes		116 (71.2)
	No		47 (28.8)
Type of surgical Complications	Facial disfigurement		66 (40.5)
	Malocclusion		56 (36.2)
	Numbness		13 (8.0)
	Recurrence		20 (12.3)
	Continuity defect		80 (49.1)
	Other		4 (2.5)

Table 7 Bivariate analysis of complication after surgery for odontogenic tumor treatment and different factors at St. Paul's referral hospital, Addis Ababa, Ethiopia

Variables		Complication after surgery		Crude OR	Adjusted OR	*P*-value
		Yes	No			
Gender	Female	55 (33.7%)	20 (12.3%)			0.97
	Male	61 (37.4%)	27 (16.6%)	0.82 (0.42,0.82)	1.02 (0.48,2.14)	
Age	0–19	27 (16.6%)	7 (4.3%)			0.16
	20–39	60 (36.8%)	22 (13.5%)	0.71 (0.27,1.85)	2.18 (0.74,6.42)	0.41
	> = 40	29 (17.8%)	18 (11.0%)	0.42 (0.15,1.16)	1.42 (0.61,3.28)	
Place of residence	Urban	53 (32.5%)	14 (8.6%)			0.05*
	Rural	63 (38.7%)	33 (20.2%)	1.98 (0.96,4.09)	2.13 (0.98,4.6)	
Tumor size	0–3 cm	23 (14.1%)	20 (12.3%)			0.186
	4–6 cm	28 (17.2%)	14 (8.6%)	1.74 (0.72,4.18)	1.86 (0.74,4.66)	0.001*
	> = 7 cm	65 (39.9%)	13 (8.0%)	4.35 (1.87,10.12)	4.24 (1.76,10.21)	
Time of OT presentation	<1 year	32 (19.6%)	19 (11.7%)			0.17
	> = 1 year	84 (51.5%)	28 (17.2%)	1.78 (0.88,3.63)	1.71 (0.8,3.67)	

maxillofacial related health problems. Thus, the use of traditional medicines among our study participants, in the context of maxillofacial problems, might increase the risk of transforming benign tumor into malignant tumor. Besides, most of our study patients sought dental and maxillofacial treatments at late stages of disease. This alone could contribute a lot to the transformation of benign OTs into malignant OTs [15, 17].

In the current study, ameloblastoma was the most frequent type of OTs accounting for about 46% of all OTs. This finding is consistent to reports from Nigeria [14, 15], India [16], Pakistan [18], Kenya [19], and Tanzania [20]. Primary IOSCC was found to be the second most common type of OTs (16%). This finding is lower than reports from Pakistan [2] and China [4], and higher than another report from China [3]. The observed variation in the distribution of primary IOSCC could probably be due to small sample size in the current study. Likewise, odontogenic myxoma was found to be the third most common type of OT in the current study which accounted for about 8.6%. This finding is consistent with a report from Nigeria [21]. Furthermore, the remaining OTs types such as KCOT, odontogenic fibroma, ameloblastic fibroma, odontoma, CCOT, cementoblastoma, malignant ameloblastoma, clear cell odontogenic tumor and gouts cell odontogenic tumor accounted for about 29.4% of the total OTs.

In the present study, most of OT cases were seen in males than females. This finding is in accordance with other reports from Pakistan [18], and Nigeria [9, 15]. In contrary, reports from Ceará, Brazil [7], Rio Grande do Norte, Brazil [10] and Mumbai, India [16] revealed a predominance of OTs among females than males. With respect to the distribution of specific OT types, the majority (56%) of ameloblastoma cases were seen among males. This finding is similar to different reports from Nigeria [9, 15, 21], India [16], and Argentina [22]. In addition, primary IOSCC was found to be the most frequent type of OTs in males 16 (61.5%), a finding consistent with two different reports from China [3, 4].

OTs were more frequent during the second and third decades of patients life. Previous reports from Ceará, Brazil [7], Rio Grande do Norte, Brazil [10], Pakistan [18], and Argentina [22] revealed similar results. In the present study, 40 (53.3%) ameloblastoma cases were identified within the age group of 20–39 years, a finding comparable to reports from Brazil [13], Nigeria [14, 15], India [16], and Pakistan [18]. Moreover, 19 (73.1%) of primary IOSCC were seen among patients with age of 40 years and older. This finding is in line with reports from China [3, 4].

About 77.3% of OTs were observed in the mandible, whereas the remaining 22.7% were located in the maxilla. This finding is similar to reports from Ceará, Brazil [7], Rio Grande do Norte, Brazil [10], Nigeria [14, 15], Mumbai, India [16], Pakistan [18], Kenya [19] Tanzania [20] and Buenos Aires, Argentina [22]. Mandible was found to be the most common site in about 89.3% of ameloblastoma cases in this study. This finding is comparable with reports from Nigeria [9, 15, 21], India [16], and Brazil [23, 24]. In addition, predilection of mandible was observed among the primary IOSCC, a finding consistent with reports from Pakistan [2] and China [3, 4].

Complication after surgical treatment of OTs is a commonly encountered phenomenon [14]. Unsurprisingly, about 71.2% of patients had complication after surgery. Of note, a patient could have more than one form of complications. About 12.3% of the cases had history of recurrence, a finding which is higher than a report from Nigeria [14]. In addition, the present study showed statistically significant association between two independent variables; place of residence and tumor size with complication after surgery. This shows that living in the rural areas lead to have higher chances of having complication after surgery than living in the urban areas. In addition, an increase in the size of tumor increased the chance of having complication after surgery. This association could be explained by the fact that dental services in general and maxillofacial services in particular are extremely scarce in Ethiopia, moreover in the rural parts. Thus, patients from the rural area would have a late presentation to dental and/or maxillofacial clinics. The late presentation of cases in turn could result in large sizes of OTs. As a consequence, necessitates a wide surgical procedures to be carried out for the treatment. Hence, patients will have a higher chance of having complications after surgery.

Conclusions

The vast majority of patient's medical records were incomplete and handled in appropriately. Therefore, the record archiving of the hospital needs to be improved, for instance, providing written data recording protocols, implementing a sustainable digital data archiving system, and providing continuous training and audit. Different patterns of OTs and their distribution among different age groups and genders were observed. Intriguingly, posterior mandible was the commonest site involved in OTs. Complication after surgery had a statistically significant association with tumor size and place of residency. Though the profession of dentistry is at the early stage of development in Ethiopia, the community has to bring behavioral changes in having habit of regular visit to dentists.

Acknowledgements

The authors are grateful to all staff members of Dentistry and Maxillofacial Surgery Department, and archive officers of St. Paul's referral hospital, Addis Ababa, Ethiopia for their support during data collection.

Funding

This work was supported by the Postgraduate office of College of Health Sciences, Jimma University, Ethiopia to [BK]. The funding institute has no role in the design of the study and collection, analysis, and interpretation of data and in writing the manuscript.

Authors' contributions

Conceived and designed the study: BK, DT, and FA. Collected data: BK and BB. Analyzed the data: BK and FA. Wrote the paper: BK, DT, BB and FA. All authors read and approved the final manuscript.

Competing interests

The authors declare that they have no competing interests.

Consent for publication

Not applicable as secondary data was used.

Ethics approval and consent to participate

Ethical approval was given by the ethical review board of College of Public Health and Medical Sciences, Jimma University, Ethiopia.

Author details

[1]Oral and Maxillofacial Surgery case team, Department of Dentistry, Jimma University, Jimma, Ethiopia. [2]Department of Surgery, Jimma University, Jimma, Ethiopia. [3]Department of Dentistry, Millennium Medical College, St. Paul's Referral Hospital, Addis Ababa, Ethiopia. [4]Department of Epidemiology, Jimma University, Jimma, Ethiopia.

References

1. Abdulai AE, Nuamah IK, Gyasi RK. Jaw Tumors in Ghanaian Children and Adolescents: A Retrospective Study. World J Surg Med Radiat Oncol. 2012;1:83–90.
2. Akram S, Naghma AMA, Shakir MM. Prevalence of Odontogenic Cysts and Tumors in Karachi, Pakistan. J Dow Uni Health Sci. 2013;7:20–4.
3. Luo HY, Li TJ. Odontogenic tumors: A study of 1309 cases in a Chinese population. Oral Oncol. 2009;45:706–11.
4. Jing W, Xuan M, Lin Y, Wu L, Liu L, Zheng X, et al. Odontogenic tumours: a retrospective study of 1642 cases in a Chinese population. Int J Oral Maxillofac Surg. 2007;36:20–5.
5. Thompson L. World Health Organization classification of tumours: pathology and genetics of head and neck tumours. Ear Nose Throat J. 2006;85:74.
6. Moridani SG, Shaahsavari F, Adeli MB. A 7-year retrospective study of biopsied oral lesions in 460 Iranian patients. RSBO. 2014;11:118–24.
7. Avelar RL, Antunes AA, Santos Tde S, Andrade ES, Dourado E. Odontogenic tumors: clinical and pathology study of 238 cases. Braz J Otorhinolaryngol. 2008;74:668–73.
8. UNDP. Human Development Report. Work for Human Development. 2015. http://hdr.undp.org/sites/default/files/2015_human_development_report.pdf. Accessed 4 Nov 2016.
9. Lawal AO, Adisa AO, Popoola BO. Odontogenic tumours in children and adolescents: A review of forty-eight cases. Ann Ibadan Postgrad. 2013;11:7–11.
10. Santos JN, Pereira Pinto L, de Figueredo CRL, de Souza LB. Odontogenic tumors : analysis of 127 cases. Pesqui Odontol Bras. 2001;15:308–13.
11. Sharif FN, Oliver R, Sweet C, Sharif MO. Interventions for the treatment of keratocystic odontogenic tumours (KCOT, odontogenic keratocysts (OKC)). Cochrane Database Syst Rev. 2010; doi:10.1002/14651858.CD008464.pub2.
12. Senel FC, Dayisoylu EH, Ersöz S, Yilmaz Altintaş N, Tosun E, Ungör C, et al. The relative frequency of odontogenic tumors in the Black Sea region of Turkey: an analysis of 86 cases. Turk J Med Sci. 2012;42:1463–70.
13. da Costa D-O-P, Mauricio A-S, de Faria P-A-S, da Silva L-E, Mosqueda-Taylor A, Lourenco S-Q-C. Odontogenic tumors: a retrospective study of four Brazilian diagnostic pathology centers. Med Oral Patol Oral Cir Bucal. 2012; 17:e389-94.
14. Anyanechi CE, Saheeb BD. A review of 156 odontogenic tumours in Calabar, Nigeria. Ghana Med J. 2014;48:163–7.
15. Ladeinde AL, Ajayi OF, Ogunlewe MO, Adeyemo WL, Arotiba GT, Bamgbose BO, et al. Odontogenic tumors: A review of 319 cases in a Nigerian teaching hospital. Oral Surgery. Oral Med Oral Pathol Oral Radiol Endodontology. 2005;99:191–5.
16. Varkhede A, Tupkari JV, Mandale MS, Sardar M. Odontogenic tumors: A review of 60 cases. J Clin Exp Dent. 2010. doi:10.4317/jced.2.e183.
17. Nagi R, Sahu S, Rakesh N. Molecular and genetic aspects in the etiopathogenesis of ameloblastoma: An update. J Oral Maxillofac Pathol. 2016;20:497–504.
18. Naz I, Mahmood MK, Akhtar F, Nagi AH. Clinicopathological evaluation of odontogenic tumours in pakistan - A seven years retrospective study. Asian Pacific J Cancer Prev. 2014;15:3327–30.
19. Butt FMA, Ogengo J, Bahra J, Chindia ML, Dimba EAO, Wagaiyu E. 19-year audit of benign jaw tumors and tumor-like lesions in a teaching hospital in Nairobi, Kenya. OJST. 2012;2:54–9.
20. Simon ENM, Stoelinga PJW, Vuhahula E, Ngassapa D. Odontogenic tumours and tumour-like lesions in Tanzania. East Afr Med J. 2002;79:3–7.

21. Ajayi OF, Ladeinde AL, Adeyemo WL, Ogunlewe MO. Odontogenic tumors in Nigerian children and adolescents- a retrospective study of 92 cases. World J Surg Oncol. 2004;2:39.
22. Guerrisi M, Piloni MJ, Keszler A. Odontogenic tumors in children and adolescents. A 15-year retrospective study in Argentina. Med Oral Patol Oral Cir Bucal. 2007;12:E180–5.
23. Deepthi PV, Beena VT, Padmakumar SK, Rajeev R, Sivakumar R. A study of 1177 odontogenic lesions in a South Kerala population. J. Oral Maxillofac. Pathol. 2016;20:202–7.
24. Kowkabi M, Razavi SM, Khosravi N, Navabi AA. Odontogenic tumors in Iran, Isfahan: A study of 260 cases. Dent Res J (Isfahan). 2012;9:725–9.

24

Validation of the Arabic Version of the Early Childhood Oral Health Impact Scale (ECOHIS)

Nada J. Farsi[1*], Azza A. El-Housseiny[2,3], Deema J. Farsi[2] and Najat M. Farsi[2]

Abstract

Background: Assessment of the adverse effects of oral health problems on oral health-related quality of life (OHRQoL) is essential to ensure the well-being of children. The Early Childhood Oral Health Impact Scale (ECOHIS) is an instrument that was designed to assess caregivers' perceptions of OHRQoL in preschool children. Although it has been translated into many languages, it has yet to be validated in Arabic. Therefore, this study aimed to translate this questionnaire to Arabic (A-ECOHIS) and test its psychometric properties.

Methods: Questionnaire responses from three samples of caregivers of preschool children ≤ 6 years of age were collected: (i) community-based ($n = 422$), from preschools selected as a stratified random sample; (ii) clinic-based, from those seeking pediatric dental care at a university clinic ($n = 246$); and (iii) a test-retest sample ($n = 68$), a clinic-based group of caregivers who completed questionnaires twice about siblings who were not receiving dental care. Children received a dental examination to assess their decayed, missed, filled teeth (dmft) scores. Convergent validity was evaluated by assessing the A-ECOHIS scores in relation to the response to a global question. Discriminant validity was evaluated by comparing the scores of children with varying levels of oral disease. Internal consistency was assessed by calculating Cronbach's alpha, and the test-retest reliability was assessed using intra-class correlation coefficients (ICCs).

Results: The A-ECOHIS scores of the questionnaire sections and the global oral health rating were significantly correlated; Spearman correlation coefficients were, $r = 0.55$, $P \leq 0.01$ (overall score), $r = 0.54$, $P \leq 0.01$ (child section), and $r = 0.51$, $P \leq 0.01$ (family section). The mean A-ECOHIS scores were also statistically significantly higher in children with higher dmft scores compared with lower dmft, and in the clinic-based sample compared with the community sample. The Cronbach's alpha value of the the child, family sections and overall questionnaire were, 0.80, 0.78, and 0.85, respectively. The intra-class correlation coefficient (ICC) of A-ECOHIS was 0.86.

Conclusion: The A-ECOHIS performed well on all psychometric tests to which it was applied. Thus, it is a valid and reliable instrument that can be used in Arabic-speaking caregivers of preschoolers aged 2 to 6 years.

Keywords: Quality of life, Validation, ECOHIS, Preschool children

* Correspondence: njfarsi@kau.edu.sa
[1]Department of Dental Public Health, Faculty of Dentistry, King Abdulaziz University, P.O. Box 80200, Jeddah 21589, Saudi Arabia
Full list of author information is available at the end of the article

Background

Children younger than six years of age are especially vulnerable to oral health problems [1]. These problems include temporary teething discomfort, trauma to the teeth and supporting structures, and early childhood caries [2]. Caries, despite recent preventive regimes and advanced early diagnosis methods, remains a prevalent childhood disease around the world. In fact, dental caries is the most common chronic disease in children [3]. In the US, 1 in every 4 children between 2 and 5 years of age has had caries in the primary teeth [4]. The prevalence of caries is also high in most Arabi countries including Saudi Arabia [5, 6]. In Saudi Arabia, the prevalence of caries was estimated to be 73% [7], and a meta-analysis by Khan et al. found a mean decayed, missing, filled teeth (dmft) score due to caries of 5.38 in primary dentition [8].

Oral health problems can have a negative effect on a young child's functional, psychological, and social well-being and, in turn, on the family as a whole. The impact of such problems can be manifested as pain, loss of function, psychological effects, problems with proper weight gain and growth, restriction of daily activities, and disruption of the normal family functioning [9–12].

Although clinical manifestations are of pivotal importance, the physical and psychosocial impact of oral disease cannot be assessed by these parameters alone [13]. Recently, healthcare professionals have begun to incorporate into the oral health assessment the patients' perceptions of how their oral health affects their quality of life (QoL) [14].

A number of oral health-related QoL (OHRQoL) instruments have been designed to assess the impact of oral health problems, some of which focus on the pediatric population. These include the Parental-Caregiver Perceptions Questionnaire (P-CPQ) [15], the infantile and toddler QoL (ITQoL), child oral health impact profile (COHIP), child oral impact daily performance (child-OIDP), child perception questionnaire (CPQ) [16–20] and Caries-QC [21]. However, it was not until 2007, when Pahel et al. developed the Early Childhood Oral Health Impact Scale (ECOHIS), that an instrument was designed especially for young children [22].

The ECOHIS tests the impact of oral health problems on both young children and their families. Because preschoolers have not reached a developmental and psychological level that allows them to accurately recall past events and give accurate accounts of personal experiences, the questionnaire is designed for adult caregivers, who can better relate the impact of oral health on the child's life [22].

The ECOHIS has performed well and has shown good reliability and validity. The scale has been translated into several languages and has been tested and validated on diverse populations with promising results [23–28]. The first translation was into French [23], followed by Chinese [25], Brazilian Portuguese [24, 27], Spanish [26], Lithuanian [29], and Malay [28]. In the Middle East, it has been translated into Farsi and Turkish [30, 31]. In this study, we aimed to translate ECOHIS into the Arabic language (A-ECOHIS) and test its psychometric properties on an Arabic-speaking population.

Methods

The questionnaire

The original ECOHIS questionnaire was developed in English by Pahel et al., who demonstrated its validity and reliability [22]. It comprises 13 questions and is divided into child and family impact sections. The child impact section includes nine items and comprises four domains: child symptoms, function, psychology, and self-image and social interaction. The family impact section contains four items and comprises two domains: parental distress and family function.

Development of A-ECOHIS

The English version of the ECOHIS was translated into Arabic using the well-recognized forward-backward translation technique [32]. Two native Arabic speakers, who speak English fluently, independently translated the original English version of ECOHIS. The Arabic versions were revised with the aid of one of the authors and the two translators, from which one preliminary Arabic version was produced. This version was translated back to English by two bilingual professionals. Finally, the two back-translated English versions were compared with the original English version, and minor adjustments were made to the final Arabic version by adjusting the translation of the words "trouble" and "upset" in questions 6 and 10, respectively (Fig. 1). As with the English version [22], response options for A-ECOHIS were coded as follows: 0 = never, 1 = hardly ever, 2 = occasionally, 3 = often, 4 = very often, and 5 = don't know; and subjects were asked to answer the questions based on the whole life span of the child. To test the questionnaire's comprehensibility, a pilot study was conducted with 10 caregivers not involved in the main study, and the questionnaire was simplified.

The total score was calculated by summing the scores of all questions, and separate scores were calculated for each of the questionnaire sections. The range of the child section scores was 0 to 36, and the range of the family section was 0 to 16. Missing values were handled as described in the original study [22]; "don't know" responses were treated as missing. For maximum utilization of the data, for subjects with ≤ 2 missing values in the child impact section, or ≤ 1 missing value in the family impact section, the missing values were

إن مشكلات الفم والأسنان وعلاجها قد تؤثر على جودة الحياة اليومية للطفل وأسرته.

الرجاء اختيار الرقم الذي يعبر عن تجربة الطفل أو تجربتك، مع الأخذ في الاعتبار حياة الطفل كاملة منذ ولادته حتى الآن أثناء الإجابة على كل سؤال . إذا كان السؤال لا ينطبق عليك فاختار "إطلاقاً"

		اطلاقا 0	نادرا 1	احيانا 2	كثيرا 3	كثيرا جدا 4	لا اعلم 5
الطفل	1 ما مدى تكرار حدوث ألم بأسنان أو فم أو فكي طفلك؟						
	ما مدى تكرار حدوث التالي لطفلك نتيجة مشكلات الفم والأسنان؟						
	2 صعوبة في شرب المشروبات الباردة أو الساخنة						
	3 صعوبة في تناول بعض الأطعمة						
	4 صعوبة في نطق أي كلمات						
	5 تغيب عن الحضانة أو الروضة أو المدرسة						
	6 مشاكل في النوم						
	7 أصبح محبطا أو سريع الانفعال						
	8 تجنب الابتسام أو الضحك في وجود أطفال اخرين						
	9 تجنب التحدث مع أطفال آخرين						
العائلة	**ما مدى تكرار حدوث التالي لك أو لأحد أفراد العائلة كنتيجة لمشكلات فم وأسنان طفلك؟**						
	10 الشعور بالانزعاج						
	11 الشعور بالذنب						
	12 أخذ إجازة أو إذن من العمل						
	13 تأثير مادي على العائلة						

Fig. 1 The Arabic version of the Early Childhood Oral Health Impact Scale (A-ECOHIS)

imputed by using the mean of the rest of the values of each section accordingly. Therefore, subjects could be included in the analysis of one section but not the other, as was done in the original study [22]. Subjects with > 2 missing values in the child impact section and with > 1 missing value in the family impact section were excluded.

Study subjects

In this study, community-based and clinic-based samples were collected. For participants to be included, Arabic had to be the native language of the caregivers, and they had to be able to fill in the questionnaire independently. They also had to be living with the child for ≥ 50% of the time. Their children had to be healthy, not on long-term medications, and with no physical, learning, or mental disabilities. The participants of the community-based sample (n = 425) were caregivers of preschool children ≤ 6 years of age. The targeted population included all Saudi and non-Saudi children who were registered in kindergarten schools in Jeddah according to the Ministry of Education (population, 14,808 children). The sampling method of the study was multistage stratified random sampling from the preschool children in Jeddah. There were 7448 male and 7360 female children distributed among 34 public and 181 private preschools.

It was determined to choose the school as a unit of sample selection using a numbered list that was previously prepared. Preschools were randomly selected using Random Number Generator [33]. Two numbers representing a private and a public school were selected in each of Jeddah's main four districts (North, East, South, and West). Approval to visit the selected preschools and collect data from the children was obtained from the Ministry of Education in Jeddah, and approval of the school principal was obtained prior to the school visit.

During the first preschool visit, consent forms with information about the study were distributed to the children. Children were encouraged to bring back the signed consent forms the next morning. At the next school visit, examinations were performed on the children who brought back a signed consent.

The clinic-based group (n = 246) comprised caregivers of a convenience sample of children 6 years old or younger seeking dental care in the pediatric dental clinics of King Abdulaziz University. The A-ECOHIS was given to the participating caregivers for completion while they were at the clinic. Socio-demographic information on the caregivers and children was also collected. In total, 750 questionnaires were distributed, and the response rate was 89.5%. The recruitment period was from September 2013 to April 2014.

Children in the community and clinic-based samples received a dental examination by one examiner who used an agreed-upon rubric and was trained and calibrated in the Faculty of Dentistry of King Abdulaziz University for the detection of caries in 2 to 6 year-old children using the World Health Organization 1997 criteria [34].

Children were seated on a chair with a back rest; a knee to knee position was used with very young children. Caries experience as decayed, missed and filled teeth (dmft) were diagnosed using a blunt Community Periodontal Index (CPI) probe (Nordent, Elk Grove Village, IL, USA), disposable plane mirror and adequate light using standard infection control measures. Teeth were examined visually and the CPI probe was used to remove debris and confirm visual evidence of caries. Teeth were recorded as sound, if they showed no evidence of treatment or caries into dentin. Teeth with white, discolored or rough spots, stained pits or fissures without cavitations or softening were also recorded as sound. Teeth were recorded carious, if there was a visible cavity, undermined enamel or detectably softened floor or wall. Teeth only extracted due to caries were recorded as missing [34]. A confidential report was given to the caregivers of the community-based sample with advice to seek dental care in any dental facility if needed.

Ethical approval for the study was obtained from the Research Ethics Committee, Faculty of Dentistry King Abdulaziz University (#036-13). Informed consent was obtained from all participating caregivers.

Validation of A-ECOHIS

Convergent validity

To test the convergent validity for the community-based sample, the following global oral health question was added: "In general, how would you rate the overall oral health of your child?" This question had five response options: 0 = excellent, 1 = very good, 2 = good, 3 = fair, and 4 = poor. The mean A-ECOHIS scores of each group of respondents, according to their global question response were compared. We hypothesized that caregivers with a response of "excellent" on the global question would have a low A-ECOHIS score, and that the score would increase as the global question responses became lower. Furthermore, ratings of "excellent", "very good" and "good" in the global question were combined into "good health", while "fair" and "poor" ratings were combined into "poor health", and the mean A-ECOHIS scores for both levels were compared with a *t*-test, which is robust against non-normality when the sample size is ≥ 40 [35].

Spearman's rank order correlations were used to assess correlations between the responses to the global question and each of the A-ECOHIS section scores.

Discriminant validity

In the community-based sample, the A-ECOHIS scores for each of the sections between children with varying dmft scores (none, 1–5, >5) were compared. We hypothesized that children with higher dmft scores would have higher A-ECOHIS scores. To further assess the discriminant validity of A-ECOHIS, we compared the A-ECOHIS scores of each questionnaire domain between the community-based and clinic-based samples. Because children in the clinic-based sample probably had worse oral health, we hypothesized that they would have lower A-ECOHIS scores.

Internal consistency

Spearman's rank order correlations were used to assess the correlations between the child and family impact section scores in the community-based sample, and to estimate the inter-item correlations. Cronbach's alpha was also produced for each of the scale sections and for the whole scale. We hypothesized that the child and family scores as well as the scale items would be correlated.

Test-retest reliability

A sample was collected ($n = 78$) to assess the test-retest reliability of the questionnaire. The caregivers of children seeking treatment at the Pediatric Dental Clinics in King Abdulaziz University, who were accompanied by siblings aged 0 to 6 years, were approached, and consenting caregivers were asked to complete the questionnaire about the sibling who was not receiving dental treatment. They were given the questionnaire again after 2 to 3 weeks, when they came for a follow-up appointment. It was verified that the participating subjects did not report changes in their child's oral health condition or treatments during this period. The intra-class correlation coefficient was used to assess the test-retest reliability in the sample for each of the questionnaire sections and for the questionnaire as a whole.

Sample size calculation

Using the tables developed by Saunders and Huynh, a sample size of 245 subjects was determined for reliability testing [36], given the assumption that the ECOHIS is a 13-item test of a moderate degree of difficulty and low variability. The calculation was made considering the degree of precision to be 0.05%.

Results

Of the 425 community-based participants, three subjects who had missing values for more than two items of the child section and more than one item of the family section were excluded from the analyses. One participant of the clinic sample with more than 2 missing values in the child section and no missing values in the family section was included in the score calculation for the family section, but not the child section. In addition, 20 participants from the community sample with more than 1 missing value in the family section and no missing values in the child section were included in the child section analyses only.

Table 1 presents the demographic characteristics of the participants. The mean age of the community-based

Table 1 Demographic characteristics of the study participants

Variable	Community-based sample	Clinic-based sample	*P*-Value
	n = 422 (%)	*n* = 246 (%)	
Age, mean (SD)	4.5 (0.6)	4.6 (1.2)	0.246
Gender			
Male	181 (42.9)	117 (47.6)	0.242
Female	241 (57.1)	129 (52.4)	
Nationality			
Saudi	263 (63.2)	123 (50.0)	<0.01
Non-Saudi	153 (36.8)	123 (50.0)	
School type			
Private	343 (81.3)	–	–
Public	79 (18.7)	–	
dmft score			
0	136 (32.2)	11 (4.5)	<0.01
1-5	161 (38.2)	40 (16.3)	
> 5	125 (29.6)	195 (79.3)	
dmft score, mean (SD)	4.0 (4.4)	9.9 (5.0)	<0.01

SD standard deviation, *dmft* decayed, missing, filled teeth

sample was 4.5 ± 0.6 years, whereas the mean age of the clinic-based sample was 4.6 ± 1.2 years. Females comprised 57 and 52% of the community and clinic samples, respectively. Of the community sample, 81% attended private schools, while 19% attended public schools. The clinic sample had statistically significantly higher dmft scores compared with the community sample (9.9 ± 5.0 and 4.0 ± 4.4, respectively).

The distribution of the A-ECOHIS responses is presented in Table 2. Among the community-based subjects, pain was the most reported item (35%), followed by irritability or frustration (24%), and difficulty eating (24%), in the child section. Caregivers being upset was the most reported item in the family section (31%). There was one response of "don't know" to three items (pain, irritability or frustration, and avoid talking) and missing values, which ranged from 0.2% for the pain item to 5.5% for the financial impact item. Among the clinic-based subjects, in the child section, the most commonly reported item was pain (65%), followed by eating difficulty (57%), and difficulty in drinking hot or cold drinks (46%). Most commonly reported in the family section was a caregiver being upset (65%), followed by feeling guilty (53%) about the child's perceived oral health condition. It was evident that subjects in the clinic sample were experiencing a greater impact on QoL compared to those in the community sample. There were 2% of subjects who answered "don't know" to the school absence item, whereas 0.8% reported this for the pronunciation difficulty, avoid smiling or laughing, and avoid talking items. Missing values ranged from 0.4% for feeling guilty, and for irritability and frustration, to 2.8% for the school absence item.

Convergent validity was assessed using the community-based data. The mean A-ECOHIS overall score was much lower for subjects who responded "excellent" (3.9 ± 4) compared with those who responded "poor" (19.1 ± 6.8) to the global health rating question. Similar trends were observed in the child and family sections. When responses to the global question were dichotomized into good and poor health, A-ECOHIS scores in the scale overall and in both of its sections were statistically significantly higher in the latter. The Spearman correlation coefficients between the global oral health rating and the total A-ECOHIS score ($r = 0.55$, $P \le 0.01$), as well as those for the child ($r = 0.54$, $P \le 0.01$) and family section ($r = 0.50$, $P \le 0.01$) scores, were moderate (Table 3).

To test discriminant validity, the A-ECOHIS scores among the community-based data for each of the questionnaire sections were stratified by dmft score (Table 4). The mean A-ECOHIS scores of each section were higher in the higher dmft groups. However, the differences between dmft scores of 0 and 1–5 were not statistically different in some of the domains. The mean A-ECOHIS scores for subjects with a dmft score of zero in the child section, family section and total score were 4.2 ± 4.2, 2.1 ± 2.7, and 6.3 ± 6.2, respectively, whereas they were 4.7 ± 4.3, 2.2 ± 2.9, and 6.6 ± 5.9, respectively, among participants with a dmft score of 1–5. Among subjects with a dmft above 5, the A-ECOHIS scores were 7.8 ± 5.0, 3.6 ± 3.0 and 11.2 ± 7.1, respectively.

When the A-ECOHIS scores were compared between the two samples, the A-ECOHIS mean scores were significantly higher among the clinic-based subjects for each of the questionnaire domains (Table 5). In the community sample, floor effects were observed in 19 and 40% of the participants in the child and family sections, respectively. However, they were observed only in 13% each of the child and family sections in the clinic sample. No ceiling effects were observed in either of the questionnaire sections in the community sample, and they were observed only in the family section in 2.9% of the clinic-based subjects (data not shown).

In the community-based sample, the Spearman correlation coefficient for the relationship between the child and family section scores was of a moderate magnitude but was statistically significant ($r = 0.56$, $P \le 0.01$). As presented in Table 6, Cronbach's alpha values for the child section, family section, and overall questionnaire were 0.80, 0.78, and 0.85, respectively. The inter-item correlations between the 13 items of the A-ECOHIS ranged from 0.1 to 0.7; all were positive and statistically significant ($P \le 0.01$–0.03).

Table 2 Distribution of A-ECOHIS responses in the two study samples

	Community-based sample ($n = 422$)			Clinic-based sample ($n = 246$)		
	Never/hardly ever n (%)	Occasionally, Often, Very often n (%)	Don't know n (%)	Never/hardly ever n (%)	Occasionally, Often, Very often n (%)	Don't know n (%)
I] Child impact section						
i) Symptoms						
Q1 Pain	274 (64.9)	147 (34.8)	1 (0.2)	86 (35.0)	160 (65.0)	0
ii) Function						0
Q2 Difficulty drinking hot or cold beverages	337 (80.2)	83 (19.8)	0	132 (53.7)	114 (46.3)	0
Q3 Difficulty eating	319 (76.1)	100 (23.9)	0	105 (43.2)	138 (56.8)	
Q4 Pronunciation difficulty	351 (84.2)	66 (15.8)	0	193 (78.8)	50 (20.4)	2 (0.8)
Q5 Missed school or daycare	346 (82.4)	74 (17.6)	0	195 (79.9)	44 (18.0)	5 (2.1)
iii) Psychology						
Q6 Trouble sleeping	368 (88.5)	48 (11.5)	0	178 (73.3)	65 (26.8)	0
Q7 Irritability or frustration	317 (75.3)	103 (24.5)	1 (0.2)	172 (70.2)	73 (29.8)	0
iv) Self-image and social interaction						
Q8 Avoid smiling or laughing	378 (90.2)	41 (9.8)	0	199 (81.6)	43 (17.6)	2 (0.8)
Q9 Avoid talking	367 (89.5)	42 (10.2)	1 (0.2)	205 (84.0)	37 (15.2)	2 (0.8)
II] Family impact section						
i) Parental distress						
Q10 Been upset	286 (69.4)	126 (30.6)	0	85 (34.8)	159 (65.2)	0
Q11 Felt guilty about child's oral health	329 (79.9)	83 (20.2)	0	116 (47.4)	129 (52.7)	0
ii) Family function						
Q12 Taken time off work	351 (87.3)	51 (12.7)	0	154 (63.4)	89 (36.6)	0
Q13 Financial impact	345 (86.5)	54 (13.5)	0	165 (67.1)	81 (32.9)	0

A-ECOHIS Arabic version of the Early Childhood Oral Health Impact Scale

Test-retest reliability was assessed on the sample of subjects who were administered the questionnaire twice ($n = 78$); however, 10 of these subjects were excluded because of missing data. The pre-test A-ECOHIS scores of the child and family sections were 6.8 ± 6.5, and 5.1 ± 4.2, respectively, and were 7.4 ± 7.1 and 6.3 ± 4.2, respectively, at the post-test. The mean of the total A-ECOHIS score was 11.9 ± 9.3 at the pre-test and 13.7 ± 10.3 at the post-test. The estimated intra-class correlation coefficients are presented in Table 6.

Table 3 Evaluating the difference in mean A-ECOHIS scores by oral health status rating category

Global health rating question response	Child impact section				Family impact section				Overall scale			
	n	Mean (SD)	r^a	*P*-value	n	Mean (SD)	r^b	*P*-value	n	mean (SD)	r^c	*P*-value
Correlations												
Excellent	147	2.85 (3.3)	0.54	–	146	1.05 (1.8)	0.50	<0.01	146	3.87 (4.1)	0.55	–
Very good	144	4.96 (3.7)			140	2.63 (2.6)			140	7.56 (5.2)		
Good	57	8.04 (4.9)			57	4.56 (3.6)			57	12.60 (7.6)		
Fair	43	8.92 (4.7)			31	3.39 (2.5)			31	10.85 (5.5)		
Poor	22	12.62 (5.5)			21	6.21 (2.6)			21	19.14 (6.8)		
Differences in mean scores												
Good oral health	348	4.57 (4.1)	–	<0.01	343	2.28 (2.8)	–	<0.01	343	6.83 (6.1)	–	<0.01
Poor oral health	65	10.17 (5.2)			52	4.53 (2.9)			52	14.20 (7.3)		

A-ECOHIS Arabic version of the Early Childhood Oral Health Impact Scale

Excluded from this analysis were 27 subjects who had > 1 missing item on the family section ($n = 18$), missing information on the global question ($n = 7$), and missing both > 1 item on family section and information on the global question ($n = 2$). Spearman correlation coefficients between [a]child impact section score and the global question, [b]family impact section score and the global question, and [c]total A-ECOHIS score and the global question

Table 4 Discriminate validity of the A-ECOHIS among the community-based sample

	Number of items	Range	Number of decayed, missed and filled teeth			Multiple ANOVA comparisons
			None	1–5	>5	
Child symptoms	1	0–4				0 vs. 1–5*
Sample size			136	161	125	1–5 vs. ≥5*
Mean score (SD)			0.5 (0.8)	0.9 (1.0)	1.6 (0.9)	0 vs. ≥5*
Child function	4	0–16				0 vs. 1–5
Sample size			136	161	125	1–5 vs. ≥5*
Mean score (SD)			2.1 (2.1)	2.1 (2.2)	3.7 (2.7)	0 vs. ≥5*
Child Psychology	2	0–8				0 vs. 1–5
Sample size			136	161	125	1–5 vs. ≥5*
Mean score (SD)			1.0 (1.4)	1.0 (1.3)	1.5 (1.5)	0 vs. ≥5*
Self-image and social interaction	2	0–8				0 vs. 1–5
Sample size			136	161	125	1–5 vs. ≥5*
Mean score (SD)			0.6 (1.2)	0.6 (1.1)	1.1 (1.5)	0 vs. ≥5*
Child impact section	9	0–36	4.2 (4.2)	4.7 (4.3)	7.8 (5.0)	0 vs. 1–5
						1–5 vs. ≥5*
						0 vs. ≥5*
Parental Distress	2	0–8				0 vs. 1–5
Sample size			134	153	115	1–5 vs. ≥5*
Mean score (SD)			1.2 (1.7)	1.4 (1.8)	2.3 (2.0)	0 vs. ≥5*
Family function	2	0–8				0 vs. 1–5
Sample size						1–5 vs. ≥5*
Mean score (SD)			134	153	115	0 vs. ≥5*
			0.9 (1.4)	0.8 (1.5)	1.4 (1.6)	
Family impact section	4	0–16	134	153	115	0 vs. 1–5
			2.1 (2.7)	2.2 (2.9)	3.6 (3.0)	1–5 vs. ≥5*
						0 vs. ≥5*
Overall scale	13	0–52	6.3 (6.2)	6.6 (5.9)	11.2 (7.1)	0 vs. 1–5
						1–5 vs. ≥5*
						0 vs. ≥5*

A-ECOHIS Arabic version of the Early Childhood Oral Health Impact Scale, *SD* standard deviation
Excluded from the family section and total ECOHIS analyses were 20 subjects with > 1 missing item in the family section. **P*-value ≤ 0.05, Tukey multiple comparisons test

Table 5 Comparison of A-ECOHIS scores of the different domains in the two study samples

Impacts	Number of items	Range	Community-based sample			Clinic-based sample			*P*-value*
			Mean ± SD	Median	Floor effects	Mean ± SD	Median	Floor effects	
Child symptoms	1	0–4	1.0 (1.0)	1	42%	2.0 (1.3)	2	17%	<0.01
Child function	4	0–16	2.6 (2.4)	2	28%	4.3 (3.4)	4	20%	<0.01
Child Psychology	2	0–8	1.1 (1.4)	0	51%	1.9 (2.0)	1	38%	<0.01
Self-image and social interaction	2	0–8	0.8 (1.3)	0	66%	1.0 (1.7)	0	63%	0.018
Child impact section	9	0–36	5.5 (4.7)	5	19%	9.2 (7.1)	8	13%	<0.01
Parental Distress	2	0–8	1.6 (1.9)	1	44%	3.5 (2.3)	4	17%	<0.01
Family function	2	0–8	1.0 (1.5)	0	58%	2.1 (2.1)	2	34%	<0.01
Family impact section	4	0–16	2.6 (2.9)	2	40%	5.5 (3.9)	5	13%	<0.01
Overall scale	13	0–52	7.8 (6.7)	7	16%	14.6 (9.2)	14	3%	<0.01

A-ECOHIS Arabic version of the Early Childhood Oral Health Impact Scale, *SD* standard deviation
**t*-test was used

Table 6 Reliability analyses of the A-ECOHIS: internal consistency and test-retest reliability ($n = 68$)

Impacts	Internal consistency reliability (Cronbach's alpha)	Test-retest reliability ICC (95% CI)
Child impact section	0.80	0.89 (0.82–0.93)
Family impact section	0.78	0.67 (0.52–0.79)
Overall scale	0.85	0.86 (0.78–0.91)

A-ECOHIS Arabic version of the Early Childhood Oral Health Impact Scale, *ICC* intraclass correlation coefficient, *95% CI* 95% confidence interval

Discussion

Oral health problems can have a negative impact on the OHRQoL of children and their families [22]. Evaluating and describing these influences can aid dentists in assessing children's oral health needs [11, 24, 25, 30, 37], providing better oral health care services [11, 24, 26, 31], and improving the oral health outcomes of children [11, 22]. Although assessment of OHRQoL is well established in adults following several decades of use, its application in children is relatively new and less understood. Prior to Pahel et al's development of ECOHIS [22], the first documented child-specific OHRQoL scale was presented by Jokovic et al. in 2002 to assess the impact of oral conditions on QoL in children 11 to 14 years of age [38]. Proper translation and validation are important for cross-cultural adaptation of QoL questionnaires [24–26, 39] and also enable comparisons between different countries using the same measurement instrument [24–26, 31, 40]. The ECOHIS questionnaire has so far been translated into French [23], Chinese [25], Farsi [30], Turkish [31], Brazilian Portuguese [24, 27], Spanish [26], Lithuanian [29], and Malay [28]. In this study, the ECOHIS was translated into the Arabic language, and its psychometric properties were tested.

Pain was the most frequently reported negative impact measure in the child section in both of our samples, and was common in other studies [22–25, 27, 28]. However, in the Turkish [31] and Lithuanian [29] studies, difficulty in eating and irritability, respectively, were most commonly reported. Similar to some studies [23–25, 29, 31], caregivers feeling upset was the most frequently reported item in the family section in this study. Taking time off work [22] and feeling guilty [27, 28] were the most commonly reported family impacts in three other studies. Although treatment at the clinic from which our sample was recruited is provided free of charge, about a third of our clinic-based caregivers reported a financial impact, which could have been attributed to other expenses incurred, such as transportation costs or missing work.

Floor effects are expected in community-based samples because only a small percentage of subjects have oral diseases [41], which explains the higher rate of floor effects among the community sample in this study. Accordingly, in the original scale study [22] and in its French [23] and Spanish translations [26], heavy floor effects were observed. The Turkish [31], Chinese ECOHIS [25], and Malay [28] validation studies showed lower floor effects, which might indicate poorer oral health in those populations [31]. Ceiling effects were not observed in other studies [22, 28, 29, 31] and were only minimally reported in the clinic sample in the current study.

Convergent validity of the A-ECOHIS was established. Caregivers who reported poor general oral health of their children had higher A-ECOHIS scores, which indicated worse OHRQoL. Unexpectedly, caregivers who reported good general oral health had slightly higher A-ECOHIS scores than did those who reported it to be fair. This could have been due to the subjectivity of the options, especially in two consecutive categories. Overall, there was a significant correlation between the global question and each of the total, child and family A-ECOHIS scores, as reported in other validation studies [22–24, 30, 31]. The Spearman correlation coefficient that we calculated for the total A-ECOHIS score with the global question was higher than that reported in the French study (−0.20) [23], but not the Turkish (0.68) [31] or Lithuanian (0.72) [29] studies.

As demonstrated in other ECOHIS validation studies [22, 24, 25, 27–29, 31], the A-ECOHIS was able to discriminate between children affected and not affected by oral disease. The total A-ECOHIS score and those of each section of the questionnaire were significantly higher among children with higher dmft scores compared with those with lower scores. The clinic sample, which we hypothesized would have a poorer oral health status than the community (school) sample, had significantly higher A-ECOHIS scores on all sections of the scale, as observed in other studies [23, 30]. This also indicated that caregivers are able to respond accurately regarding their child's OHRQoL based on the child's visible oral health condition [22, 42, 43].

The A-ECOHIS child and family section scores in this study were significantly correlated, suggesting that the scale is related to the concept it is intended to measure [22, 31], with a correlation coefficient that was within the same range as some reports (0.54 – 0.68) [23, 24, 29, 31], but higher than that of the ECOHIS development study (0.36) [22]. The inter-item correlations observed in this study also fell within the range of correlations observed in other studies (0.005 to 0.8) [23, 28–31].

Cronbach's alpha values greater than 0.8, as were calculated for the A-ECOHIS, indicate excellent internal reliability [25, 44]. The values reported for the child section ranged from 0.79 to 0.92, in reports of the French and Turkish language versions, respectively [22–25, 27, 29–31]; in the family section, the values ranged from 0.65 to 0.95 in the Brazilian and original ECOHIS studies, respectively [22]. In this study, Cronbach's alpha estimated for the A-ECOHIS as a whole was similar to that estimated in Brazilian and Lithuanian studies (0.86) [27, 29], and slightly higher than those of the French (0.82) [23] and Malay studies (0.83) [28], but lower than those of other studies (0.91 to 0.99) [24, 25, 31].

The test-retest reliability sample showed the stability in responses to the questionnaire. The ICC values for the child section and the total questionnaire fell within the ranges observed in other studies: 0.83 to 0.98 for the child section [23, 24, 27, 31] and 0.82 to 0.98 for the total questionnaire [22, 23, 27–31]. The family section ICC score in this study (0.67) was lower than that of most of the other studies (0.81 to 0.97) [23, 24, 27, 31]. The test-retest reliability of the Chinese study demonstrated the lowest ICC scores, at 0.64, 0.44 and 0.64 for the child, family sections and total questionnaire, respectively, which might be attributable to their small sample ($n = 21$) [25].

Missing values in validation studies can indicate a lack of comprehensibility or the irrelevance of items [23]. Missing responses in this study of the A-ECOHIS were infrequent, ranging from 0.2 to 5.5% in the community sample and not exceeding 2.8% in the clinic sample, which is less than what was reported previously [41]. This is a good indication of the comprehensibility and relevance of the A-ECOHIS items [23]. Adding "don't know" options to questionnaires helps subjects answer questions thereby avoiding missing data [23]. Nevertheless, some of our respondents left some questions blank. The highest percentages of missing values were in the "financial impact" (5.5%) and "taking time off work" (4.7%) questions. It is possible that some of the caregivers were mothers unemployed outside of the home who did not have a full picture of the spouse's work status or the family's financial situation. Additionally, respondents may have felt embarrassed by or unwilling to expose their financial difficulties. Indeed, only a small percentage of subjects reported not having enough money, although it seems reasonable to assume that most of the patients who choose to visit the free clinics of King Abdulaziz University are financially insecure. The "don't know" responses did not exceed 0.2% of the community-based sample and ranged from 0.8 to 2.1% of the clinic-based sample. This was much lower than the response rate for "don't know" in the original study [22], and the French [23] and the Brazilian [24] validation studies.

A limitation of this study is that some factors hindered our planned data collection scheme; namely, the number and level of cooperation of public schools in Jeddah was very low. Furthermore, the fieldtrips coincided with the 2014 Middle-Eastern respiratory syndrome coronavirus outbreak crisis in Saudi Arabia. Many schools refused visits from healthcare providers because they were worried about the spread of infection from contaminated dentists. However, it should be noted that, in validation studies, it is acceptable to select samples based on validation needs [23, 45].

A family's socioeconomic status (SES) can affect the caregiver's perceptions regarding their child's oral health [24, 26, 46] and is related to oral health conditions [47]. The discriminant validity results in this study, which compared the A-ECOHIS scores between the community and clinic samples, could have been influenced by the families' SES differences. These differences were not accounted for because socioeconomic information was only collected for the clinic sample. Despite the potential socioeconomic differences between the samples, when an objective measure of oral health status (dmft score) was used to differentiate subjects based on their oral health status, the A-ECOHIS scale still exhibited discriminant validity.

Due to the very small number of public preschools in Jeddah, 81% of the school sample participants attended private preschools; however, Al Algili et al. demonstrated that school type is not always a good indicator of SES in this city [47]. Due to the shortage of public preschools in Jeddah, some caregivers who cannot easily afford it will enroll their children in lower cost private preschools.

Although there are many dialects of Arabic, the formal Arabic language, which is understood and read by all Arabic-speaking populations, was used in this version of the questionnaire. The questionnaire testing in our study was not restricted to the Saudi population; 50% our clinic-based sample and 37% of the community sample were from other Arabic nationalities. Therefore, it might have potential for use by other Arabic-speaking populations.

The strengths of this study are worth mentioning. The sample size was adequate for the analyses and was larger than most of the other ECOHIS validation studies [22, 23, 25–28, 30, 31]. Furthermore, the recruitment of two samples enabled the testing of more psychometric properties than studies comprised of one sample. Finally, the samples included all age groups covered by this scale.

Conclusion

The A-ECOHIS performed well on all psychometric tests to which it was applied. It demonstrated convergent validity, discriminant validity, internal consistency, and test-retest reliability. Therefore, it is a valid and reliable instrument to use for Arabic-speaking caregivers of preschool-age children.

Abbreviations

A-ECOHIS: Arabic Version of the Early Childhood Oral Health Impact Scale; CI: Confidence interval; dmft: Decayed missed and filled teeth; ECOHIS: Early Childhood Oral Health Impact Scale; ICC: Intra-class correlation coefficient; OHRQoL: Oral health-related quality of life

Acknowledgements
The authors acknowledge with thanks the technical and financial support of Deanship of Scientific Research (DSR). The authors acknowledge the help of Dr. Dania Bahdaila, Dr. Haneen Bakhaidar, and Dr. Reham Alamoudi in data collection. We would also like to thank Editage (www.editage.com) for English language editing.

Funding
This project was funded by the Deanship of Scientific Research (DSR), King Abdulaziz University, Jeddah (No. 319/165/1433). This fund was used to purchase the examination instruments, print questionnaires, transport the investigators to and from the schools, cover the allowance of the research secretary, and manuscript editing services.

Authors' contributions
NJF conducted the statistical analyses, interpreted it, and wrote the manuscript. AAE conceived the study, participated in its design, participated in development of the questionnaire, and critically revised the manuscript. DJF participated in the study design, participated in the questionnaire development, applied for the fund, managed the study budget, collected the data, and critically revised the manuscript. NMF reviewed the translation of the questionnaire and conducted the research, and reviewed the manuscript. All authors read and approved the final manuscript.

Competing interests
The authors declare that they have no competing interests.

Consent for publication
Not applicable.

Ethics approval and consent to participate
Ethics approval was obtained from the Research Ethics Committee, Faculty of Dentistry, King Abdulaziz University (#036-13). Informed consent was obtained from all participating caregivers.

Author details
[1]Department of Dental Public Health, Faculty of Dentistry, King Abdulaziz University, P.O. Box 80200, Jeddah 21589, Saudi Arabia. [2]Department of Pediatric Dentistry, Faculty of Dentistry, King Abdulaziz University, Jeddah, Saudi Arabia. [3]Department of Pediatric Dentistry, Faculty of Dentistry, Alexandria University, Alexandria, Egypt.

References
1. American Acdemy of Pediatric Dentistry. Policy on Early Childhood Caries (ECC): Classifications, Consequences, and Preventive Strategies. 2014; Available from: http://www.aapd.org/media/policies_guidelines/p_eccclassifications.pdf.
2. Vargas CM, Crall JJ, Schneider DA. Sociodemographic distribution of pediatric dental caries: NHANES III, 1988–1994. J Am Dent Assoc. 1998; 129(9):1229–38.
3. Benjamin RM. Oral health: the silent epidemic. Public Health Rep. 2010; 125(2):158–9.
4. Dye BA, Thornton-Evans G, Li X, Iafolla TJ. Dental caries and sealant prevalence in children and adolescents in the United States, 2011–2012. NCHS Data Brief. 2015;191:1–8.
5. The World Oral Health Report. Continuous improvement of oral health in the 21st century - the approach of the WHO Global Oral Health Programme. Geneva: Oral Health Programme Noncommunicable Disease Prevention and Health Promotion. World Health Organization; 2003.
6. Al Agili DE. A systematic review of population-based dental caries studies among children in Saudi Arabia. Saudi Dent J. 2013;25(1):3–11.
7. Al-Malik MI, Holt RD, Bedi R. Prevalence and patterns of caries, rampant caries, and oral health in two- to five-year-old children in Saudi Arabia. J Dent Child (Chic). 2003;70(3):235–42.
8. Khan SQ, Khan NB, Arrejaie AS. Dental caries. A meta analysis on a Saudi population. Saudi Med J. 2013;34(7):744–9.
9. Acs G, Lodolini G, Kaminsky S, Cisneros GJ. Effect of nursing caries on body weight in a pediatric population. Pediatr Dent. 1992;14(5):302–5.
10. Casamassimo PS. Relationships between oral and systemic health. Pediatr Clin North Am. 2000;47(5):1149–57.
11. McGrath C, Broder H, Wilson-Genderson M. Assessing the impact of oral health on the life quality of children: implications for research and practice. Community Dent Oral Epidemiol. 2004;32(2):81–5.
12. Alkarimi HA, Watt RG, Pikhart H, Sheiham A, Tsakos G. Dental caries and growth in school-age children. Pediatrics. 2014;133(3):e616–23.
13. Allen PF. Assessment of oral health related quality of life. Health Qual Life Outcomes. 2003;1:40.
14. Broder HL, Wilson-Genderson M. Reliability and convergent and discriminant validity of the Child Oral Health Impact Profile (COHIP Child's version). Community Dent Oral Epidemiol. 2007;35 Suppl 1:20–31.
15. Jokovic A, Locker D, Stephens M, Kenny D, Tompson B, Guyatt G. Measuring parental perceptions of child oral health-related quality of life. J Public Health Dent. 2003;63(2):67–72.
16. Gherunpong S, Tsakos G, Sheiham A. Developing and evaluating an oral health-related quality of life index for children; the CHILD-OIDP. Community Dent Health. 2004;21(2):161–9.
17. Prosser LA, Corso PS. Measuring health-related quality of life for child maltreatment: a systematic literature review. Health Qual Life Outcomes. 2007;5:42.
18. Thomas CW, Primosch RE. Changes in incremental weight and well-being of children with rampant caries following complete dental rehabilitation. Pediatr Dent. 2002;24(2):109–13.
19. Anderson HK, Drummond BK, Thomson WM. Changes in aspects of children's oral-health-related quality of life following dental treatment under general anaesthesia. Int J Paediatr Dent. 2004;14(5):317–25.
20. Higginson IJ, Carr AJ. Measuring quality of life: using quality of life measures in the clinical setting. BMJ. 2001;322(7297):1297–300.
21. Gilchrist F. Development of a child-centred caries specific measure of oral health related quality of life 'CARIES-QC'. The University of Sheffield. [cited Sep 1, 2016]; Available from: https://www.sheffield.ac.uk/dentalschool/research/create/teethanddentists.
22. Pahel BT, Rozier RG, Slade GD. Parental perceptions of children's oral health: the Early Childhood Oral Health Impact Scale (ECOHIS). Health Qual Life Outcomes. 2007;5:6.
23. Li S, Veronneau J, Allison PJ. Validation of a French language version of the Early Childhood Oral Health Impact Scale (ECOHIS). Health Qual Life Outcomes. 2008;6:9.
24. Scarpelli AC, Oliveira BH, Tesch FC, Leao AT, Pordeus IA, Paiva SM. Psychometric properties of the Brazilian version of the Early Childhood Oral Health Impact Scale (B-ECOHIS). BMC Oral Health. 2011;11:19.
25. Lee GH, McGrath C, Yiu CK, King NM. Translation and validation of a Chinese language version of the Early Childhood Oral Health Impact Scale (ECOHIS). Int J Paediatr Dent. 2009;19(6):399–405.
26. Bordoni N, Ciaravino O, Zambrano O, Villena R, Beltran-Aguilar E, Squassi A. Early Childhood Oral Health Impact Scale (ECOHIS). Translation and validation in Spanish language. Acta Odontol Latinoam. 2012;25(3):270–8.
27. Martins-Junior PA, Ramos-Jorge J, Paiva SM, Marques LS, Ramos-Jorge ML. Validations of the Brazilian version of the Early Childhood Oral Health Impact Scale (ECOHIS). Cad Saude Publica. 2012;28(2):367–74.
28. Hashim AN, Yusof ZY, Esa R. The Malay version of the Early Childhood Oral Health Impact Scale (Malay-ECOHIS)–assessing validity and reliability. Health Qual Life Outcomes. 2015;13:190.
29. Jankauskiene B, Narbutaite J, Kubilius R, Gleiznys A. Adaptation and validation of the early childhood oral health impact scale in Lithuania. Stomatologija. 2012;14(4):108–13.
30. Jabarifar SE, Golkari A, Ijadi MH, Jafarzadeh M, Khadem P. Validation of a Farsi version of the early childhood oral health impact scale (F-ECOHIS). BMC Oral Health. 2010;10:4.
31. Peker K, Uysal O, Bermek G. Cross - cultural adaptation and preliminary validation of the Turkish version of the early childhood oral health impact scale among 5-6-year-old children. Health Qual Life Outcomes. 2011;9:118.

32. Guillemin F, Bombardier C, Beaton D. Cross-cultural adaptation of health-related quality of life measures: literature review and proposed guidelines. J Clin Epidemiol. 1993;46(12):1417–32.
33. Bouchard GA BD, Carlson DA, Varadharajan A. Random number generator. Google patents. 2005.
34. Oral health surveys: basic methods. 4th ed. Geneva: World Health Organization; 1997.
35. Oral health surveys: basic methods. 4th ed. Geneva: World Health Organization; 1997. Available from: http://apps.who.int/iris/bitstream/10665/41905/1/9241544937.pdf. [cited Sep 1, 2016].
36. Saunders J, Huynh H. Consideration for sample size in reliability studies for mastery tests. Washington DC: Publication Series In Mastery Testing South Carolina University Colombia, School Of Education National Inst of Education (DHEW); 1980.
37. Broder HL. Children's oral health-related quality of life. Community Dent Oral Epidemiol. 2007;35 Suppl 1:5–7.
38. Jokovic A, Locker D, Stephens M, Kenny D, Tompson B, Guyatt G. Validity and reliability of a questionnaire for measuring child oral-health-related quality of life. J Dent Res. 2002;81(7):459–63.
39. Herdman M, Fox-Rushby J, Badia X. A model of equivalence in the cultural adaptation of HRQoL instruments: the universalist approach. Qual Life Res. 1998;7(4):323–35.
40. Allison PJ. Health-related quality of life comparisons in French and English-speaking populations. Community Dent Health. 2001;18(4):214–8.
41. Landis JR, Koch GG. The measurement of observer agreement for categorical data. Biometrics. 1977;33(1):159–74.
42. Filstrup SL, Briskie D, da Fonseca M, Lawrence L, Wandera A, Inglehart MR. Early childhood caries and quality of life: child and parent perspectives. Pediatr Dent. 2003;25(5):431–40.
43. Barbosa TS, Gaviao MB. Oral health-related quality of life in children: part III. Is there agreement between parents in rating their children's oral health-related quality of life? A systematic review. Int J Dent Hyg. 2008;6(2):108–13.
44. Cronbach LJ, Warrington WG. Time-limit tests: estimating their reliability and degree of speeding. Psychometrika. 1951;16(2):167–88.
45. Streiner DL, Norman GR. Health measurement scales: a practical guide to their development and use: oxford medical publications. 1995.
46. Wandera M, Kayondo J, Engebretsen IM, Okullo I, Astrom AN. Factors associated with caregivers' perception of children's health and oral health status: a study of 6- to 36-month-olds in Uganda. Int J Paediatr Dent. 2009; 19(4):251–62.
47. Al Agili DE, Alaki SM. Can Socioeconomic status indicators predict caries risk in schoolchildren in Saudi Arabia? a cross-sectional study. Oral Health Prev Dent. 2014;12(3):277–88.

Permissions

All chapters in this book were first published in OH, by BioMed Central; hereby published with permission under the Creative Commons Attribution License or equivalent. Every chapter published in this book has been scrutinized by our experts. Their significance has been extensively debated. The topics covered herein carry significant findings which will fuel the growth of the discipline. They may even be implemented as practical applications or may be referred to as a beginning point for another development.

The contributors of this book come from diverse backgrounds, making this book a truly international effort. This book will bring forth new frontiers with its revolutionizing research information and detailed analysis of the nascent developments around the world.

We would like to thank all the contributing authors for lending their expertise to make the book truly unique. They have played a crucial role in the development of this book. Without their invaluable contributions this book wouldn't have been possible. They have made vital efforts to compile up to date information on the varied aspects of this subject to make this book a valuable addition to the collection of many professionals and students.

This book was conceptualized with the vision of imparting up-to-date information and advanced data in this field. To ensure the same, a matchless editorial board was set up. Every individual on the board went through rigorous rounds of assessment to prove their worth. After which they invested a large part of their time researching and compiling the most relevant data for our readers.

The editorial board has been involved in producing this book since its inception. They have spent rigorous hours researching and exploring the diverse topics which have resulted in the successful publishing of this book. They have passed on their knowledge of decades through this book. To expedite this challenging task, the publisher supported the team at every step. A small team of assistant editors was also appointed to further simplify the editing procedure and attain best results for the readers.

Apart from the editorial board, the designing team has also invested a significant amount of their time in understanding the subject and creating the most relevant covers. They scrutinized every image to scout for the most suitable representation of the subject and create an appropriate cover for the book.

The publishing team has been an ardent support to the editorial, designing and production team. Their endless efforts to recruit the best for this project, has resulted in the accomplishment of this book. They are a veteran in the field of academics and their pool of knowledge is as vast as their experience in printing. Their expertise and guidance has proved useful at every step. Their uncompromising quality standards have made this book an exceptional effort. Their encouragement from time to time has been an inspiration for everyone.

The publisher and the editorial board hope that this book will prove to be a valuable piece of knowledge for researchers, students, practitioners and scholars across the globe.

List of Contributors

Rahul Naidu
School of Dentistry, The University of the West Indies, Saint Augustine, Trinidad and Tobago

June Nunnand Erica Donnelly-Swift
School of Dental Sciences, Trinity College Dublin, Dublin 2, Ireland

Maha A. Bahammam
Department of Periodontology, Faculty of Dentistry, King Abdulaziz University, P. O. Box 80209, Jeddah 21589, Kingdom of Saudi Arabia

Zhifei Zhou and Xiaojing Wang
State Key Laboratory of Military Stomatology, National Clinical Research Center for Oral Diseases, Department of Pediatric Dentistry, School of Stomatology, Fourth Military Medical University, Xi'an, People's Republic of China

Fen Liu
State Key Laboratory of Military Stomatology, National Clinical Research Center for Oral Diseases, Department of Pediatric Dentistry, School of Stomatology, Fourth Military Medical University, Xi'an, People's Republic of China
Department of Oral Medicine, Northwest Women's and Children's Hospital, Xi'an, People's Republic of China

Shuning Shen
1State Key Laboratory of Military Stomatology, National Clinical Research Center for Oral Diseases, Department of Pediatric Dentistry, School of Stomatology, Fourth Military Medical University, Xi'an, People's Republic of China
Department of Oral Medicine, PLA 261 Hospital, Beijing, People's Republic of China

Linjuan Shang
State Key Laboratory of Military Stomatology, National Clinical Research Center for Oral Diseases, Department of Pediatric Dentistry, School of Stomatology, Fourth Military Medical University, Xi'an, People's Republic of China
Department of Pediatric Dentistry, Foshan Stomatological Hospital, Foshan, People's Republic of China

Lei Shang
Department of Health Statistics, School of Public Health, Fourth Military Medical University, Xi'an, People's Republic of China

P. Wetselaar, A. Faris and F. Lobbezoo
Department of Oral Kinesiology, Academic Centre for Dentistry Amsterdam (ACTA), University of Amsterdam and VU University Amsterdam, MOVE Research Institute Amsterdam, Gustav Mahlerlaan 3004, 1081 LA Amsterdam, The Netherlands

Myung-Soo Cho
Department of Health Policy and Management, Graduate School of Public Health, Yonsei University, Seoul, Republic of Korea
Division of Management & Planning, Korea Health Promotion Foundation, Seoul, Republic of Korea

Kyu-Tae Han
Department of Public Health, Graduate School, Yonsei University, Seoul, Republic of Korea
Institute of Health Services Research, Yonsei University College of Medicine, Seoul, Republic of Korea

Sohee Park
Department of Biostatistics, Graduate School of Public Health, Yonsei University, Seoul, Republic of Korea

Ki Tae Moon
National Evidence-Based Healthcare Collaborating Agency, Seoul, Republic of Korea

Eun-Cheol Park
Institute of Health Services Research, Yonsei University College of Medicine, Seoul, Republic of Korea
Department of Preventive Medicine, Yonsei University College of Medicine, Seoul, Republic of Korea.

Shuo Yang, Quan Shi, Jinglong Liu and Juan Xu
Department of Stomatology, Chinese People's Liberation Army General Hospital, 28 Fuxing Road, Beijing 100853, China

Jinru Li
Department of Stomatology, Chinese People's Liberation Army 322 Hospital, 2 Yunzhong Road, Datong 037000, China

Changxiang Wang, Anthony J. Smith and Paul R. Cooper
Oral Biology, School of Dentistry, University of Birmingham, 5 Mill Pool Way, Edgbaston, Birmingham B5 7EG, UK

Robert Lucas
GlaxoSmithKline Consumer Healthcare, St. George's Avenue, Weybridge, Surrey KT13 ODE, UK

Jae-Hong Lee
Department of Periodontology, Daejeon Dental Hospital, Wonkwang University College of Dentistry, Daejeon 35233, South Korea

Jung-Seok Lee and Seong-Ho Choi
Department of Periodontology, Research Institute for Periodontal Regeneration, Yonsei University College of Dentistry, 50 Yonsei-ro, Seodaemun-gu, Seoul 03722, South Korea

Jung-Kyu Choi
Department of Health Insurance Research, Ilsan Hospital, National Health Insurance Service, Goyang 10444, South Korea

Hye-In Kweon and Young-Taek Kim
Department of Periodontology, Ilsan Hospital, National Health Insurance Service, 100 Ilsan-ro Ilsan-donggu, Goyang 10444, South Korea

Sarra Jawad and Craig Barclay
Department of Restorative Dentistry, University Dental Hospital of Manchester, Higher Cambridge Street, Manchester M15 6FH, UK

William Whittaker
Division of Population Health, Health Services Research and Primary Care, School of Health Sciences, University of Manchester, Manchester, UK

Martin Tickle and Tanya Walsh
Division of Dentistry, Faculty of Biology, Medicine and Health, University of Manchester, Manchester, UK

Honghu Liu, Marvin Marcus, Ian Coulter, Carl Maida, Vladimir Spolsky, Jie Shen and James Crall
1Division of Public Health & Community Dentistry, School of Dentistry, University of California, Los Angeles (UCLA), Los Angeles, CA, USA

Ron D. Hays
UCLA Department of Medicine, David Geffen School of Medicine, Los Angeles, CA, USA

Francisco Ramos-Gomez
UCLA Section of Pediatric Dentistry, Los Angeles, CA, USA

Yan Wang
UCLA Department of Biostatistics, Los Angeles, CA, USA

Steve Lee
UCLA Section of Restorative Dentistry, Los Angeles, CA, USA

Li Cai
UCLA Department of Education, School of Education and Information Studies, Los Angeles, CA, USA

Ye Tao, Yan Zhou, Qing Hui Zhi and Huan Cai Lin
Department of Preventive Dentistry, Guanghua School of Stomatology, Guangdong Provincial Key Laboratory of Stomatology, Sun Yat-sen University, 56 Ling Yuan Road West, 510055 Guangzhou, Guangdong Province, China

Rong Min Qiu
Department of Preventive Dentistry, Guanghua School of Stomatology, Guangdong Provincial Key Laboratory of Stomatology, Sun Yat-sen University, 56 Ling Yuan Road West, 510055 Guangzhou, Guangdong Province, China
Department of Pediatric Dentistry, College of Stomatology, Guangxi Medical University, Nanning, China

Dorota T. Kopycka-Kedzierawski and Cyril Meyerowitz
Eastman Institute for Oral Health, University of Rochester, 625 Elmwood Ave, Rochester, NY 14620, USA

Mark S. Litaker, Gregg H. Gilbert and National Dental PBRN Collaborative Group
University of Alabama at Birmingham, Birmingham, AL, USA

Sidney Chonowski
Private practice of general dentistry, Morristown, NJ, USA

Marc W. Heft and Valeria V. Gordan
University of Florida, Gainesville, FL, USA

Robin L. Yardic
Health Partners, Minneapolis, MN, USA

Theresa E.Madden
Private practice of periodontics, Olympia, WA, USA

Stephanie C. Reyes
University of Texas Health Science Center at San Antonio, San Antonio, TX, USA

Weini Xin
Dental Care Center, The First Affiliated Hospital of Shantou Medical College, Shantou, China

Katherine Chiu Man Leung
Prosthodontics, Faculty of Dentistry, The University of Hong Kong, Hong Kong SAR, China

Edward Chin Man Lo
Dental Public Health, Faculty of Dentistry, The University of Hong Kong, Hong Kong SAR, China

Mo Yin Mok
Department of Biomedical Sciences, City University of Hong Kong, Hong Kong SAR, China

Moon Ho Leung
Department of Medicine, Queen Elizabeth Hospital, Hong Kong SAR, China

Andreas Hellak
Department of Orthodontics, University Hospital Giessen and Marburg, Campus Marburg, Georg-Voigt-Strasse 3, Marburg 35039, Germany
Abt. für Kieferorthopädie, UKGM Standort Marburg, Georg-Voigt-Strasse 3, 35039 Marburg, Germany

Nicola Schmidt, Michael Schauseil, Steffen Stein and Heike Maria Korbmacher-Steiner
Department of Orthodontics, University Hospital Giessen and Marburg, Campus Marburg, Georg-Voigt-Strasse 3, Marburg 35039, Germany

Thomas Drechsler
Private practice, Wiesbaden, Germany

Jens C. Türp
Department of Reconstructive Dentistry and Temporomandibular Disorders, University Center for Dental Medicine Basel, University of Basel, Basel, Switzerland

Anna Schlenker
Department of Prosthodontics, University of Heidelberg, Heidelberg, Germany

Johannes Schröder
Section of Geriatric Psychiatry, University of Heidelberg, Heidelberg, Germany

Marco Essig
Department of Radiology, University of Manitoba, Faculty of Medicine, Winnepeg, Canada

Marc Schmitter
Department of Prosthodontics, Dental School of the University of Würzburg, Würzburg, Germany

Ping Ye
Institute of Dental Research, Oral Health, Westmead Hospital, Westmead, Australia
Affiliation of Faculty of Dentistry, the University of Sydney, Sydney, Australia

Hong Yu
Microscopy Laboratory, Westmead Institute for Medical Research, Westmead, Australia

Mojgan Houshmandi
Institute of Dental Research, Oral Health, Westmead Hospital, Westmead, Australia

Young-Suk Kim
Department of Dental Hygiene, U1 University, Yeongdong, Korea

Mina Ha and Ho-Jang Kwon
Department of Preventive Medicine, Dankook University College of Medicine, 119 Dandae-ro, Dongnam-gu, Cheonan, Chungnam 31116, Republic of Korea

Hae-Young Kim
Department of Health Policy and Management, College of Health Science, and Department of Health Science, Graduate School, Korea University, Seoul, Korea

Youn-Hee Choi
Department of Preventive Dentistry, School of Dentistry, Kyungpook National University, Daegu, Korea.

Makiko Nishi, Máiréad Harding and Virginia Kelleher
Oral Health Services Research Centre, University College Cork, Wilton, Cork, Ireland

Helen Whelton
The School of Dentistry, University of Leeds, Leeds, UK

Finbarr Allen
Faculty of Dentistry, National University of Singapore, Singapore, Republic of Singapore

Adriana Santamaría-Villegas and Claudia Restrepo-Serna
CES-LPH Research Group, Universidad CES, Calle 10A. No. 22-04, Medellín, Colombia

Rubén Manrique-Hernandez and Emery Alvarez-Varela
Universidad CES, Calle 10A. No. 22-04, Medellín, Colombia

Masako Fujioka-Kobayashi
Department of Cranio-Maxillofacial Surgery, Bern University Hospital, Inselspital, Bern, Switzerland.
Department of Oral Surgery, Institute of Biomedical Sciences, Tokushima University, Tokushima, Japan

Heinz-Dieter Müller and Adrian Lussi
Department of Preventive, Restorative and Pediatric Dentistry, School of Dental Medicine, University of Bern, Bern, Switzerland

Andrea Mueller and Patrick R. Schmidlin
Clinic of Preventive Dentistry, Periodontology and Cariology, Center of Dental Medicine, University of Zurich, Zürich, Switzerland

Anton Sculean
Department of Periodontology, School of Dental Medicine, University of Bern, Bern, Switzerland

Richard J. Miron
Department of Preventive, Restorative and Pediatric Dentistry, School of Dental Medicine, University of Bern, Bern, Switzerland
Department of Periodontology, College of Dental Medicine, Nova Southeastern University, Fort Lauderdale, FL, USA
Cell Therapy Institute, Center for Collaborative Research, Nova Southeastern University, Fort Lauderdale, FL, USA
Department of Periodontics and Oral Medicine, University of Michigan School of Dentistry, Ann Arbor, MI, USA

Rajesh V. Lalla
Section of Oral Medicine, MC1605, University of Connecticut Health, 263, Farmington Avenue, Farmington, CT 06030-1605, USA

Leslie Long-Simpson and James S. Hodges
Division of Biostatistics, School of Public Health, University of Minnesota, 2221 University Ave SE Suite 200, Minneapolis, MN 55414, USA

Nathaniel Treister
Division of Oral Medicine and Dentistry, Brigham and Women's Hospital, 1620 Tremont Street, 3rd Floor, Boston, MA 02120, USA
Department of Oral Medicine, Infection and Immunity, Harvard School of Dental Medicine, 188 Longwood Avenue, Boston MA 02115, USA

Thomas Sollecito
Department of Oral Medicine, University of Pennsylvania School of Dental Medicine, 240 South 40th Street, Philadelphia, PA 19104, USA

Brian Schmidt
Department of Oral & Maxillofacial Surgery and Bluestone Center for Clinical Research, New York University College of Dentistry, 421 First Avenue, New York, NY 10010, USA

Lauren L. Patton
Department of Dental Ecology, School of Dentistry, University of North Carolina, Chapel Hill, NC CB 7450, USA

Michael T. Brennan for the OraRad Study Group
Department of Oral Medicine, Carolinas Medical Center, 1000 Blythe Blvd, Charlotte, NC 28203, USA

Leena Merdad
Department of Dental Public Health, Faculty of Dentistry, King Abdulaziz University, P.O. Box 80209 1589 Jeddah, Saudi Arabia

Azza A. El-Housseiny
Department of Pediatric Dentistry, Faculty of Dentistry, King Abdulaziz University, Jeddah, Saudi Arabia
Department of Pediatric Dentistry, Faculty of Dentistry, Alexandria University, Alexandria, Egypt

Bruktawit Kebede
Oral and Maxillofacial Surgery case team, Department of Dentistry, Jimma University, Jimma, Ethiopia

Dawit Tare
Department of Surgery, Jimma University, Jimma, Ethiopia

Birke Bogale
Department of Dentistry, Millennium Medical College, St. Paul's Referral Hospital, Addis Ababa, Ethiopia

Fessahaye Alemseged
Department of Epidemiology, Jimma University, Jimma, Ethiopia

Nada J. Farsi
Department of Dental Public Health, Faculty of Dentistry, King Abdulaziz University, P.O. Box 80200, Jeddah 21589, Saudi Arabia

Azza A. El-Housseiny
Department of Pediatric Dentistry, Faculty of Dentistry, King Abdulaziz University, Jeddah, Saudi Arabia
Department of Pediatric Dentistry, Faculty of Dentistry, Alexandria University, Alexandria, Egypt

Deema J. Farsi and Najat M. Farsi
Department of Pediatric Dentistry, Faculty of Dentistry, King Abdulaziz University, Jeddah, Saudi Arabia

Index